The Mind/Brain Connection

As the Pendulum *Swings*

If It Isn't Hypnosis... Then What Is It?

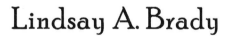

Lindsay A. Brady

Foreword by Steve Chandler, Author of *Fearless*

Robert D. Reed Publishers • Bandon, OR

Robert D. Reed Publishers
P.O. Box 1992
Bandon, OR 97411
Phone: 541-347-9882; Fax: -9883
E-mail: 4bobreed@msn.com
Website: www.rdrpublishers.com

Cover Designer: Cleone L. Reed
Book Designer: Debby Gwaltney

ISBN 13: 978-1-934759-36-3
ISBN 10: 1-934759-36-8

Library of Congress Control Number: 2009928232

Manufactured, Typeset, and Printed in the United States of America

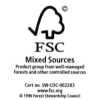

FSC

Mixed Sources

Product group from well-managed
forests and other controlled sources

Cert no. SW-COC-002283
www.fsc.org
© 1996 Forest Stewardship Council

DEDICATION

To:

Darlene

    Shannon

    Heather

    Kristen

    Patrick

    Laurel

    Amber

        Their Children

           And their Children

               Ad infinitum

ACKNOWLEDGMENTS

Darlene for allowing me the seclusion to write this book

Steve Chandler my real live Socrates

Kathy Eimers Chandler for making my writing sensible

Cleone Lyvonne and Robert Reed for creative publication guidance

Carol Adler for publishing consultation

To all of my colleagues who inspired and challenged my ideas

To my clients for their insight and feedback

TABLE OF CONTENTS

Foreword.. 9

Preface 11

Introduction 13

THE STORY - PART ONE

Chapter 1.......... Curiosity 21

Chapter 2.......... The Door Opens 29

Chapter 3.......... The Search 35

Chapter 4.......... The Discovery... 45

Chapter 5.......... A New Direction 51

Chapter 6.......... Moving Forward 59

Chapter 7.......... An Emotional Experience 65

Chapter 8.......... Crickets.. 75

Chapter 9.......... The Sage 85

Chapter 10........ Eric... 95

Chapter 11........ The Teaching 105

Chapter 12........ The Corporation 115

Chapter 13........ The Stage 123

Chapter 14........ Stage-Show Lesson One 133

Chapter 15........ The Second Performance 139

Chapter 16........ Lesson Two 147

Chapter 17 .... Back on Stage 155

Chapter 18........ Bombshell Performance 165

Chapter 19........ Lesson Three and Meeting Socrates....... 173

Chapter 20........ My Premiere Performance 183

Chapter 21 .... My Second Performance 195

Chapter 22........ Parting of the Ways 205

Chapter 23........ Preface to Regressive Hypnotherapy 213

Chapter 24........ Regressions This Life............................. 215

Chapter 25........ Regressions Past Lives........................... 227

Chapter 26........ A Menagerie of Strange Requests
                     and Memorable Sessions........................ 251

Chapter 27........ Finding Stuff 265

THE THEORY - PART TWO

Chapter 28........Organization and
            a Move Back to Phoenix........................ 273
Chapter 29........University Enlightenment..................... 281
Chapter 30........Arizona Society for
            Professional Hypnosis 291
Chapter 31........Simplifying the Induction 297
Chapter 32........The Pendulum Swings........................... 311
Chapter 33........No Altered States of Consciousness 319
Chapter 34........"Sleep" and Receptiveness..................... 325
Chapter 35........The Recording................................. 333
Chapter 36........Regression Revisited.......................... 335
Chapter 37........Perceptionism 349
Chapter 38........The Mind-Brain Connection 355
Chapter 39........One Mind...................................... 361
Chapter 40........Now! 369
Chapter 41........Perception Revisited 377
Appendix I... 393
Appendix II 434
Appendix III 438
Appendix IV... 442
Appendix Study Data... 445
Bibliography 447

FOREWORD

This book is not a book about hypnotism as much as it is a book about finding peace of mind through joy of consciousness.

Lindsay Brady has been my hypnotherapist over the last ten years. Under his guidance I have rid myself of some nasty habits, addictions and fears that were plaguing me. Rid myself forever! But more than my therapist, he has become my friend. We have spent many hours discussing the universe and the human mind, and I've never met anyone with such a passion for understanding both.

For years I'd wished he would write a book. He had always been so enthusiastic about my own books and writing and so self-deprecating about his abilities with words that I never thought it would happen. But now it has, and am I ever glad it did.

Because this book is great. Not just good, but great. And what makes it great is Lindsay's ability to entertain. His stories are so compelling that one reads about the first part of his life and hypnotic misadventures like one reads a fun novel... a hilarious, heartbreaking, page-turner of a novel.

Lindsay's first encounters with "hypnosis" (a term he never fully endorses) are funny and eventually uplifting. I laughed so hard in the early parts that I thought this book might not ever get to the brilliance of Lindsay Brady because it was too funny... and he is so humble and innocent telling these stories on himself. How will he later deliver the profound insights I've come to learn from him? But I had nothing to worry about.

The book just keeps getting deeper and better because through these funny stories he has been building his case, or I'd rather say his structure of light... his illumination of how the human mind really works... where our mental limitations and dysfunctional behavioral habits come from, and how the mind holds the key to its own liberation.

Hypnosis is not really the subject of this book, although there isn't a hypnotist in the world who won't want a copy of this book to read more than once. In fact, in our years of conversations on the mind Lindsay has never said the word "hypnosis" without making quote marks with his fingers in the air to show me that it isn't really his preferred word.

What he has discovered is bigger than that. It is more universal, and therefore more helpful. It is about relaxation, peace of mind and perception and how the mind really and truly controls the brain, the body and emotions... and therefore the *life*, yes the whole life, of the individual, which is to say you and me.

You and I have a lot to learn from this book. Take a deep breath and relax all the tension in your body because you are about to read some things that will make you very happy. The key to a mentally healthy and fulfilling life is yours to use... it's in you already, the search is over. The key is yours to locate and then project, just as you would a projection camera. And this book explains it better than any I have read.

And we're not talking new age woo-woo stuff here either. Because Lindsay Brady is the ultimate scientific skeptic. He trusts nothing he cannot verify with rigorous inquiry and reasoning. So the journey here is quite exciting intellectually! Lindsay asserts nothing without challenging it himself. The dialogues he has with himself in this book have the riveting quality of great courtroom drama. And in the end, we win. We, the readers, win big. We win a fresh understanding of how and why we generate problems in our lives—why we do what we really *don't want to do*—and how gentle and simple the solution really is.

For Lindsay, hypnosis is nothing more than a clear understanding of how to operate your mind efficaciously, so that you can have the life you want. How you perceive and picture what you want initiates the process that actually results in immediate and dramatic behavioral change. And there is no mysticism to believe in. No creepy spiritual synchronicities to hang your heart on. This is simply how the mind uses the brain to motivate and operate your body and your emotions.

Yet the effect of reading his explanation is pure magic.

The stories in this book are unforgettable. The characters are too amazing to have been made up, and the beauty is in the telling. This man who never thought he was good with words has masterfully used words to weave a tapestry of fresh and useful reality.

Once you are finished with this book you'll be moved to 1) read it again and 2) tell your friends to get their copies. Because this is a book about you. You'll notice that halfway into it. It's about how you think, how you worry, how you dream and how you act and feel. With all the scary mystery taken out, piece by piece. Lindsay Brady has done a great service for us by sharing the details of his life and his work in this way, and no matter how popular the book becomes with the general public, it will always be a very personal experience for each reader; it will always feel like it's written just for me and for you in an act of pure generosity.

Steve Chandler
Phoenix, Arizona
January, 2009

PREFACE

This book is not *only* a book about "hypnosis," but also a memoir about how my life has been transformed from one of fear, low self-esteem, guilt and self-doubt into one of confidence, joy and peace of mind by using the process **called** "*hypnosis*"—a process more accurately described by the word *perceptionism*. It is a story about my personal crusade to overcome the manacles of tradition, bigotry, closed-mindedness and self-imposed limitation that eventually led to being at peace with myself and pleased with who I am.

It is a tale of becoming a hypnotherapist and developing a unique approach to effectively help my clients rid themselves of unwanted habits and self-destructive behavior. It is a book that tells stories about the lessons I learned from thousands of clients that, in turn, compelled me to scrap obsolete terms, techniques, methods and even some of my most cherished concepts. It is a book about having to adjust my approach and methods in order to effectively help my clients more easily achieve their goals, engage in healthy behavior, be free from guilt and find happiness and peace of mind. It is a story about solving the puzzle of how to demonstrate to my clients that *perception* is the means by which the human mind, brain and body communicate with each other. It explains how human consciousness can intentionally instruct *its* brain to bring about healthy behavior and create an emotional state of well-being that is independent of past experiences, present conditions and the uncertainty of the future. And it is a story that validates the power and the dynamics of taking charge of **now**.

This book is a treatise intended to dispel outmoded ideas about "hypnosis" as being something a person goes into or under, or that it is a trance in which a person is unaware. It tells the story of how the vague, stale term, *hypnotism* (which implies nothing about a process), is transformed into the definitive dynamic term, *perceptionism*... the driving force behind the "hypnotic process" *and* human behavior.

INTRODUCTION

Look into my eyes... My gaze is making you relax, and causing you to feel very tired. You are getting so very tired and sleepy now. Your eyes are getting heavier and heavier. Your arms and legs are getting heavier and heavier. Your entire body is getting heavier and heavier with relaxation.

In a moment I will count down from the number five to the number one. Each number I count down you will feel yourself getting even more tired and sleepy. Each number I count, your eyelids will get heavier and heavier as you sink into a deeper and deeper sleep.

When I reach the number one I will snap my fingers, and when I do, your eyelids will spontaneously close and your head will drop onto your chest. You will fall into a deep sleep, and at that moment the only thing that will matter to you will be my voice and what I am saying. From that moment on you will follow and carry out every instruction I give and do exactly as I command.

Still gazing into my eyes:

Five...   Your arms are getting very heavy and relaxed now.

Four...   Your legs are getting very heavy and relaxed now.

Three...   Your entire body is getting very heavy and relaxed now.

Two...   Your mind is relaxed now. The only thing mattering to you now is my voice.

One...   [Snap!] SLEEP NOW! Following and carrying out my every command, NOW!

Automatically, ten pairs of eyes snap closed and ten heads drop to their owners' chests.

———

In a moment I am going to snap my fingers again; when I do, you will try to open your eyes but be unable to do so; and the harder you try to open your eyelids, they will just stick tighter and tighter shut, and all you will be able to do is raise your eyebrows. When I snap my fingers you will try to awaken yourself, but the harder you try to awaken yourself you just sink into a deeper and deeper sleep.

[Snap!]

Ten pairs of eyelids are stuck shut and ten pairs of eyebrows raise, as ten people attempt to open their eyes and try to awaken themselves. [Laughter, amazement, skepticism and disbelief from the audience.]

———

Now, place your arms straight out in front of your body at shoulder height. Twenty arms stick straight out at shoulder height.

On the back of your right arm there is a large and heavy dictionary. You feel the weight of that dictionary pushing your right arm down now and the harder you try to hold your right arm up, the weight of that dictionary just pushes your right arm down... lower and lower... lower and lower.

Around your left wrist is tied a giant bunch of helium-filled balloons–like you would see at a carnival. Those balloons are now pulling your left arm up higher and higher... higher and higher. All of the muscles in your left arm are relaxed now and your arm is just floating up into air, higher and higher. When I snap my fingers your right arm will be so very tired, you will be unable to hold it up, so you just let it fall to your side and your left arm will float straight up in the air.

[Snap!]

Ten right arms drop and hang loosely down at each person's side and ten left arms comfortably float straight up, as though suspended by a giant bunch of helium-filled balloons. [Laughter, amazement, skepticism and disbelief from the audience.]

——

The person whose head I am touching now is a Martian. You are an Alien from Mars. The only language you speak and understand is Martianese. When I next snap my fingers you will be able to only speak and converse in Martianese.

The person whose head I am touching now, you are a renowned journalist. As a renowned journalist you are fluent in speaking and understanding Martianese.

When I snap my fingers, Journalist, you will interview our Martian visitor. I will then have a few questions for you to ask the Martian. You will translate my questions to Martianese, and in Martianese you will ask our Martian guest the same questions. Since only you and the Martian can speak and understand Martianese, your job is, in English, to interpret his answers.

[Snap!]

Me: Ask the Martian how he got to earth.

Journalist: Jabuls kroloba nobillisenpmba?

Martian: Roulo Jegagnemas agl ydarb yasdnil nu kloggagga. Nualla ereg zziel raeaez.

Journalist's translation: He says you must really be an idiot to ask such a stupid question. Of course he got to earth in a Spaceship.

Me: What does he think about Earth and the customs of us Earthlings?

Journalist: [Jabbering]

Martian: [Jabbering]

Journalist's translation: He says earth is hot and wet and he can't believe any sane creatures, even Earthlings, could have much fun drinking alcohol and breathing oxygen. He says give him a good ol' chaw of dry ice, some CO_2 and a fifth of Methane, and he'll show you a *really* good time.

Me: What does he think of us Earthlings?

Journalist: [Jabbering]

Martian: [Jabbering and doing some obvious gestures with his hands.]

Journalist's translation: He says that the males of our species are as ugly as [jabbering and looking at the Martian, who is pushing up on his nose]... as ugly as pigs. But, but the females of your species are... well... [As he gropes for the right words he looks at the Martian, who is signifying a shapely hourglass figure with gestures, licking his lips, and turning his eyes heavenward to express signs of ecstasy, and gesturing with his hands to show a woman's well-endowed bust line] ...are highly, ah... sexy! [Laughter, amazement, skepticism and disbelief from the audience.]

————

In a moment I'm going to snap my fingers and you will open your eyes. When you do you will stand up, look around and act as though you have lost something. When I ask, "Have you lost something–Is something missing?"–you will realize it is your bellybutton that is missing. First you will check to see if your suspicions are correct, and discover that your bellybutton is missing. You will begin looking for your lost bellybutton in every conceivable place. You may have left it in your shirt pocket. It may have slipped down in your underwear. You check out your pants pocket and your shoe. And the more you look for your lost bellybutton, the more it is amusing to you that you could have lost it; and the more you think about losing your bellybutton the more humorous it becomes.

When I snap my fingers a second time you will look at me and realize that I have your bellybutton in my open hand. Finding it amusing that I could have your bellybutton, you will come to me and select your bellybutton from my hand, reinsert it in its proper spot and return to your chair.

[Snap!] *Open your eyes now. Have you lost something–is something missing?*

Five guys stand up and start looking around. Pulling up their shirts to check out their stomach—no bellybutton where one ought to be. Looking in their shoes—no bellybutton. Turning their pockets inside out—no bellybutton. Shaking their pants leg—no bellybutton... Laughing at themselves and their companions because none of them can find their bellybutton. And the more they look for their bellybutton, the more they laugh about having lost it.

[Snap!] *Here. I have your bellybutton in my hand.*

Five guys look at my open hand and one by one, cautiously, retrieve their bellybutton and carefully insert it into its proper place... except for the last guy who says: "That ain't my bellybutton. That's an innie, and it's white!"

"Oh crap," says one of the white guys, "I took the wrong one!" As they exchange bellybuttons they joke and laugh about their blunder and explain to the audience the difference between innies and outies and, black and white bellybuttons. [Laughter, amazement, skepticism and disbelief from the audience—AND FROM ME!]

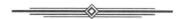

The suggestions (instructions) stated above are just a few of about 50 scripts that I created over 30 years ago, in an attempt to become a world-renowned Stage Hypnotist.[1] The responses actually occurred during my stage show performances, at least once, exactly as they are described.[2] And, without exception, while the subjects were carrying out their antics, I was wondering why! Wondering amidst my own laughter, amazement, skepticism and disbelief, what is going on in their brain?

Even though I was the hypnotist, I wondered: Why in the world are they doing these things just because I tell them to?

I wondered: What is really going on up in their head that causes them to do such absurd things just by suggestion?

I wondered: What is the process that manipulates their behavior and causes the mental processes in their brain that trigger such irrational behavior—just because I speak a few words?

I reasoned with myself: If these people were behaving this way out on the streets they would be thrown into the Loony Bin. They would be diagnosed as being mentally deranged, psychotic and insane!

The more I thought about the power of this process, what I really wondered was this: How can this process be put to use in a practical, positive way to help people change their everyday behavior? Can it be done with the same ease as it is with people on stage—causing them to lose their inhibitions, change their personality and spontaneously spark their creative imagination?

How can this process be used to cause a person to cease self-destructive behavior and switch their powers to constructive behavior? Can this power be used to cause people to enjoy good health, happiness, confidence, financial

---

1. It wasn't until much later in my hypnotherapy career that I discovered that I *could* have been a renowned Stage Hypnotist if I would have practiced being an *entertainer*. But at that time I was more interested in learning about "hypnosis" than I was interested in learning how to entertain. Renowned Stage Hypnotists such as Ormand McGill, Pat Collins, Reveen, Flip Orley, Terry Stokes, Mort Berkowitz and Don Rice are all entertainers by nature who learned to "hypnotize" people.

2. Every performance is a new experience for the Stage Hypnotist. Although the exact same suggestions are given to different subjects, the response of each subject varies as much as human personalities vary from one person to another. Unlike almost all other forms of entertainment, the Stage Hypnotist is at the mercy of the subjects who volunteer to participate. The Stage Hypnotist cannot predict exactly how a subject will respond to their suggestions beforehand. However, this is good because the most entertaining and funniest antics occur spontaneously without suggestion: "That's not my bellybutton. That's an innie and it's white!"

security and peace of mind—and change behavior and attitudes as easily and as quickly as with the snap of one's fingers?

This book is the story of a life-long curiosity. It is a tale about why we human beings behave as we do, and a commitment to exploring the answer to that and other questions. It is an in-depth query into why "hypnosis" works for some people; and why it seems to not work for others. And to share a few techniques I have discovered in almost four decades of working with well over 27,000 individual clients.

For the novice (a person who is just interested in or curious about hypnosis), it will be an enlightening adventure. But for the professional hypnotist it will probably create some eyebrow-raising questions and at times powerful disagreement since my methodology has evolved into a unique but simple approach that oftentimes flies in the face of traditional, old-fashioned theories and beliefs about our mind, our brain and hypnosis.

"Hypnosis" is a subject that gives rise to many intriguing questions. I have concluded that there are no "right" answers or "wrong" answers; there are only hypotheses based on one's perceptions and experience. The following pages describe how I arrived at my best-guessed conclusions as to the impetus that powers the hypnotic process, to explain my method of using it and to unravel many of the false perceptions about this fascinating puzzle.

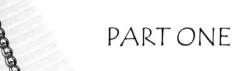

PART ONE

THE
STORY

CHAPTER 1

Curiosity

Probably from the moment I discovered the part of my brain used for rational thinking I have had a great curiosity about almost everything, and with that curiosity came endless questions. I wondered about and questioned the things that I observed; things that I heard about; things that I read; things about science; things about religion and God; things that people told me about church and God. But most of my wondering was about people: *Why do people behave as they do?*

I wondered why some people are "straight A" students (like my brother, Rodney) and why others just squeak by (like me). Why some people are popular and part of the "in crowd" (like my other brother, "K"), and why others just hover on the periphery of the "in crowd" (like me). Why some people are fearful of engaging in daring physical acts (like my brothers and my sister, Joanne) and others are dare devils (like me). Why is it that some people who miss many days of school are still A/B students, and others (like me) who are always there just barely pass? Why can some people read well and others (like me) struggle with reading? I wondered how perfectly rational people could have such differing opinions about things like ethics, politics and religion and be completely convinced that their point of view is the only right one and that everyone else's is wrong.

And I also often wondered about this thing called hypnosis—what is it, how does it work and what ability or talent does a hypnotist have that gives him the power to make people do strange things and change their behavior? But most of all, I wondered if hypnosis could be the secret to overcoming my own lack of confidence, my inhibitions and my scholastic deficits. Most people thought I was a confident person, but it was only a façade; I was just very skillful at putting on a good act. In my younger years, inside of me there was a mass of confusion and the self-perception that I couldn't (and didn't deserve to) measure up to the level of other people.

My interest in hypnosis all started as a young boy (maybe eight or nine) when I overheard a conversation in which a cousin was telling my relatives about a "stage-show hypnotist" that had come to his school and how the hypnotist made some of his classmates do strange and curious things. "I couldn't believe what I was seeing," he said. "The hypnotist made my best friend act like a dog and for five minutes he was down on the floor on hands and knees, crawling around in circles, chasing an imaginary tail and barking at it. He had another friend stretched between two chairs, like a board, balancing there just by his neck and his heels... and he even sat on him! But the strangest of all is what he made this very quiet, timid girl do. She is nice enough, but she is so shy that even our teacher can't get her to stand up at her desk and read (let alone get up in front of the class). She hardly ever speaks unless you talk to her first. But the hypnotist somehow got her up on stage and made her act like she was in a minstrel show. She was up there strumming an imaginary banjo, dancing around and singing 'Mammy,' just like she was Al Jolson. He made her do a lot of other strange stuff too, but after (when she wasn't hypnotized any more) she went right back to her old self and didn't remember what she had done or how she had acted. I couldn't believe it. It was like the Devil had gotten into her and left only when the hypnotist snapped his fingers!"

From that moment on I frequently wondered about hypnosis. I wondered about why a shy and withdrawn girl could become outgoing, even if it was just for a little while. I wondered what would have happened if he *hadn't* snapped his fingers. Would she still be outgoing or would she be possessed by some demon? I wondered if a hypnotist could hypnotize me and make me confident and remove my limitations and social fears so I could feel good about myself. I had no one I could talk to about hypnosis on a rational level (because of its "satanic and demonic" nature, I would have been severely criticized and thought of as being satanic myself), nor did I know how to find a hypnotist that could enlighten me on the subject.

My first experience with applying "hypnosis" (at least that's what my next door neighbor, Gary Asay, and I called it) was on his dad's chickens!

By laying a chicken on its back and slowly waving a hand in front of its eyes for fifteen seconds it becomes paralyzed. Once it is "hypnotized" it will just lie there for an hour if it is not disturbed.

Another way to hypnotize a chicken is to lay it on its stomach and with a finger repeatedly, from its beak outwards, draw a line on the ground about a foot long with a finger. The results are the same. The next time you have a live chicken in your hands, try it. It always works.

I had another neighbor, Lionel Brown, whose father had a small chicken ranch. One day "Liney" (that's what we called him) and I thought we'd play a joke on his dad.

Just before the time his dad's routine would take him out to tend to his flock, we "hypnotized" several of his chickens (some on their backs, feet sticking up; others on their stomachs, wings stretched outwards) and placed them in various locations in the chicken yard. When Mr. Brown walked into the yard it appeared as though some plague had struck the throng—we could hardly contain our sniggering as we witnessed his cussing.

We emerged from our hiding place and Liney told his dad what we had done. We were greatly relieved when Mr. Brown thought it was more humorous than we did. We one by one gave each of the fatalities a little nudge with our foot, which caused it to resurrect, jump up and squawk away.

I still wonder why this works. Maybe it is an inbred evolutionary process for the survival of certain snake species—like a cobra swaying before its prey.

So for a decade or more, from time to time my thoughts reflected back to my cousin's story of the hypnotist and I tried to rationalize how one person (the hypnotist) could determine another person's behavior just by talking to him. And I wondered if hypnosis would work on the hypnotist. I had so many unresolved questions and didn't know how to find the answers. Then, surprisingly, one day in the spring of my senior year in high school (1955), a discussion about hypnosis came up in my sociology class and, of course, what the teacher had to say about the topic grabbed my attention.

Our teacher, Mr. Bruce, was talking about how one person can have a profound influence on a great number of people and even sway the thinking of a nation. As an example, he recounted Hitler's rise to power and his ability to convince millions of people to support his policy of world dominance and cleansing society of "sub-human beings" (which included anyone who was not a Aryan). Mr. Bruce likened it to mass hypnosis. And that's how the topic of hypnosis came into the discussion.

In those days, to most of us students (and probably all of our parents), hypnosis was a dark, mystical power that the hypnotist had, with which he could, at will, take control of another person's mind and soul if he chose to. To dispel this notion, Mr. Bruce asked for a volunteer to demonstrate that although hypnotic suggestions can strongly influence the behavior of an individual, the hypnotized person still has his or her own capacity to choose, and they do not lose their ability to reject suggestions that would cause harm to themselves or violate their standards.

At first no one was interested in volunteering, probably because of our false conceptions about the subject. And for sure I wasn't going to volunteer and end up on the floor on all fours going around in circles chasing an imaginary tail and barking at it! Finally, Judy agreed to be the "guinea pig."

Mr. Bruce had Judy sit on a chair and instructed her to put her hands comfortably in her lap. He explained that all she needed to do was to listen to his voice and think about what he was saying. He told her that she would always be aware and soon he would be counting down from five to one two times; and that as he counted down she would feel more and more relaxed; and that with each number he counted, her eyelids would get more and more heavy, tired and sleepy. He also instructed her to try to keep her eyes open until he asked her to close them. He slipped off his wedding ring and held it about a foot in front of Judy's face and asked her to focus her gaze on the ring. Then, talking to her in a soft, rhythmical voice he began counting down:

> "Five...........you are getting very tired and sleepy."
>
> "Four..........you are getting very tired and sleepy."
>
> "Three ....you are getting very tired and sleepy."
>
> "Two ....you are getting very tired and sleepy."
>
> "One ....you are getting very tired and sleepy."

Judy's eyelids began to sag and it appeared that she was struggling to keep them open. He continued to speak in the same rhythmical voice:

> "Five...........you are so very sleepy and relaxed."
>
> "Four..........you are so very sleepy and relaxed."
>
> "Three ....you are so very sleepy and relaxed."
>
> "Two ....you are so very sleepy and relaxed."
>
> "One ....you are so very sleepy and relaxed."
>
> "Just close your eyes now and sleep now."

Judy closed her eyes and her head drooped down to her chest.

While Mr. Bruce was going through his "hypnotizing," I was frantically writing down every word he was saying. It was fortunate that he repeated each phrase five times, otherwise I couldn't have gotten the words exactly right—I was very slow at writing, too.

Mr. Bruce continued, *"Would it threaten you if I told you that you couldn't open your eyes? Would you be okay with that suggestion?"*

In a very quiet voice Judy said, "Yes."

Mr. Bruce said, *"Judy, your eyes are stuck closed and you are unable to open them now. When I ask you to try to open your eyes, try, but all you will be able to do is raise your eyebrows; your eyes will just close tighter and tighter. Try to open your eyes now, but the harder you try, your eyelids just close tighter and tighter."*

Just as Judy began trying to get her eyes open the bell rang, signaling the end of class, but Judy still just sat there trying to open her eyes and raising her eyebrows. Not as spectacular as strumming an imaginary banjo and singing "Mammy," but it left a profound impression on my psyche.

Mr. Bruce calmly said, *"Everything is fine, Judy. When I snap my fingers you will open your eyes and be wide awake feeling relaxed and feeling wonderfully refreshed, just like you have had a nice long nap."*

Mr. Bruce snapped his fingers and Judy's eyes popped open. He then asked her how she was feeling. She reported that she felt really good, relaxed and refreshed, just like she had awakened from a nice long nap.

As the classroom emptied some of my classmates and I gathered around Judy and asked her about her experience—what was it like and how did it feel? Her response was brief: "I wanted to tell him that I wasn't hypnotized because I could hear everything he was saying, but I just couldn't get the words out. I thought I would be able to open my eyes but I couldn't and when the bell rang I started worrying about being late for my next class if I didn't wake up! Then when Mr. Bruce said everything was fine, I just had this really neat feeling come over me." And she hurried off to her next class so she wouldn't be late.

For a long time after this experience I thought about what I witnessed and pondered over a few things that had impressed me:

> First: How Mr. Bruce handled the situation when the bell rang—no sense of urgency or alarm. He just kept talking in his calm soothing voice and reassured Judy that everything was fine. I've tried to emulate that demeanor from the moment I began hypnotizing people—or in the beginning, *trying* to hypnotize people.

> Second: It surprised me that Judy was aware that the bell rang and was still able to reason (concerned about being late for her next class), although she didn't wake up until Mr. Bruce instructed her to do so at the snap of his fingers. I thought you were supposed to be unconscious and unaware of what was going on around you, let alone being able to reason.

Third: Judy couldn't have been hypnotized for more than five minutes, yet she felt like she had just had a nice, long nap.

Fourth: I wondered, had the bell not rung, what kind of suggestions Mr. Bruce would have given to demonstrate to the class that a hypnotized person would not cause harm to themselves or do anything against their standards.

For the rest of the school year I wanted to engage Mr. Bruce in a discussion about hypnosis, but because of my inhibitions never did.

So! After watching Mr. Bruce hypnotize Judy; and since it didn't look all that difficult to hypnotize somebody; and since I was so impressed by the ease with which Mr. Bruce hypnotized Judy; and because she reported how good she felt afterwards (and since I had in my hot little hand a script of what to say), I thought I'd try to hypnotize someone at my earliest opportunity. *But who in the world would ever consent to letting me try to hypnotize them?* I wondered.

Judy was not the only student Mr. Bruce had hypnotized. Although I didn't witness it, my fellow students told me that in his psychology class Mr. Bruce had hypnotized Eddie and had him stretched out like a board between two chairs (just like I heard from my cousin many years earlier) and also gave him a "post-hypnotic" suggestion that after class he would go directly to the principal's office door and loudly hoot like an owl until the door began to open, and when it did he would calmly walk away and pretend that it was someone else who had done the hooting... which he did. Principal O. D. Ballard was affectionately (or for many of us not so affectionately) referred to as "The Owl"— he had a hooked nose on which was always perched a pair of large, perfectly round, dark-rimmed glasses that magnified the size of his eyes by at least two, creating the appearance of an owl. I never heard whether the parties involved in pulling off this antic were discovered, but I'm sure that if they were, the consequences were not pleasant. O.D. Ballard was not one for any kind of horseplay, although Benny Bruce was.

For the next few evenings I practiced memorizing the exact words that Mr. Bruce had said while hypnotizing Judy. For the next week or so, every day, for at least an hour, I sat facing an empty chair imagining that someone was sitting on it, and I began to practice. I practiced making my voice soft yet with an air of authority. And I practiced emulating the rhythmical cadence that Mr. Bruce had used. And I imagined myself becoming the world's greatest hypnotist. But I needed a real live person to try it on.

It was just couple of weeks after Mr. Bruce's demonstration that the opportunity to try out my newly acquired skill arose.

I was on a double date with my friend, Kent, his date, Evelyn, and my date, DeAna. Kent was driving and DeAna and I were sitting in the back seat and I directed the conversation to the experience of watching Mr. Bruce hypnotize Judy. All three seemed to be very interested in the topic so I asked DeAna if she would be willing to be my very first hypnosis subject. To my surprise she consented. So Kent pulled in to a grocery store parking lot, turned off the radio and said in a questioning skeptical voice, "This is going to be very interesting."

I asked DeAna to put her hands comfortably in her lap. I slipped off my class ring and held it about a foot in front of her face and asked her to focus her gaze on the ring (trying to talk to her in my soft, rhythmical, practiced, Mr. Bruce voice) and began counting down:

"Five...........you are getting very tired and sleepy."

"Four..........you are getting very tired and sleepy."

"Three........you are getting very tired and sleepy."

"Two ....you are getting very tired and sleepy."

"One... ....you are getting very tired and sleepy."

I continued speak to her, as best I could, in a rhythmical voice.

"Five...........you are so very sleepy and relaxed."

"Four..........you are so very sleepy and relaxed."

"Three........you are so very sleepy and relaxed."

"Two ....you are so very sleepy and relaxed."

"One ....you are so very sleepy and relaxed."

"Just close your eyes and sleep now."

DeAna closed her eyes momentarily, but then opened them and looked squarely at me as she unsuccessfully suppressed a giggle that burst into a full-fledged laugh that was echoed in perfect concert from the front seat... So much for becoming the world's greatest hypnotist!

I know now that I had a couple of big things going against me from the start.

First, I had not talked to DeAna about what to expect... mostly because *I* didn't know what to expect myself. But mostly, I didn't know that to successfully hypnotize a person, the pre-hypnotic talk is more important than the "induction" itself. Although Mr. Bruce's pre-hypnotic talk was very short, he had explained to Judy what to expect and what was going to happen. Also,

I did not even *try* to dispel any of her preconceived notions about hypnosis. I am sure DeAna still had the concept (just as most of our contemporaries) that hypnosis is a dark, mystical power that the hypnotist has and can use to take control over another person's mind and soul at will, if he chooses to. She knew that *I* had no such power.

Second was the setting: A grocery store parking lot, the back seat of a car, next to a busy street with cars, busses and trucks rumbling by and two people gawking from the front seat scrutinizing her reaction with every word I spoke. Come on!

CHAPTER 2

The Door Opens

After my red-faced fiasco of trying to hypnotize DeAna, my vision of *being* a hypnotist was shattered, not to mention what it did to an already low self-esteem: Just one more failure to add to my repertoire of self-worth reducing experiences.

Therefore, I gave up the matter actively until well after my high school days. But it was always in the back of my mind.

But the more I thought about my cousin's story of the "stage-show hypnotist"—and what I had observed firsthand in Mr. Bruce's class—the more my curiosity intensified. My interest now was not to become a hypnotist but rather that hypnosis might be the key for my own self-improvement and unlock a hidden potential. I always felt that bottled up, just under the surface, simmered the potential to excel at something. Anything!

Maybe if I could just find a hypnotist, he could hypnotize me and make me confident and outgoing, I thought. The problem was I didn't have the confidence to call one. I found the number of a hypnotist in the telephone book (only one was listed) but when I went to dial the number I couldn't get the phone off the hook. What a double bind: *I needed a hypnotist to conjure up the courage to call a hypnotist!*

I wondered, *What is getting in my way?* And further reasoned with myself, *There is no rational reason I shouldn't just pick up the telephone and dial the number. I know that he would like me to call; that's why he put an ad in the phonebook. Is it that I am afraid of hypnosis itself, or afraid of admitting to someone that I need help? Or maybe it's that I'm just afraid to use the telephone? I know I have a hard time returning calls from customers, even when they call to give me an order, and I'm terrified to make cold calls to prospective buyers. But this is different: I'm not trying to sell somebody something; I'm trying to give him an order, buy his services. Maybe I'll just put it off until tomorrow, when I feel more like doing it*, I decided with a sigh of relief. Of course "tomorrow" never got here!

I went on thinking, *Well if I don't have the courage to call a hypnotist, maybe I can learn how to hypnotize myself* (I remembered that Mr. Bruce had mentioned that people could do that). But then some demon thought from the past terrorized my thinking: *I don't have the intellectual capacity, education, resources or self-worth to pursue such a thing....* So I gave up on that idea, too.

Just as a side note: As illogical as it seems now, I thought a person needed an education before they could pursue scholastic interests. I remember thinking when I was in high school (even more illogically), *smart people are smart first and because they are smart they study, and dumb people's basic nature is dumbness so they don't study.* It didn't dawn on me until later in life that the reason smart people are smart was because they studied and the dumb ones were the way they were because they didn't. Talk about dumbness (in retrospect)!

In the ensuing years I made only one half-hearted attempt to expand my knowledge about hypnosis—I sent away for a mail-order book on hypnosis. The advertisement in the "Personals" section of a tabloid type newspaper said:

LEARN HOW TO HYPNOTIZE
PUT PEOPLE UNDER YOUR SPELL
Get whatever you want

Back in the mid sixties, hypnosis was still a taboo and advertisers had to use discretion as to what they put in their ads to avoid sanctions from the *Board of Ethical Advertising* (or some agency with a name something like that).

The short tag that followed the bold heading was so vague that I didn't know for sure what I was sending for.

When it arrived, it turned out to be a five-page booklet on how to entice a woman into your bedroom, with only one mention about hypnosis: "Hypnotists do it all the time, and you can too," and then an address where you could send to get the *real thing*!

To me this had no appeal whatsoever, especially since at the time I had an attractive, spectacular wife and three beautiful daughters. So the results of my endeavor (and the $5 shipping and handling fee) ended up in the trashcan.

At the time (1964) I was living in Phoenix, Arizona with my wife Darlene and daughters Shannon, Heather and Kristen. But I was born in 1936 in my parents' home in Sandy, Utah, a suburb of Salt Lake City. I attended Sandy Elementary School, Sandy Jr. High School and Jordan High School, also in Sandy.

My profession, for most of my early adulthood, was selling—everything from construction tools to memberships in a flying club. I always earned enough money to pay my bills, but little beyond that. I was good at selling things, once I conjured up the courage to make a sales call, but most of my effort was spent figuring rational reasons to avoid making them—the car needs servicing or I'll design a new gadget to put on my boat and make my calls tomorrow.

Then in 1970 we moved back to the Salt Lake City area and I became an "Associate" of Dell Rogers, the distributor for Success Motivation Institute (SMI). SMI produced albums of phonograph records that a person could listen to with the intent of getting motivated to become successful. When I first started with SMI, cassette tapes (and of course CD's) hadn't hit the market yet, so all of the programs were on 33 1/3 phonograph records.

An "Associate" meant that I bought an SMI program at the associate price from Dell and then either sold it to someone for full retail price, or used it to recruit another person to be my Associate... who would either sell his or her purchased program to someone at retail price, or use it to recruit someone to be their Associate... a true pyramid-marketing scheme that worked quite well and held the potential for making a sizable amount of money. (At the time, pyramid marketing like this was legal.)

When Dell Rogers gave me his "sales pitch" and told me that just listening to positive self-improvement, motivational and success-oriented records would change my thinking, improve my self-esteem and make me self-confident, I was sold! I was interested not only for the obvious reasons of self-improvement and the potential of earning money, but because now I could acquire knowledge about how to overcome my limitations and I didn't have to read to do it.

Immediately after unpacking my *Formula for Success* program I began listening to the recorded messages and using them in accordance with the enclosed printed material. It took a couple of weeks before I noticed any change in how I felt and how I felt about myself, but there was definitely *some* change in my disposition—slower than I had hoped for, but enough so that I was motivated to religiously listen to the recordings.

SMI marketed a number of different programs to help a person excel in specific professions (insurance sales, real estate sales, business administration, public speaking, academic endeavors, etc.). In addition to those structured programs there was a catalog of other individual recordings that included many of the popular motivational and self-improvement books of the time: *Think and Grow Rich*, Napoleon Hill; *Psycho-Cybernetics*, Maxwell Maltz; *The Power of Positive Thinking*, Norman Vincent Peale; *How to Win Friends and Influence People*, Dale Carnegie; *The Magic of Believing*, Claude Bristol; Earl Nightingale's *The Strangest Secret*; and many more. I spent many hours listening to these recordings; a "platter" version of books on tape—books that I would have never read, or even heard about for that matter, had it not been for SMI.

Because of my reading difficulties I had read very few books from cover to cover (maybe four), and when I did it took forever! But now I could begin to satisfy my curiosity and thirst for knowledge without having to read.

The idea behind the recordings was that a person could listen to the same messages over and over, with a period of time between each listening so that the ideas on the recording could "sink in" (a process that SMI called "spaced repetition"). All you needed to do was listen, and eventually the message would get into your subconscious mind and your subconscious mind would automatically change your behavior. That sounded great to me!

Although listening to SMI recordings and rubbing shoulders with positive-minded people helped to raise my self-confidence, the greatest benefit that came out of my affiliation with SMI was that I met Art Baker—not the Art Baker of radio and early television notoriety, but Art Baker the hypnotist.

But I am getting a little ahead of my story.

As I listened to my recordings I quickly became aware that hypnosis was mentioned often. Hypnosis was used to illustrate the powers of the subconscious mind, and to show how suggestions can facilitate changes in behavior and even cause those changes to happen quickly. So my interest in hypnosis had a "jump start" and I began looking for books on the subject, to no avail.

Then one evening at a weekly SMI recruiting/training meeting, one of the prospective recruits stood up and introduced himself as Art Baker, who worked for Western Airlines, but who was also a part-time professional hypnotist. Bingo!

Art and I became friends. Not close friends (he was much older than I), but he was willing, and even eager, to share with me much of his knowledge about hypnosis. He even let me sit in (for a fee) and watch him hypnotize some of his clients.

It appeared to me that almost all of his subjects went "under" hypnosis, because they "looked" like they did, but I was never really sure. I observed that *some* of the people he hypnotized made marked improvement in the area of life for which they had been hypnotized; but I also observed that most of them didn't—it appeared to me that hypnosis was a hit or miss process, and I wondered what made the difference. Art defended this by arguing that *they* just weren't ready to change their behavior, or didn't want to in the first place.

Art didn't know about my own self-confidence issues because I was still putting on my act. I often considered having him hypnotize me and "make" me be more successful. (I use the term "make" because that's what I thought a hypnotist did—*make* a person do something.)

I thought, *Maybe he could "make" me be confident and remove my reading limitation and "make" me be free of my inhibitions... Or, "make" me lose some weight*—I am 5'6" and at the time I weighed almost 250 pounds! The thing that got in the way of my pursuing being hypnotized was my fear of "blowing my cover" of *looking* self-confident. I wasn't going to let anyone know what was really going on inside of me. And for sure, I wasn't going to let somebody hypnotize me who knew me—and have them witness me spill my guts and reveal all of my deep, dark hidden secrets.

I know now that a person will not divulge anything that they choose not to reveal, but I didn't know it then. I even thought of finding another hypnotist who didn't know me, but decided that wouldn't be any better.

Art had instructed me earlier: *In order to make any kind of a significant change in a client's present behavior, it is necessary to go back in one's life and dredge up long-forgotten experiences. Every experience a person has ever had is stored in their subconscious mind and it has to be removed in order for a person to resolve present conflicts.*

I interpreted this to mean, *you have to dig up all of the garbage of the past, analyze it, dissect it, and re-experience all of the emotions related to it before you can change it.* I was wrong!

But I am getting *far* ahead of my tale.

Then one day, Art invited me (for a fee) to join in on a "group" hypnosis session that he was conducting for a few people who wanted to lose weight. Perfect! I could kill two birds with one stone: Lose some of the excess energy that had been stored on my body in the form of body fat, and experience what it was like to be hypnotized at the same time. Also, I rationalized, *if I was part of a group I'd be less likely to be spilling my guts.*

So, when the designated time arrived I showed up at his office and was introduced to six other rather portly individuals. Art invited me to sit in the remaining chair and went through his pre-hypnotic talk. He had everyone place their hands comfortably on their lap and asked us to focus our gaze on a ring that he had just slipped off of his finger (déjà vu!), but his introduction varied significantly from that of Mr. Bruce:

"*I want you to look at the ring I am holding and clear your mind. I want you to take in a very deep breath and hold it in while I count down...5,4,3,2,1 and exhale.*"

Art waited for everyone to empty their lungs.

"*Now take in another deep breath and hold it in... 5,4,3,2,1 and exhale.*"

Everyone did just as he instructed... including me.

"*And now take in one last deep breath and hold it in... 5,4,3,2,1 and exhale.*"

He continued in his rhythmical almost sing-song voice: "*While still looking at the ring, I want you to relax. Just relax and listen to my voice. I want you to let your mind be free of all of your worries. Just relax; nothing can harm you. I want you to start with your finger tips, just think about your finger tips, your finger tips are relaxing now, your finger tips are relaxed. I want you to relax your hands; your hands are relaxed now. I want you to relax your wrists; your wrists are relaxed now. And now I want you to relax your lower arms; your lower arms are relaxed now...."*

His method was a process of telling us what he wanted us to relax and then telling us that it had happened.

Art went on in a very slow, methodical voice making the same kind of suggestions for different parts of our anatomy: *Upper arms, shoulders, neck, the scalp of your head, the little muscles in your face, neck, chest, back, stomach, hips, upper legs, lower legs, ankles, feet, and toes.*

From time to time throughout his relaxing instructions, he slipped in the suggestion: *"Your eyes are getting heavy, tired and sleepy."* It took at least 15, maybe 20, minutes for Art to go through all of the body parts that he "wanted" us to relax.

And then he said, *"Just close your eyes now and sleep!"*

Momentarily I closed my eyes, but immediately opened them and looked directly into Art's eyes, and with some difficulty managed to suppress a giggle (déjà vu again). I shrugged my shoulders and held up my hands in defeated resolution and then looked around the room. I saw six people sitting comfortably in their chairs with their eyes closed and their heads resting on their chests. *I guess I am not a good candidate for being hypnotized,* I disappointingly surmised.

But I was not ready to give up just yet. *Well, since I am not a good prospect for having someone else hypnotize me,* I thought, *maybe I can learn how to hypnotize myself.* And I renewed my search for a book on self-hypnosis.

After the group session, Art explained, "Because of your 'defensive nature,' self-hypnosis would probably work better for you than being hypnotized by someone else." *At least,* I philosophized, *I won't have to share my deep, hidden secrets with anyone but myself.*

Out of desperation, I special-ordered a little skinny book (120 pages) on self-hypnosis from a local bookstore. "Skinny" and "little" because I was still wrestling with reading difficulties and figured that I'd have a better chance of completing it if it was skinny and little. A week later, *A Practical Guide to Self-Hypnosis,* by Melvin Powers, was in my hand and an exciting, but challenging, adventure began: A personal evolution—a transformation from being interested in hypnosis to becoming a "hypnotist."

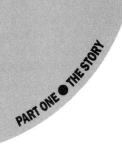

CHAPTER 3

The Search

My affiliation with SMI was short-lived. I thought I had found a home for life—selling a product in which I eagerly believed and one that provided people a means to improve the circumstances in their lives and to be successful and a resource to continue on my own quest for self-improvement.

But the bubble burst! A national law was enacted that prohibited pyramid marketing schemes such as the one used by SMI. And the bottom fell out of my financial security basket.

Thinking that SMI would continue on forever, I had made several sizable purchases on credit and I was soon financially over-extended. With the added burden of my newly acquired obligations, my monetary situation became very grave in short order.

Although I needed to find a means to meet my commitments, hypnosis as a legitimate source of income didn't even enter my mind. Besides, Art Baker, who had many years of experience, needed to work at another job in order to pursue his interest in hypnosis. Even if I had *thought* of being a hypnotist to earn money, my still fledgling self-confidence, inexperience, and limited resources would have made it impractical. My only interest in hypnosis was learning how to use it for my own self-improvement.

Having no other marketable skill, I went back to selling industrial products with about the same level of success that I had had before SMI—on the short end of mediocrity.

Even though I had learned many important principles about personal achievement and goal setting from listening to SMI recordings, applying them to real life performance was a different story. I still fell far short of my potential to make a good living and I just kept falling further and further behind with my financial obligations. I tell people that my circumstances were so grave that when the bill creditors came banging on my door demanding their money, with "...or we will take your kids," I quipped, "That would be great. You take them and feed them!" In reality, my children never did go hungry. No one knew the severity of my financial situation (not even my wife, Darlene). I was still very good at creating a façade and putting on a good act.

Not only was my financial situation in shambles but my personal life had become exceedingly complicated, confused and in disarray. At one point, my circumstances became so grave and my anxieties so great that I seriously considered ending it all. *If I can just make it look like an accident, at least my wife and children would be okay financially,* I told myself—double indemnity life insurance.

In fact, one day I sat for a very long time considering the consequences of moving on to what comes after *this* life—if anything does. I philosophized that no matter the outcome, it would be more pleasurable than the misery and gloom I am experiencing now. *If death is like my parents have taught me (when I die I go back to God's presence and I can visit with all my ancestors and the other great people who lived before me) that would be wonderful. On the other hand if it is as I had personally observed, witnessed and experienced (when we die we spend a very long time in a state of peaceful unawareness) that would be okay too.* Either way I would be out of my miserable state of being. A third alternative did not dawn on me at the time: Reincarnation. But the *wondering* about what happens after death *seemed* very familiar.

At the time I had no knowledge of the narration Plato gave in the *Apology*, recounting how Socrates philosophized about his pending departure from this life, having been condemned to death by drinking the poison hemlock. It was several years later that I discovered Socrates' thoughts on the matter were almost identical to the alternatives that I had just been considering.

Having made the decision to be out of my miserable state and to discover what happens next, I revved up the engine and called to mind the spot a mile down the freeway where there was a gap in the guard railing and a three-hundred foot cliff beyond. As I sat there with the engine still revving, I reconsidered: *If I drive off that cliff and I end up down there dead, tomorrow morning when the sun comes up nothing will matter to me—that is exactly what I want, to have nothing matter.* I gave no consideration to how my decision might affect other people. All I was interested in was ridding myself of my wretched state of mind. I further reasoned with myself: *But what if I am not dead and am just crippled for the rest of my life? Well, that would be okay too, because I would then have an excuse for being a failure!*

And then there came a voice into my consciousness (it was as though someone else was speaking but I knew that the words came out of one of those folds deep in my rational brain): *If I am down there dead and nothing matters, then why should they matter if I am alive!*

And then came some words from one of my SMI recordings: The brain cannot distinguish the difference between a real experience and one that is vividly imagined. *If that is true why not imagine that I am dead, and if my brain cannot tell the difference then nothing should matter if I am alive!*

So in my imagination I drove off the cliff and saw myself down there dead.... And all of a sudden I felt a great burden lift from my being and a sense of freedom like I had never before experienced. My body and my mind felt like I had just emerged from a dark cold cave into the warm sunlight of a new experience and could clearly see my place in the scheme of things. I felt that I was no longer shackled by the thoughts and opinions of other people or the restraints of tradition.... And then I noticed the engine was still revved-up.

It was not a "spiritual experience" as a person would normally think of it, but in that moment I gained a wonderful sense of relief and an unexplained peace of mind. But I knew that it all happened as the result of something that went on between my conscious mind and my physical brain. Interesting!

Fortunately, I had only *mentally* followed through with the scheme of ending it all. But embedded in the futility of my situation—and with the somber consideration of initiating the discontinuation of this life's experience and the peace of mind that I experienced about still being alive—were the seeds from which sprung some major transitions in my life.

Well, since I'm not going to end it, I reasoned, *I guess I had better find a way to do something with it.* So with my newly acquired state of emotional freedom I engaged all of my energies to learning how to hypnotize myself. Learning self-hypnosis seemed to hold the greatest possibility to gain the confidence and the self-esteem necessary to enjoy being on this planet. So I picked up my book on self-hypnosis and began to study and practice again.

Interestingly, I thought that it was necessary to get my attitude and self-confidence fixed *first,* before I could engage in productive activities. It was the same kind of erroneous thinking that I'd had when I'd concluded that smart people were smart first and that's why they studied; I thought that successful people by nature were confident and success-oriented *first,* so they engaged in activities that brought them success. In reality, the opposite is true: The action of engaging in successful behavior *first* (even in the face of being fearful of doing so) breeds confidence and success. But this principle had not yet dawned on me.

Although I did force myself to go out and make a few sales calls, my primary interest was learning how to get myself hypnotized. *If I can just learn how to hypnotize myself, I can then give myself a post-hypnotic suggestion that I am successful. And then I will be successful. And since I am successful, I will do the things that successful people do that make them successful,* I illogically reasoned. So I spent a good deal of time studying and trying to hypnotize myself rather than making sales calls.

Because of my persistent reading deficiency, I laboriously struggled through *A Practical Guide to Self-Hypnosis* several times, word by word. I had located a remote corner in the city park where I would be out of the way and undisturbed. For two or three hours a day (over the course of several months) I sat staring at a ring I had glued to the ceiling of my car in an attempt to hypnotize myself.

Although I really "believed" that hypnosis was a powerful resource for developing my potential, I still had many false perceptions about it—the same ones many people still have today. The greatest one was that I thought a hypnotized person was asleep, and that because they were asleep they were unconscious and oblivious to what was going on. Apparently, I had forgotten about Judy back in high school being able to know that the bell had rung. But that was several lifetimes ago, it seemed.

Once I had memorized Melvin Powers' self-hypnosis "induction" procedure I began to practice doing exactly what he had instructed. But when I reached the point in the process where I was supposed to make a "test" to confirm that I was hypnotized, I didn't even try the test because I thought: *I am not hypnotized because I am not unconscious. I can still hear the swings clanging over there in the playground, so how can I be hypnotized? Oops, there goes another siren off in the distance.*

I seriously wondered: *If I do get myself hypnotized, and I go unconscious, how am I going to wake myself up?* I even worried, *If I hypnotize myself and I go unconscious and can't wake myself up, maybe six months from now someone will stumble upon a car parked in an isolated part of the park and find a skeleton sitting there with its hollow gaze fixed on a ring stuck on the ceiling!*

Obviously, Mr. Powers' method wasn't working. So I decided to go to the Salt Lake City Public Library and see if I could find some additional information on self-hypnosis that would give me some insight into what I was doing wrong.

Up until then, I really wasn't aware of the "evil" and "satanic" reputation hypnosis had managed to acquire over its 250 years of notoriety. Nor was I prepared for the intolerance that some people have for those of us who didn't take full advantage of our learning opportunities.

Many people, unless they have personally experienced a fear or phobia, may have difficulty understanding or sympathizing with those of us who have, so not everyone will be able to grasp the reality of my fear of institutions and feelings of inferiority when in the presence of people who are in a position of authority; those with titles and those who appear to be highly educated.

Although I "wanted" to go to the library, just the thought of it churned my stomach. It took a few days to muster up the courage to even get my car pointed in that direction, let alone get out and venture inside.

Consciously I knew the exact event from which my "Library Phobia" stemmed: Misbehaving at the Sandy City Public Library one day back in the fourth grade.

Shortly after arriving at the library that day, I found myself being grabbed by the hair on the back of my head, dragged in front of the other students and severely scolded by our teacher, Miss Howard, for having misbehaved and creating a ruckus. "A library is not a place for that kind of behavior. A library is a place where people come because it is quiet. It is not a place for horseplay. Lindsay, you really don't deserve to be here...." When finished with her "humiliation" ritual, Miss Howard marched me back to school (it was just a short walk from the library) and straight into the principal's office, where I spent the next two hours sitting on a three-legged stool, facing a familiar barren corner and fuming over the injustice of it all—I only pulled *hard* on Joan's pigtail once. This was not the only time my body had adorned this corner of the principal's office!

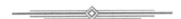

The Salt Lake City Public Library was, of course, much larger than the Sandy City Library so it was all the more imposing, but I finally conjured up the courage, drove to the library, took a deep breath, got out of my car, walked to the entrance and froze there for what seemed to be ten minutes while reasoning with myself: *There is nothing in there that is threatening. Besides that, even if there is it can't hurt me since I am already dead at the bottom of a cliff!* So I pulled open the imposing door and stepped into the house of dread. After looking around I spied a volunteer type person sitting behind a well-polished counter under the "HELP" sign.

I had had limited experience (as I think of it now, none!) in finding my way around a library and I needed some help to find the location of the books that I was looking for. When I asked the elderly, very prim, yet pleasant, grandmotherly woman how to find books in "her" library, she kindly smiled and said, "You can find any book you want if you will just look in the reference card files." When I asked her, "Where do I find the reference card files?" she less kindly pointed a slightly arthritic finger to a very large bank of cabinets right behind me that contained what to me looked like thousands of little drawers.

I said quizzically, "Okay, so how do I use the reference file?" Rather than coming down from her perch and *showing* me how to use the card file, she responded with even less kindliness. "Haven't you ever used a library reference card file before? I can't believe it! How can it be that someone your age doesn't know how to find a book in a library?" Not giving me time to answer she continued to question me. "Didn't you go to school? Didn't your teachers take you to the library and teach you how to find books when you were a child?"

I wanted to tell her, *No my teacher didn't. And the last, and only, time I was in a library I got kicked out and haven't been in one since.*

She hardly took a breath before continuing. "Second and third graders come in here every day and easily find any book they want! And here you are—what are you, twenty-five years old? (She was wrong, I was thirty-five—little consolation that she didn't know *everything*!) And you don't even know how to find a book in a library. I can't believe it!"

Her demeanor had switched from disparaging to contempt as she slowly and deliberately mouthed every word as though I was hearing-impaired and, pointing her gnarled, deformed finger, said, "Go over to that case with all the little drawers; find the drawer that has a reference card for the book you want." Again without a breath she continued, giving me no time to respond. "The drawers are arranged alphabetically. The "A's" start at the left end of the case and the "Z's" end up on the right. It is just like reading—from left to right."

Do I really appear to be so dim-witted that she thinks that I don't know that you read from left to right? I remember thinking.

She further advised me, "You can find the book you want by looking it up by the topic, the book title or the author's name." She explained that after I found the right drawer, I would find a card containing information about the book I wanted and that there would be some reference numbers on the card that corresponded with a number on one of the shelves in the library. She also explained that the books were arranged generally by either fiction or nonfiction—"Do you know the difference?"—and finally stopped talking for a moment.

Either she is just having a bad hair day, or she is trying to provoke me into doing something stupid so she can have me kicked out of "her" library. I was seething.

But she started up again. "After you find the right section, just look at the plaques at the end of each row of the bookcases to find the number that matches up with the numbers on the reference card. It is that easy," she said a little more softly. As I walked away from her "judicial bench," I heard her say under her breath, "*I just can't believe it!*"

She was right. It was easy. I found with little difficulty the drawer labeled "Hir" to "Hyp," and with less difficulty found three cards with the heading of "hypnosis." I wrote down the information on a 3x5 card and headed towards the sign that indicated nonfiction. But when I arrived at the shelf where the hypnosis books were supposed to be, there was only empty space.

I was still a little peeved by the way I was "helped" by my grandmotherly volunteer, and because the books weren't where they were suppose to be, my mood had not improved. I thought, *Maybe the topic of hypnosis is so popular that all three have been checked out. Or maybe an incompetent library staffer put them in the wrong place. But most likely it's my own lack of experience in library protocol.* Whatever the reason, I was reluctant to ask for any more "help."

Finally, out of desperation, I found a person who looked like a "real" librarian and asked if she could help me find the books that I was looking for.

"I need help. The books I want are not on the shelf where they are supposed to be. I don't know if I am not looking in the right place or if maybe they have been put on the wrong shelf?" I articulated carefully as I spoke to "Ms. Librarian" in an effort to sound like I was not simple-minded.

It turned out that getting help from a "real" librarian wasn't much better.

"I am sure, young man, that the books you want are exactly where they are supposed to be. Maybe they are all checked out, but if they are not they will be precisely where they should be; you just don't know where to look." As it turned out, she was right; *I* didn't know where to look because *she* had them hidden!

She continued on with her lecture: "Our people here are well-trained and they don't just throw books willy-nilly onto any shelf. Let me see what you have there."

I handed her my 3 x 5 card and when she looked at the titles there was a long, agonizing pause. Then she looked at me over her half-moon glasses, glared, and said unapologetically—with more than just a hint of disdain—"Oh, *those* books! We keep *those* kinds of books in a safe place. We keep them in a special cabinet in the back room under lock and key so they don't fall into the wrong hands."

In wise-guy mode (typical for me when having been provoked), I questioned her. "Wrong hands? Who are the people whose hands are the wrong ones?"

She looked at me with a "Don't get smart with me, sonny" look and said, "You know... young people, people who are deranged, people who are mentally ill, people who are evil and would use hypnosis to control the minds of innocent people and make them do bad things—those kinds of people."

I thought to myself, *This is truly bizarre. Are there really people who think of hypnosis as being so evil that they have to censor books about it?* And I retorted, "How do you know if someone is mentally ill, deranged or evil?"

She glared at me again and said, "I can just tell."

I said, "Would you show me where you safely keep them so I can check them out? Or do I look evil, deranged and satanic?"

"How old are you, sonny?" she questioned me. "To check them out you have to be over 21 years old, you know... and in good standing."

"What do you mean by 'in good standing?' In good standing with whom?"

Obviously agitated, she blurted out, "Show me your driver's license and then I'll take you to the head librarian."

I am sure that she led me off to the head librarian's office *not* because I looked like a person who was in "good standing," but because she was sick and tired of dealing with this smart aleck kid!

Once the head librarian had scrutinized my driver's license and had given me the once over, I was escorted to a locked glass bookcase in a storage room. As she was unlocking the case with what looked like a cell-door key, she curtly said, "You can check out only one of these at a time, you know."

I didn't know, but I did wonder why.

The bookcase contained about twenty books, none of which looked dangerous to me, but I am sure they were there so they wouldn't fall into the wrong hands. "Madame Librarian" kept an evil eye over my shoulder as I examined the three books about hypnosis. They looked brand new and had probably never been checked out. None of them dealt with *self*-hypnosis; and as I pondered which one might best fit my needs, I heard a scratchy voice coming from just behind my left ear: "Well, get on with it and choose one. Don't just stand there gawking. Just get on with it, so I can get back to doing something useful."

After hurriedly choosing one without paying much attention to its title, I was marched off to the checkout desk (where my reputation apparently had preceded me); and I was issued a library card by the "jailhouse matron" they had hired. Just before leaving I was sternly advised, "Make sure you keep good track of that book so it doesn't fall into the wrong hands."

With George Estabrooks' HYPNOSIS: *Current Problems* in hand, I walked out of the "dungeon" wondering, *Is the mentality of even the learned (library administrators and librarians) so distorted and irrational that they think books about hypnosis are dangerous? 'A dark, mystical power that the hypnotist has and can use to take control of another person's mind and soul, if he chooses to!' How could that kind of bigotry still be going on in the last half of the Twentieth Century?*

Estabrooks' book turned out to be exactly what I *didn't* want; it was written in a vocabulary geared for academia. Even with a pocket dictionary in one hand and his book in the other, it was beyond my full comprehension. So, after maybe 20 pages, I gave up. Not because of the difficult reading but because its content was not at all what I was looking for or needed.

I didn't know where else to look to find the information I was looking for, but I knew one thing for sure: I wasn't going to go back to the dungeon of dread and face the vultures again! So I picked up my copy of *A Practical Guide to Self-Hypnosis* and started studying and practicing again. With little noticeable progress, I gave up, dejected.

Then one day, several weeks later, just by pure chance (although people in my circle of acquaintances would have attributed it to Divine Intervention: "God led me to it") I stumbled upon a book at a rummage sale: *The New Self-Hypnosis*, by Paul Adams, and my interest in self-hypnosis was rekindled.

With a different approach, I thought, *maybe I can get self-hypnosis to work.* So I returned to my secluded park sanctuary and started studying and practicing once again.

The New Self-Hypnosis, although a full-sized book, turned out to be fairly easy reading. It was well organized and used logical reasoning rather than straightforward instructions on what to do. In Chapter Two, Adams attempted to dispel many of my false perceptions about hypnosis, and on page 20 he summarized each point:

1. Hypnosis is not sleep.

2. All the phenomena of hypnosis can be produced in the so-called "waking state."

3. An intelligent individual is easer to hypnotize than a not-so-intelligent person.

4. You will not violate your moral beliefs or lose your will while under hypnosis.

5. Hypnosis does not weaken the mind or will.

6. Hypnosis is a normal state.

7. Most of your daily functions are accomplished on a subconscious level.

8. All hypnosis is self-hypnosis.

9. Hypnosis is "an altered state of consciousness."

10. Hypnosis is a state of hyper-suggestibility.

11. The conscious mind possesses a "critical faculty."

12. The unconscious mind possesses a feedback mechanism.

13. Most people need to be de-hypnotized.

14. Self-hypnosis is the most effective way to effect change in your life.

Wow! This is just what I have been looking for... especially number 14: "Self-hypnosis is the most effective way to effect change in your life." Or maybe number 13; after thirty-six years of negative thinking I had unknowingly "hypnotized" myself into thinking that I couldn't or shouldn't achieve success and happiness and now I just needed to get myself "de-hypnotized." But then I wondered about number three: *Was I one of those "not-so-intelligent" people? Maybe that was why I couldn't hypnotize myself!*

CHAPTER 4

The Discovery

What Adams had to say about the nature of hypnosis was logical, made good sense and was relatively simple. But the "induction" process was so long and drawn out that it took at least 30 minutes to get through it. However, he assured the reader that, "When you finish this 'self-hypnosis induction' you *will* be in hypnosis."

The written instructions were not all that complicated, but it took me several days of *not* making sales calls before I had it memorized word for word.

When I was confident that I had it down—when I was sure I was using the very words that Adams told me to use—I began to practice:

As I close my eyes, I enter into a complete state of relaxation. I pay attention only to the thoughts I am giving myself. Any noises or sound I hear will not distract or disturb me. In fact, they will actually deepen my hypnosis. Each time I go into hypnosis I will go into it more deeply and quickly than the previous time. I will now feel perfectly comfortable and at ease. My breathing is easy, normal, and gentle. Every breath I take puts me more deeply into hypnosis. I feel the stream of air in my nostrils, and I feel my pulse beat, and every beat of my pulse puts me more and more deeply into relaxation.

This first part of the induction was really the only hard part to commit to memory. From here on it was redundant:

I now center my attention on my right foot. My right foot begins to relax more and more. The muscles in my toes relax more and more. This relaxing feeling moves into the arch of my foot and into my heel. My entire right foot feels enveloped in relaxation. My right foot is loose and limp and totally and completely relaxed. It has the sensation that it is being gently massaged.

Now I center my attention on my left foot. My left foot begins to relax....

The induction process was similar to the method that Art Baker used, except Art started with your fingertips.

Essentially the same words were used to relax my ankles (left and right), calves (left and right), knees (left and right)... and so on, progressively stopping at every muscle and joint and "centering my attention" on every part of my body up to my neck. And then starting with my fingers, wrists... and ending up with my scalp.

Even after I had "centered my attention" on every imaginable individual appendage, joint and muscle of my body, I was instructed to continue suggesting to myself that my body as a whole was relaxed; that took five minutes or so... And then my mind was relaxed for another five minutes. Ending up with, *I am now going deeper and deeper into relaxation. As I count down from ten to zero I will go deeper with every number that I count. Ten–I am relaxing more and more, and I am going deeper and deeper. Nine–I am relaxing more and more and going deeper and deeper. Eight... Seven... Six... Five... Four... Three... Two... One... Zero–now I am totally and completely relaxed, and my subconscious is now ready to receive suggestions.*

As with Art Baker and Powers, Adams said that I needed to make a "test" to determine if I had successfully hypnotized myself. So I chose to use *my eyes are stuck and I can't open them,* as a test. Art Baker had used this suggestion to "see" if he had successfully hypnotized his client.

Hence, after having spent thirty minutes hypnotizing myself I thought it was time to do the "test." So I said to myself, *My eyes are stuck closed and I cannot open them. When I try to open my eyes I will be unable to do so and my eyes will stick tighter and tighter shut. Now try to op...* and my eyes popped open. Damn! It didn't work.

All of my resources about hypnotizing myself (Baker, Powers and now Adams) said that I may not be successful the first time I tried, but if I would persist eventually I would be successful. So I started at the beginning: *As I close my eyes, I enter into a complete state of relaxation....*

Thirty minutes later I said to myself, *My eyes are stuck closed and I cannot open them. When I try to open my eyes I will be unable to and my eyes will stick tighter and tighter shut and no matter how I try to open them they will not open. Now try to op...* "Damn" again!

Two or three times a day for the next few weeks, I "persisted" with no better results. Each failure brought greater anxieties and frustrations; I was dejected, depressed, angry (I didn't know with whom I was angry, I was just angry) and so disappointed that I screamed to myself: *What am I doing wrong? Why can other people be hypnotized or hypnotize themselves and I can't do either?*

I continued to wonder, *What am I going to do now? Am I going to spend my whole life fearful of people and feeling self-conscious? Will I ever be able to feel good about myself? Is there any hope that I will be able to earn enough money to support my family and have a few of the extra things like other people have? Why does it seem that everything has to be so hard for me? Why can other people be happy and successful in their job, in their family life, and learn easily and I can't? Maybe I should have physically driven off of the cliff and ended it all!*

And then a voice came from some deep recess in my brain: *Lindsay, you have within you every quality, every attribute, every talent, every ability and everything that is needed to become, to achieve, to be, or to acquire anything you choose. It's about time to get off of your duff and start using it in spite of your fears.* Those were words Dell Rogers spoke to me a few weeks after he had recruited me into SMI.

And then came some other words: *Whatever the mind of man can conceive and believe he can achieve.* Those were Napoleon Hill's words right out of *Think and Grow Rich.*

And then: *We are what we think about most of the day.* Earl Nightingale, *The Strangest Secret.*

And bursting into my consciousness: *By changing a person's self-perceptions their behavior automatically changes. Psycho-Cybernetics,* Maxwell Maltz.

Maxwell Maltz was a plastic surgeon who found that performing cosmetic surgery to change a patient's physical appearance also changed their personality. The patient was the same person with the same talents and intellect, and possessed the same abilities as before the surgery, but just by changing their self-image their behavior changed. Apparently, having some physical attribute about which they were self-conscious and which they found unacceptable (and thinking that other people thought the same) caused them to be withdrawn and inhibited. But by removing or changing that physical attribute so they perceive themselves as acceptable to themselves and others, they become confident and outgoing.

And then came into my consciousness: *Your brain cannot distinguish the difference between a real experience and one that is vividly imagined.* Of course, those are the very words that came to me just before "not" driving off of the cliff. *Maybe that is the element I have been missing in my quest to hypnotize myself: I have not been "seeing" in my mind what I was saying with my mind. I was just saying words without visualizing what I was saying.*

With this idea in mind I went through my well-rehearsed self-hypnosis induction ceremony, but this time "pictured" in my mind the *meaning* of each word and phrase that I said—seeing the *images* that the words and phrases represented, not just *saying* the words.

So I started at the top: *As I close my eyes, I enter into a complete state of relaxation....* Rather than just saying the words I pictured myself "*entering into a complete state of relaxation.*"

...I will now feel perfectly comfortable and at ease. I not only said the words, but I imagined *I feel perfectly comfortable and at ease.*

...Now I center my attention on my left foot. My left foot begins to relax.... Rather than *saying My foot is beginning to relax,* I chose to "*see*" it relaxing.

...As I count down from ten to zero I will go deeper with every number that I count. Ten—I am relaxing more and more, and I am going deeper and deeper. (With each suggestion I made, I pictured that it was true.) *Nine—I am relaxing more and more and going deeper and deeper. Eight... Seven... Six... Five... Four... Three... Two... One... Zero—now I am totally and completely relaxed, and my subconscious is now ready to receive suggestions.*

When I reached zero I not only said to myself, *My eyes are stuck closed*, I "pictured" them stuck! I continued, *When I try to open my eyes I will be unable to and my eyes will stick tighter and tighter shut and no matter how hard I try to open them they will not open.* Remembering what I had observed with Art's clients, I imagined myself experiencing the same condition.... I pictured myself *trying* to open my eyes but only being able to raise my eyebrows.

Now try to open your eyes, I told myself, but I kept the mental picture of my eyes being stuck. When I tried to open them, they didn't open!!

This is really dumb, I thought, but continued to hold the image of my eyes being stuck. *I know that I can open my eyes but why don't I?* I continued to question, *I wonder what would happen if I changed the picture and "saw" my eyes open?* So I changed the image and "saw" them open, and they popped open!!!

I am sure this experience contained one of the greatest, if not the greatest, discoveries of my life: Limitations are created by "seeing" ourselves as limited—like me "seeing" my eyes as stuck limited me from opening them— and just by changing the image, we get out of our own way and the limitation disappears—when I pictured my eyes as open, they opened easily. *Can it be that simple?* I hoped yes!

So rather than trying to change my behavior directly while hypnotized— that is, rather than trying to force a behavior with pure willpower—I practiced "seeing" myself behaving as I chose to behave.

For example: Rather than thinking (as I had for all of my selling experiences) that I had to *make* myself make sales calls, whether I wanted to or not (I thought I had to use willpower or force myself to make them), I "pictured" myself peacefully making sales calls. And for some unexplainable reason, making sales calls seemed easier.

By setting aside *only* an hour each day to practice self-hypnosis (rather than *most* of the day as I had been doing over the previous several months) there began to be some very noticeable changes in my performance and confidence. I continued to use my newly discovered weapon of the innate powers of my mind and began overcoming (one by one) the limitations that I had accumulated over the first thirty-six years of my life.

Slowly I began to confidently make sales calls. As a matter of fact, within three months my sales volume was sufficient to often put my name at the top of the company's weekly sales report.

My financial circumstances started to improve, I found it easer to read, I started losing weight, I became more comfortably involved in social activities and I started feeling good about myself. I began to experience observable, measurable, changes in myself and in circumstances just as a result of hypnotizing myself and while in hypnosis giving myself suggestions (by "seeing" in my imagination) that the behavior and conditions I chose to possess were true. I knew I still had a long way to go to reach the confidence and self-esteem level I wanted to reach but, for sure, I had *discovered* the key to cause it to happen. But, unbeknownst to me, there were some major changes in the offing.

CHAPTER 5

A New Direction

From the moment I failed to hypnotize DeAna back in high school I had no intention whatsoever of *being* a hypnotist. All of my interests were directed toward using self-hypnosis to rid myself of my own inhibitions and inadequacy.

I had been practicing self-hypnosis for almost a year and was progressively removing many of my self-imposed hang-ups. Not *all* by any stretch of the imagination, but enough so that I felt like I was emerging from a deep, dark cave of ignorance and failure, and was beginning to see some light at its entrance.

One day I happened upon Richard. A few years earlier Richard and I had been selling burglar alarms for a company called Gardsite. Gardsite was one of the first (if not the first) companies to develop, manufacture and distribute motion-detecting burglar alarm systems. More accurately put, Richard was selling burglar alarms and was very good at it, and I was trying to conjure up the courage to sell burglar alarms.

Richard was one of those "old pros" who had zero call reluctance and who could probably sell anything to anyone. He was also one of those people willing to help anyone who he thought wanted or needed help to improve their selling skills.

He did a very good job of imparting his knowledge and philosophy about what it takes to be a top rate salesperson, but he had little success conveying to me (what I thought of as) his pure nerve and pushiness. I know now what it really was: a combination of self-confidence, an inborn comfort with meeting and talking with strangers and the use of logic and assertiveness to manipulate customers into buying what he was selling.

In an attempt to get me over my fear of asking customers for an order, he explained to me how *he* thought of it: "I just convince the customer that the product or service I am selling has greater value to them than their money. But sometimes I just have to push them into making the decision to part with some of it so they can enjoy the benefit of my product or service."

Richard explained, "The only time money has value is when a person is spending it. Money that is just sitting in a checking account or in someone's wallet is useless and has no value until it is given to someone else—until they take it from its hiding place and give it away in exchange for something that makes them feel good. So all I do is talk people into giving me their money in exchange for an alarm system so they and their property are safe—and that makes them feel good. Making the customer feel good by taking their money also makes me feel good. So why, Lindsay, would you ever hesitate to assertively ask your customer to part with some of their money, when by doing so you get an order and both of you feel good?"

My only answer was, "I don't know. I never thought of it that way before!"

I knew he was frustrated with my shyness, lack of motivation and fear of making phone calls to set up appointments and even making the calls after the appointments had been made. Even when he gave me some of his "sure sale" leads, I managed to make only an occasional sale. It wasn't that I couldn't have done much better, but more often than not I either made an excuse about why I couldn't make the call or just plain didn't show up at all. In spite of Richard's frustration over my inhibitions, we developed a good friendship.

The use of motion-detecting equipment (rather than the standard "hard-wired" circuit breaker method) as a means of keeping one's person and property safe, with its ability to automatically dial the police if there *was* an intruder, was in its infancy. As with many newly developed products, the Gardsite systems had some very serious technical problems. For example, the police might be called just because a loose piece of metal-backed insulation was blowing in the breeze at the lumberyard. Or a cat might unwittingly call the police for assistance as it crept around protecting a Big O tire store from mouse intruders. Almost every installation was plagued with false alarms and malfunctions, so not only were the customers upset but also the police were enraged. Gardsite was out of business in less than six months. So Richard went his way and I went mine.

Anyway, when I happened upon Richard again a few years later, he was as friendly and as genuine as I remembered him.

He greeted me with a hearty, "Well, hello, Lindsay, you old rascal, I hardly recognized you, you must have lost a ton of weight!" I had. Well, not a ton, but about 75 pounds. When I told him that I was selling industrial supplies and was doing quite well—and that much of my success was because I was using a few "tricks of the selling trade" that he had taught me a couple of years earlier—he thanked me for the compliment and said, "It was not your selling technique that got in the way of your being a good salesman; it was your pure terror of using the telephone, making sales calls and asking the customer for some of their money. I always knew you had it in you. What made the difference?"

"I have been hypnotizing myself and while hypnotized I give myself suggestions about being confident; that it is fun to make prospecting telephone calls, that being assertive and asking them to give me some of their money is a service to my customers—it makes both of us happy. Just as you taught me," I told him.

"Do you mean that hypnosis can make that kind of a change in a person? How does it work?"

I explained to him what I did to hypnotize myself and the kind of suggestions I gave to myself while hypnotized, but said that I didn't "know" how it worked. "I just visualize how I choose to be and eventually something inside of me just causes it to happen. I'm still trying to get rid of a lot of bad attitudes, unwanted habits and limitations, but self-hypnosis has certainly caused making sales a whole lot easier... and sometimes even fun!"

"I have heard that a hypnotist can "make" someone stop smoking. Is that true?" he asked.

"I know of a number of people who have successfully stopped smoking by being hypnotized, but I don't think that the hypnotist 'made' them do it. I do know that they stopped smoking after they were hypnotized, but I think it happened as the result of something inside themselves; it wasn't the hypnotist that 'made' it happen," I told him.

"I really want to stop smoking," he said. "I've tried about everything I can think of to get rid of this nasty habit. Oh, I've been able to quit for a day or two at times but I go right back to it and the more I try to stop, the harder it gets, and when I think about stopping I just smoke all the more." Without giving me a chance to respond (just as he did when selling burglar alarms to a prospective customer), he said, "I've been smoking since I was a kid and I wish I'd listened to my parents and the Bishop, who told me that smoking was a sin. I know that it is bad for me and that my wife and family hate the smell. It's expensive, too—I mean, they're up to 35 cents a pack and it's breaking me. Do you think you could hypnotize me and 'make' me stop smoking?"

When he stopped talking long enough for me to respond, I told him that I had never hypnotized anyone else before and that I didn't even know if I could. "I tried to hypnotize my date back in high school and it turned out be something far less than a great experience, but if you are willing I'll give it a try."

In addition to selling industrial supplies, a friend and I had rented a small office/warehouse and started an environmental products supply company that we called ECOLOGY II. I arranged to meet Richard at the office the next day and after moving a bunch of "stuff" around, I cleared enough space to set up a couple of chairs that faced each other.

Richard showed up right on the dot and after explaining what I thought he would be experiencing (with a very short pre-hypnotic talk) I slipped my wedding ring off and held it about a foot in front of his face. *"Just focus your gaze on my ring. In a moment I'm going to count down from five to one and with each number I count down your eyes will get more tired and sleepy. Five... Four... Three... Two... One... now just close your eyes."* He closed his eyes and for thirty minutes I went through essentially the same scenario that I used to hypnotize myself, to "induce" hypnosis in Richard. (I asked him to visualize that each part of his body was relaxed, and suggested to him that he was in a deep sleep and would be receptive to my suggestions.) When he "looked" hypnotized, I asked him to "see" himself as a non-smoker and to "picture" himself as healthy and being comfortable around his family. I told him that he no longer needed to feel self-conscious about how his clothing smelled and asked him to "visualize" himself with more money in his pocket. I went on for another thirty minutes with similar suggestions.

I said, *"I am going to count up from one to five and when I reach the number five, just open your eyes."* I counted up, suggesting to him with each number that he was waking up, feeling fine and following the suggestions that I had given him. When I reached the number five I said, *"Open your eyes now and you are wide awake!"*

"Well, what do you think?" I asked.

Richard said, "I don't think I was hypnotized because I was conscious all of the time, but I feel more relaxed right now than I have in a very long time. I feel like I just woke up from a nice nap. I really feel great. But I was never unconscious..."

He might have gone on and on about how wonderful an experience it had been, had I not interrupted him to ask, "But do you feel like you want to smoke??"

He stopped for a moment and after some obvious introspection said, "Right now I don't feel like I need a cigarette. I didn't even think about smoking until you mentioned it. It's really strange. I always feel like I need a cigarette when I wake up. I feel like I just woke up, but I truly don't feel like smoking. I don't remember much of what you said, but whatever it was I guess it worked. It really is weird that I have been trying to stop smoking for years and those few times I quit for a day or two I always *wanted* to smoke, but now, after just five minutes of hypnosis, I really don't want a cigarette—at least right now. This is truly great!"

I was very much surprised by his enthusiastic response and even more surprised that he thought it had been only five minutes, when in fact it had been an hour or more! And then I thought, *There seem to be some inconsistencies in what Richard just said:* "I was never unconscious the whole time, but I don't remember much of what you said." *That's something I need to think about. How can a person be asleep, say they heard everything that was said, and then not remember much of what was said afterwards? And not only that, think that an hour was five minutes!*

I had been indoctrinated by Art Baker (and by the authors of the books that I had read about hypnosis) to believe that getting a client to stop smoking was one of the most difficult issues to deal with and one of the hardest habits to break; that for a person to stop smoking it would take several sessions; that the longer a person had been smoking the more sessions it would take to break the habit; that it takes a few weeks for the nicotine to get out of one's system; and that even with hypnosis it is a long, drawn-out process to get a person to stop smoking for good. But when I asked Richard when he wanted his next session he responded, "Why would I need another session?"

I explained to him that the experts had told me that it would take about five sessions to make it "stick." So he agreed and we set up one session for three days hence and another one in a week.

At the end of the third session I asked when he would like to make his next appointment and, again, his answer was, "Why?" He, in his natural assertive way, said, "For over a week I haven't had or wanted a cigarette; I have had no cravings or even a hint of a desire to smoke. I love everything that has happened since I have been a non-smoker, as do my wife and children, and I think that having any more sessions would be a waste of my time as well as yours. Don't you remember me telling you a couple of years ago that once the sale is made, 'Shut up and leave'?"

I had no rational response, and began to question what I had been told by those who should be in the know. And I wondered if some people didn't need multiple sessions to achieve the desired results.

That a client might need only one session was only the first of hundreds of lessons I would learn from my clients over nearly four decades. This lesson was loud and clear: Don't do in five sessions what can probably be accomplished in one! The additional time and expense constitute a disservice to the client.

From that moment on, my objective has been to accomplish the desired change in a person's behavior in a single session. Some people may require more than one session, but I can't tell beforehand which ones will. If they do need additional sessions I'll see them more than once, but I have no intention of having people come back multiple times just for the sake of having more sessions, if they don't need them.

It appears to me that the hypnosis session begins the moment I first speak to the prospective client—that's when the pre-hypnotic talk begins. If I tell a prospective client that I want to see them three, four or five times, that plants in their mind the "suggestion" that it is going to take three, four or five times. So, by telling them that most of the time I see my clients only once, but that if they need additional sessions I'd be happy to work with them, I send an entirely different message.

Because of Richard's positive response and apparent success I began considering the possibility of getting into hypnosis as a profession. But I wasn't in a financial position yet to have hypnosis as my sole source of income. Even Art Baker, who had been hypnotizing people for twenty years or more, needed to keep his position at Western Airlines so he could afford to pursue his love of helping people with hypnosis. *Besides, maybe Richard's success was just a fluke*, I thought to myself. *Maybe he was just at a point in his life where he would have stopped smoking anyway and hypnosis had nothing to do with it*—some of my old negative thinking creeping back into my consciousness.

I hoped it was the hypnosis, but I really didn't know. *And besides that*, I questioned myself, *didn't a person need experience, training or some kind of schooling to be a hypnotist?* At the time I didn't know that there is no such thing as a degree in hypnosis, and although I tried, I could find no institution that offered hypnosis training or certification. So I decided that I would just have to learn how to do it on my own. All I needed was to find some people to practice on.

I didn't have to wait long. A few days after my last session with Richard, one of his friends called and asked if I could "do" to him what I had "done" to Richard. "I want to stop smoking, too," he said.

I informed him that I had had very little experience hypnotizing other people. "In fact, Richard was my very first subject. I don't know if I can help you or not, but if you want to try I'd be happy to accommodate you. Besides, I have been looking for people to practice on. Would you like to try anyway?"

Rob said, "Yes."

After he arrived at my office, I asked him to sit down on one of the two chairs in the "clearing" in the center of my office. I led him through a short pre-hypnotic talk, using a few ideas that I had gleaned from Art Baker—an expanded version of the pre-hypnotic talk I had used with Richard. I figured that if I was going to be a professional hypnotist I ought to begin a session like the pros did.

"Hypnosis is not being asleep," I told him. "It's kind of like when you are driving your car home from work and you end up in your driveway but don't remember making any turns or stopping for red lights. I don't know how hypnosis works, all I know is that self-hypnosis has made a big difference in my life, and that after being hypnotized Richard stopped smoking. Under hypnosis you can't be made to do something that you normally wouldn't do, or do anything that would threaten you or cause you harm," I explained.

I then said, *"Just put your hands in your lap and look at the ring I am holding...."*

An hour or so later I counted up from one to five and said, *"Open your eyes, you are wide awake!"*

Rob opened his eyes and almost word for word echoed Richard's comments after he had been hypnotized. I suspected that Richard had told Rob about his experience and retold several times how he felt after his session. I even had to stop him from talking on and on to ask, "Yes, but do you feel like you need a cigarette?"

He thought for a moment and said, "No. Right now I really don't want a cigarette. I feel like I just woke up and I always feel like I need a cigarette when I wake up. I guess this stuff really works."

I thought I'd take my chances and see if maybe only one session was all that would be needed, so I asked, "Do you think that you will need another session or do you think that one is all that it will take?"

He answered, "No, I don't think I'll need another session." Remembering what Richard told me to do when the sale is closed, I "shut up" and sent Rob out the door.

I never did hear back from Rob, so I assumed that he had successfully stopped. However, there was a sense of relief when he didn't call back, because if he had, and had said that he was smoking again and that it hadn't worked, it would have been an affront to my still fragile ego.

Now I just need some more people to practice on, I thought to myself. *But how can I find them?*

I knew that I couldn't ask any of my friends or family to be practice subjects; they were still in the "hypnosis is evil and the work of the Devil" mode. So I just kept hypnotizing myself and hoping that I would stumble onto someone else that was open to being hypnotized.

CHAPTER 6

Moving Forward

Over the next several months I had kept up with my self-hypnosis regimen and had special-ordered a couple of books about hypnotizing other people, but could find no one to practice on. It was difficult to find people who even wanted to *talk* about hypnosis (on a rational level), let alone willing to let me practice on them. *The "evil" reputation is still floating in the ether around the whole of Salt Lake City, and not just with people I know,* I contemplated.

But then all of that changed. Not the evil part, but interest in and curiosity about hypnosis. It was like an evangelical revival.

For as long as I could remember, and probably since the day Brigham Young looked out over the Salt Lake Valley and announced, "This is the Place," never had there been such an advertising blitz as the one that announced: *Reveen is coming.*

Reveen was an internationally renowned stage-show hypnotist who was touring the United States and Canada. For a month on every major thoroughfare there was at least one billboard announcing his arrival. And for two weeks on radio stations and in every newspaper there were blurbs informing the population of SLC that: *Reveen the Hypnotist is coming.*

Of course I could hardly wait. On the day of his premier performance I showed up at Highland High School along with (I am guessing) two thousand other people.

Every one of his six performances was a sell-out and I attended three of the six. All were superbly orchestrated and choreographed. Reveen and his support people were true professionals at their various trades.

With few exceptions, the format of each show was identical, but in reality they were all exceedingly different because of the way in which the different volunteers responded to the same suggestions.

It was everything, and more, that I could have ever imagined. My cousin's story of the stage-show hypnotist back when I was a kid was tame compared to what I witnessed.

After demonstrating some of his psychic and memory skills, Reveen asked for volunteers to come up on stage to be hypnotized. Within seconds the stage was flooded with willing subjects. I wondered to myself, *Where did all of these people come from? How is it that there are thousands of people that are not only interested in hypnosis, but hundreds willing and anxious to be hypnotized?* In six months I had found only two!

After weeding out all but about twenty of the volunteers, within ten minutes he had five or six different scenarios going on simultaneously. How he kept track of them all I'll never know.

He had two shirtless guys with robust abdomens strutting around the stage showing off their belly dancing skills, and two more fellows doing the hula with exaggerated rolling of their hips. A teenage girl and boy were crawling around on all fours among the other volunteers, hissing and barking at each other. There was a starry-eyed guy romancing a microphone. There was another chap who *really* needed to go to the restroom; halfway to the exit sign, however, he forgot where he was going and went back to the stage, only to find when he reached the stage that the urge hit him again and he headed off for the exit sign once again.

There was a really studious looking fellow (I'm sure Reveen picked him because of his looks) who could not remember or say the number six. Reveen asked him to count the fingers on both of his hands. He counted, "One... two... three... four... five... seven... eight... nine... ten... eleven!" He looked at his hand with the extra finger, obviously frustrated, and contemplated where that spare finger could have come from. Reveen told him to keep working on it until he got it right. He never did, until the end of the show when Reveen snapped his fingers.

After having been suggested to do so, a jealous girl began trying, to no avail, to win over the affection of the lover who was enamored with the microphone; and there were two competing Elvises trying to out-do one another with songs and gyrations.

As one scenario had run its course, Reveen would engage the volunteers in a different routine. To a select few volunteers, so it would be obvious to the audience but so only the subject could hear him, he whispered some additional suggestions (creating some suspense and anticipation within the audience). And all of a sudden Reveen bellowed, *"Everyone look at me!"* And then, so all of the volunteers could see, he raised his hand high above his head, snapped his fingers and commanded, *"Wide awake!"*

They all stopped in their tracks and looked around, puzzling at what they were doing on a stage in front of an auditorium full of people laughing at them—wondering what had been going on. The "swooner" looked at the microphone with embarrassment and then at the audience and snuck off of the stage, while the girl who had been pursuing him slithered off, red-faced, in a different direction. The extra finger was reconciled and the Elvises congratulated each other on having conducted a fine performance—all just as they had been suggested to do.

The stage was now empty—except for a few people whose left foot had apparently been glued to the floor. And as they were struggling to un-stick themselves, from the seats in the auditorium came the shouts of some of the volunteers, who, when they sat down in their seats, immediately jumped up and cried, "The redcoats are coming! The redcoats are coming!"

After letting the volunteers do their suggested tasks for a few moments, Reveen clapped his hands and shouted, "*Everyone* wide awake!" The left-foot-stuck-to-the-floor people walked off of the stage with no difficulty and the volunteers in the audience stopped warning everyone about the impending advance of the British.

But the restroom guy was still tromping from stage to aisle and back to stage again. When Reveen walked up to him and asked what he was doing, he said, "I *really* feel like I need to go to the bathroom but when I get halfway there I don't need to go anymore, so I go back to the stage and it starts all over again. I've been doing this all night and I can't figure it out. Reveen placed one hand on the young man's shoulder and with his other hand snapped his fingers in front of his face and said, "*Wide awake!*" The young man blinked his eyes, looked at Reveen, said, "Who are you?" and turned around and returned to his seat.

There were many more routines that I have not recounted and the ones I have may not have been told *exactly* as they happened, but my account is close enough to make my point: I was stunned, amazed and curious!

I wondered, *How can people almost immediately be "talked into" doing such irrational things by another person? I wonder if, in everyday life, people get "suggested" into irrational behavior by another person, with neither the "suggestor" nor the "suggestee" being aware that hypnosis was involved. Or is it something other than hypnosis?* I continued to analyze. *Why did the volunteers seem to be perfectly conscious and aware while doing such crazy things on stage and then seem to not remember afterwards? Reveen had told them to "sleep" when he was hypnotizing them and when he snapped his fingers said "Wide awake," but were they ever really asleep?* I further pondered: *What was going on in the subject's brain that automatically transformed a hypnotic suggestion into the very behavior that had been suggested?* I wondered if *I* would ever develop enough courage, confidence and skill to be a stage hypnotist.

And then Napoleon Hill's voice oozed up out of one of those deep brain folds: "When a need or desire arises in the human mind, the means by which to fulfill the need or desire will surely appear!" I wondered if what he said was true!

As a result of Reveen's advertising blitzkrieg and the media stories that followed, people began to openly talk about hypnosis. I often initiated the conversation about the topic, hoping that someone might be interested enough to be my next practice subject.

It surprised me that almost everyone I talked to had either heard of Reveen or had attended at least one of his shows.

When I told them that *I* had hypnotized a "few" people (I should have been truthful and said two) and was looking for people to practice on, their first reaction was skepticism that I actually had, and then they would respond, "Even if you *can* hypnotize people, for sure I don't want to be one of them!" I suspected that what they really meant was that they didn't want to head off to the bathroom and halfway there forget where they were going.... Or fall in love with a microphone!

But in a roundabout way, Reveen did bring me my next subject.

A week or so after the stage-shows, I received a call from another acquaintance of Richard's. She said her name was "Sonnie Shine," and that she worked as a counselor (salesperson) at an employment agency. She admitted that Sonnie Shine wasn't her real name; it was just an alias she used when at work. "My clients seldom forget my name!"

She said that earlier in the day she had been talking with Richard when the topic of hypnosis came up. She told me that she had been to see Reveen do his hypnosis stage-show-comedy-act thing, and had asked Richard if he had ever seen a person hypnotized. "He told me that he hadn't *seen* anyone hypnotized, but that he had *been* hypnotized several months earlier to stop smoking and hadn't smoked a cigarette since. And then he told me that you had been using self-hypnosis to get over the fear of making prospecting telephone calls and being assertive when it came time to close the sale.

"I was just wondering if you could hypnotize me and *make* me be better at my job?" she asked.

When I asked her what exact part of her job she wanted to get better at, she said, "I want to improve my performance in "selling" my clients on making a good impression when applying for a job and "selling" the prospective employer to hire them. But I am also interested in maintaining a positive attitude, staying motivated, keeping focused, having the courage to be assertive, improving my self-esteem, trimming some weight, not being so sensitive to criticism, being happy and having more patience with my husband and kids...." She took in a deep breath and then let it out. "That's all," she said with a chuckle.

I gave her my story about being very new at hypnotizing people but told her that if she wanted to try I'd be happy to work with her. (Besides, I needed people to practice on.) "Do you want to try anyway?" I asked her.

As with Richard and Rob, my inexperience was not an issue and she answered, "I don't care how long you have been hypnotizing people, I just want to get better at what I am doing and feel good about myself. Yes, I want to try."

CHAPTER 7

An Emotional Experience

Sonnie was a neatly dressed, thirty-five-year-old, well-spoken, mature young woman who, from all outward appearances, was confident and self-assured. To me, it appeared she should have no difficulty whatsoever confidently selling herself and successfully selling her "people" clients on making a good impression when interviewing for a job, or selling her "company" clients on hiring the people she sent in to fill a position. But I could relate to her problem because for most of my life the first impression most people had of me was that I was self-confident and outgoing, while in reality they didn't have even an inkling of what was going on under the façade.

As we conversed about what specifically she wanted to change (being confident and assertive), I thought, *She must be as good at putting on an air of self-confidence as I am.*

The session with Sonnie went smoothly, with seemingly good success, and when she left my office she commented on how good she felt and that she was looking forward to being free from being stressed-out about everything and being rid of her self-imposed limitations.

A few weeks later she called and said she had increased her weekly client job placement rate in each of the last two weeks and that her relationship with her husband and children had greatly improved since our session. "But there still seems to be something holding me back," she said. "Do you think that another session might help to improve my performance even more?

"My manager says that I am just not assertive enough with my clients. He says that it's as though I am afraid that someone might get angry with me if I assert myself. I *want* to be more assertive, but even thinking about being pushy makes my stomach ache. Do you think you can help me?" she pleaded.

I told her that I didn't know if I could help her or not, but that those were the same feelings that I used to get just thinking about making sales calls, and that if she wanted to give it a try, I'd be willing.

Because I was still very much unsure of my hypnotizing skills, and wanted to get more knowledgeable about hypnotizing other people, I had been reading some new mail-order hypnosis books. (Two of them were not much more than pamphlets; the third one was Arnold Furst's *Post-Hypnotic Instructions*.) Although each author's approach was different, when dealing with emotional issues all three were of the same opinion: You have to "regress" the subject back to the "sensitizing" event (the "core experience") that was the cause of their unwanted emotion. Once the core experience has been found, all the hypnotist needs to do is suggest to the client that they will no longer feel the emotions, since they now know the event that created them. All three authors cited convincing case histories resulting in the client being "cured" as a result of having used this method.

Art Baker had alluded to this same approach, but I had not witnessed the procedure in real life. So, since the experts said that this method was effective, I thought that this must be the way it was supposed to be done.

The next morning Sonnie showed up. After a modified pre-hypnotic talk in which I explained to her what I had learned from those in the know, and after going through my thirty-minute "induction"—and when I thought Sonnie was hypnotized—I was ill-prepared for her reaction when I said, "*Go back to the experience that causes you to have your fear of asserting yourself when dealing with your clients.*"

Without warning, Sonnie broke out into a wild display of uncontrollable emotions! Although she had opened her eyes they were seemingly fixed on some unseen image, as though she was in some sort of a fit, and she began sobbing uncontrollably, with her fists clenched tight and her body shaking while saying over and over, "It wasn't my fault, it wasn't my fault...."

Although her outburst triggered a heightened state of anxiousness in *me*, I tried my best to do a "Mr. Bruce" act and attempted to stay calm, but in reality my insides were roiling. As calmly as I could I said over and over, "*Everything is fine. You are perfectly safe. Just relax....*"

Having had zero experience handling this sort of an emotional outbreak, I was at a loss to know how to properly deal with her state of hysteria.

I wondered, *What have I turned loose in her? Maybe hypnosis does open up one's soul and give the Devil an opening to take possession of a person's being! If not some evil spirit, at least I must have revealed some deep, dark, long-hidden secret that had been lurking in her subconscious mind just waiting for an opportunity to be released. I wonder if causing her to expose some traumatic experience that occurred in her past could have a serious consequence on her psyche for the rest of her life?*

Not knowing what else to do, I just kept on assuring her that everything was fine, she was safe, and she should relax and think of something pleasant.

Eventually she calmed down to the point where she stopped her sobbing and could speak. "I have always remembered that experience but I didn't know that it was tied up with those kinds of intense emotions. I'm okay now, but I am still fuming inside about the injustice of the whole thing. I have always known my mom's response was reasonable because she didn't know all of the facts—she didn't know what really happened—but from time to time when I think about it I get this shaking feeling in my body and my stomach just churns."

I was greatly relieved that she had not been possessed by an "evil spirit" and that I was not responsible for disclosing some dark, hidden, "subconscious mind" secret, yet I was still reluctant to ask her about the event since I was afraid asking might spark another round of emotional outburst! But in time, when she had calmed down considerably and my curiosity became too great, I took my chances and asked in my softest voice (and soft was difficult, considering the emotional trauma I had experienced myself!), "Is this something that you would like to talk about?"

Much to my relief Sonnie said, "Sure. I quite often talk about it with my friends, but I just never before burst out emotionally like that. To the contrary, when I talk to my friends about the event we laugh about it." She stopped and thought for a moment. "Only the first part, though. I have never talked to anyone about the last part!"

She told me that back when she eleven years old, she was goaded into telling off and confronting a "gruff, grouchy old neighbor" because he would not return a Frisbee that had sailed into his back yard. To emphasize his displeasure, he angrily spewed out a stream of vulgar expressions containing words whose meaning she had only a vague notion—but they inferred that Deity was going to damn her and her little friends to hell for a very long time, where their tiny bodies would rot forever! And then he made several references that questioned their mothers' fidelity.

"Since I was the oldest of the group," she said, "they dared me to crawl over the fence and tell him what we thought of him as a person and to do whatever it took to retrieve the Frisbee.

"To bolster my reputation as a dare-devil I calmly clambered over the fence, naively thinking all I would need to do was politely ask him to 'pleeeeze' give back the Frisbee. I walked up to him, but before I could say a word he swatted me with one solid blow right on my behind and sent me sprawling."

After a momentary chuckle about the scene in retrospect, Sonnie continued. "Something inside me snapped! Stunned, I got up off of the ground, fuming mad, and walked right up to him. Using some of the same words I had learned just moments earlier, I began cussing at him, calling him every name I could think of and stomping on his foot, I grabbed the Frisbee out of his hand and spun around to make my escape back to the sanctuary of my own yard—and this is where the funny part ends. When I looked up, there was my mom, standing on our side of the fence, hands on her hips, glaring."

Sonnie's voice and manner turned dead serious and she said, "After I crawled over the fence, my mother grabbed me by the nape of my neck and marched me to my bedroom, and with several good hard swats of her own on my already tender hind-side, expounded, 'Don't you have any respect for other people's feelings? Whatever in the world got into you? Where in the world did you learn those kinds of words? Is that how your friends talk? I didn't think that a child of mine would ever act and talk like that. Don't you know those kinds of actions and words make me and your dad look bad? Don't you care what other people think of you? You stay in your room until your dad gets home and I'll let him deal with this, and if *I* ever hear of you asserting yourself like that again there will be all hell to pay! I just don't know what we are going....'"

Sonnie stopped in mid sentence, looked at me and exclaimed, "Asserting! I have never before associated the word 'assertive' with that experience. You know, when people tell me that I need to be more assertive I get this wrenching feeling in my gut. That is the same feeling I had while I was waiting in my bedroom for whatever the consequences were going to be when my dad got home. Do you think that that has something to do with my fear of being assertive?"

"Yes," I replied, "at least from what I understand from the experts (my pamphlets, Baker and Furst). According to them, now that you know the experience associated with the fear it should go away."

I continued cautiously. "I feel better now, but when you were sobbing out of control, glassy-eyed and staring out into space, I was really anxious. I'm not sure I want to go through that again." And I left it at that.

After a short conversation about the emotional outburst, I assured her that she would be feeling better and should be able to get on with her life now and be free to be assertive without the gut-wrenching emotions.

As I sent her out the door she said, "I hope so."

Immediately after Sonnie left my office I called Art Baker and asked for some advice about how I should have handled my session with Sonnie.

He assured me that I had dealt with it just fine and went on to say, "Those kinds of emotions often just pop up when you least expect it, especially when dealing with past experiences. You just don't know what's going to leap out of a client's subconscious mind. I have found that the best way to deal with it is to let them just sit there and sob—just let them vent it all out. It may take a while for them to settle down to a point where you can talk to them rationally, but eventually they'll calm down. I've had people go on for most of an hour before they got back to their senses."

"That's good advice, Art, but what do you do after they come to their senses? How do you extract those memories from a person's subconscious mind and then wipe out the negative feelings associated with them?"

"Well, it's a rather involved process and may take several sessions," he told me. "First you need to be sure that they don't have a history of mental disorders, like severe psychosis, neurosis or attempted suicide. If they have had any of those symptoms or tendencies, send them to a psychiatrist or psychologist—you don't want to mess with them."

"But how do you find out if they have mental disorders? I have had serious thoughts about suicide," I admitted, "but I don't think that I am insane."

"Well, you are not insane," he scolded me. "Did you ever really go through with your plan or did something from inside you keep you from taking action that would have caused self-inflicted harm?"

My answer was no, I didn't and yes, it did.

"Then just ask them. Ask them if they have ever gone through psychotherapy or spent time in a mental institution. If they say yes, send them away! If they say no, help them to change whatever it is that they want to change."

"Okay. So if a person is not insane, has not been under psychiatric care, and has not seriously tried to kill himself, *then* what do I do?" I asked.

"After you have found the source of the problem, find some way to have them discard it bit by bit. Here is a method that I use: I suggest to my client to imagine himself pulling a little red wagon down the 'street of their life.' Strewn along the sides of the street are pieces of the experience that they want to get rid of. As they approach each scrap I suggest to them to pick it up and examine it, and as they consider what it means, I have them tell me what it is and how it relates to the problem. You may have to ask a few additional questions to prod them along, such as, 'What does this scrap have to do with the problem?'" he said.

"After they have scrutinized that scrap of information, I suggest to them that they chuck it into their little red wagon, and that as they do that, they are throwing away that part of their problem. I suggest to them that it is as if that scrap of the problem was never there. Then I tell them to move on to the next bit of garbage... because that is all their problem is, anyway—garbage.

"After they have gathered up all of their garbage, I have them proceed down their street of life to a bridge that spans a river. I suggest to them that when they reach the river they toss their load of garbage, wagon and all, over the side and watch every piece of their problem float away forever.

"It might take several sessions to get all of the garbage off of their street of life, but there is usually a significant improvement after the first session."

When I got off of the phone with Art, I scribbled down what he had told me as best as I could remember. I reviewed my scribblings several times and practiced saying what he had said, and began committing it to memory... just in case I ever needed it.

And two days later I did need it!

Sonnie called and said that she had had the worst two days of her life at work and at home. "All I can think about is my mom and dad yelling at me and telling me how much they were disappointed in me for asserting myself and having stomped on 'Mr. Grinch's' toe and cussing at him. I've lost my enthusiasm for work, and my husband and kids are about ready to send me back home to my mother. Can you help me get rid of these bad feelings and my crummy attitude?"

I told her that I had talked to my mentor and had received some advice on how to help people who are struggling with emotional issues related to past experiences. She said that she was ready to try anything, so I agreed to see her the next morning.

When she entered my office I remember thinking, *She looks like she has aged ten years in just a few days. Her hair looks like she tried to comb it with a square of butter (matted and greasy), her clothes are untidy and her attempt to improve her appearance by putting on make-up failed. She looks a mess!*

After a short conversation and a brief pre-hypnotic talk, I had her sit in my newly purchased recliner in my newly arranged empty-of-stuff room (rather than sitting on a folding chair amid boxes of inventory) and asked her to look at the ring I was holding....

When I thought she was relaxed and hypnotized, I asked her how she felt and she responded, "Better."

So I began. *"In a moment I will be asking you to imagine yourself pulling a little red wagon down the street of your life. Strewn along the sides of the street you will find pieces of the experience of the past that you want to get rid of—the experience of being criticized by your parents for having been assertive and treating your neighbor with disrespect. I will be asking you, as you come upon each scrap of the experience, to pick it up, examine it, and tell me how it relates to your feeling 'crummy.'"*

Art Baker had told me that it is much more effective to tell the hypnotic subject what you want them to do, and then tell them to do it.

So I continued. *"Start walking down the street of your life now, pulling your little red wagon, and when you come to each piece of the experience pick it up and tell me what it is and how it relates to the bad feeling that you have been experiencing."*

I waited for a very long time, maybe three minutes that seemed like ten, without saying anything because I could tell there was something going on in her mind by the changing facial expressions she was creating. My impatient nature finally won out and I asked, *"What is happening?"*

Startled, she bolted out of the recliner and with her eyes open said, "I was dreaming.

"I dreamed that I was walking down a street pulling a little red wagon and I came to a place where there was a little pile of garbage lying in the gutter. I thought I was supposed to pick it up but I couldn't make myself do it. I kept thinking about picking it up but I was afraid to. It was like I was responsible for the litter and if it hadn't been for me the whole street would be clean and orderly. So I just stood there looking at it feeling guilty. I had a feeling that if I picked up a single piece I would find out something I didn't want to know."

I thought, *What do I do now?* Art didn't tell me what to do if the client opens her eyes and looks at me. When she had opened her eyes and talked to me with a matter of fact, rational voice, I thought that she must have come out of hypnosis. So I improvised—remaining as calm I could—and, asking her to close her eyes, I went through my hypnosis induction again. When she looked hypnotized again, I said, *"Return to your dream and tell me why you don't want to pick up the garbage."*

She just sat there without responding and when I was about to speak, she whispered, "All of my family is standing nearby looking at me, but if I pick up the garbage it will be an admission that it was me who made the mess. It would be admitting that it was my fault and that what would have otherwise been a happy and orderly street is a mess because of me; everyone is angry at me for having made the mess. It's just one little pile but everyone thinks that it makes the whole street look messy."

Moving a little closer, so I could better hear what she was whispering, I asked, *"What does the trash in the street have to do with your having those ugly feelings you have been experiencing over the past few days?"*

Again she just sat there for what seemed to be a longer period of time than should have been necessary to come up with what, to me, should have been an obvious answer.

Finally she said, in a barely audible voice, talking as if she was actually experiencing the scenario at the moment, "The street is my life. As I look up and down the street in both directions everything is clean, orderly and bright, except for this little stack of garbage. But that small pile of garbage makes the whole street ugly. It *doesn't* really make the whole street look ugly, it just seems to *me* that it does, but it seems that everyone else sees it as a blight."

I waited for her to continue but she just sat there as motionless as a rock. So I asked, "*What does this have to do with your emotional state of the past few days? How does all of this relate to making an otherwise positive, motivated person–you–feel so miserable?*"

Again I waited, but she just sat there until I asked, "*What are you thinking about? What is going on in your mind?*"

And then she said, "It is like my life. Although I have always been an adventuresome person, my whole life has been spent doing what I thought was right–except for that one experience with my neighbor. That was the only time in my entire life that my mother ever condemned me or gave me a swat on my rump. And then when my father came home all he could do was criticize me for being..." and then she paused for a moment. "Here's that word again–for being *assertive*! At the time I really didn't know what assertive meant and I still don't know why they used it because it really doesn't seem to quite fit, but I felt that it had to be something awful."

To clarify what she had just told me I asked, "*Does the little pile of garbage in the street represent this one experience in your life, but it makes your whole life seem messy?*"

"Yes."

So I asked her if she wanted to clean up the mess, throw it away, and have that experience no longer trouble her.

Again she responded, "Yes."

"*Okay. Return back to the pile of clutter. In a moment I'm going to have you pick up each piece of garbage one by one, because that is all it is anyway–garbage. As you pick up each piece, recognize that each one represents a single part of that one event in your life and, since it serves no purpose in your life now, throw it in your little red wagon. Tell me when you have cleaned up the mess and the whole street is neat and orderly. Start picking up your garbage now.*"

To my surprise she opened her eyes, got out of the chair and began physically going through the motions of picking up imaginary scraps of garbage, examining them, and then tossing them over her shoulder into an invisible wagon!

While this was going on I was thinking that this looked just like one of the antics I saw during Reveen's stage-show. *If I ever get the courage to do stage-show hypnosis, this might be an interesting scenario to recreate,* I thought.

It took several minutes for her to get everything cleaned up, but while she was going through her charade, I was also wondering, *What is really going on in her mind? Is she, in her mind, really "seeing" garbage and a little red wagon? Why did she get out of the chair to go through this pantomime? She seems oblivious to everything else (me and her surroundings) and is behaving as though the street, the wagon, and the garbage are really real.*

I further philosophized, *How many people are running around, including me, acting as though things that aren't real are real? It is obvious to me that there is no garbage on my office floor and that there is no little red wagon to throw it into, but it appears that to her there is. I wonder what is happening up in her head?*

All of a sudden she said, "It's all cleaned up and in the wagon." And she sat back in the recliner and closed her eyes.

So I said to her, "*Okay, without getting out of the chair, and only in your imagination, look down the street and you will see a bridge that crosses a river. Can you see it?*"

"Yes I can."

I thought I had better ask her to stay in her chair because I didn't want her to get up again and take her imaginary wagon out the door looking for a bridge and a river to throw it in.

"*Pull your little red wagon down to the bridge and throw all of the garbage and the wagon into the river and watch it all float out of sight. As it does, all those bad feelings you have been experiencing also float out of sight for good. Tell me when it is all gone.*"

Again I waited, wondering, *What is going on in her brain?*

It didn't take long until she said, "I threw it in the river. I watched it float out of sight and it is all gone and I feel like I just got rid of a heavy burden."

I said to her, "*I am going to count up from one to five. When I reach five, open your eyes, and you will be wide-awake feeling fine. One, two, three, four, five, open your eyes and you are wide awake.*"

She opened her eyes, looked at me with a smile and said, "What happened? I know that something happened but I don't remember any of it, and I really feel great! It seems like I've been hypnotized for just a few minutes but I feel like I have had eight hours of sleep. It's like I just got rid of a huge burden of some kind. What happened?"

As I recounted each part of the episode that I had just witnessed, Sonnie responded with, "I remember saying that and doing that now." But what *I* was wondering was why she didn't remember it until I brought it up. Strange!

After inquiring how she was feeling and if she was okay, I told her that when she was gathering up her garbage and throwing it in her little red wagon, she looked just like those people during Reveen's stage-show. "If I ever find the courage," I told her, "I might try doing stage-shows, but I don't know anyone who could teach me stage-show hypnosis."

I sent her out the door, but continued to wonder about what I had just witnessed and wondered what effect the session would have on Sonnie's behavior in the future, good or bad. I really didn't know.

My experience with Sonnie sent me into one of my philosophical, questioning modes: *Why, while hypnotized, did she have that outbreak of emotions, but was able to talk about it with her friends without the emotions? Although she was very much aware, and understood my questions and rationally articulated her thoughts, she seemed to be oblivious of reality. When using self-hypnosis, I sometimes feel some emotions but never an outburst like Sonnie's. Nor did I ever lose track of what was real and what I imagined. I wish I could find some kind of a guru who could give me answers to all of my questions.*

I learned some very valuable lessons from hypnotizing Sonnie. I discovered that I was still ill-prepared, because of my inexperience, to feel comfortable when dealing with emotional issues. I also learned that when asking questions of a person who is hypnotized, I need to be patient because the answers seem to come slowly; and that I also need to be prepared for any emotional outbursts that might spontaneously erupt.

If Sonnie's emotional response to hypnosis is typical, I'm not sure that this is what I want to do for a living, I thought.... Then I thought about how much fun Reveen seemed to be having when doing stage-shows. *I think I might like that better.... But how would I ever conjure up the courage, let alone learn how to do it?*

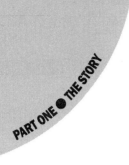
CHAPTER 8

Crickets

Two days later Sonnie called and said that she had had the best two days of her life—at work and at home. Her boss was enthusiastic about her new assertiveness and her husband and children had noticed an overnight change in her demeanor. "Oh, by the way, did I leave my sunglasses at your office?" she asked. "I've looked everywhere and I can't find them."

I told her no, and we hung up.

Although pleasant, her manner was rather matter of fact and I was disappointed that she hadn't been more enthusiastic about the change in her disposition; she didn't rave on about how great a hypnotist I was and that if it hadn't been for me she would still be carrying around all of her old "garbage".... *But then, for that matter, I reflected, except for their immediate response after being hypnotized, neither Richard nor Rob had called back to thank me for the great job I had done.... And now as I think about it, Sonnie probably wouldn't have called back either had she not been looking for her sunglasses!*

I guess I was just looking for some validation that I was a good hypnotist, after all, with three clients and apparently three success stories.

I continued to hypnotize myself and kept refining my techniques for hypnotizing other people by "hypnotizing" my new recliner (*it* didn't seem to care or even notice) but I could find no one else to sit in it while I practiced.

I thought about calling Richard, Rob or Sonnie to see if they knew anyone who might be interested in letting me practice on them, but I didn't feel quite right about asking people to help me find clients. To this day I have never *asked* for referrals from my clients; there is nothing unethical about it; it's just not in my nature.

But I did wonder how Reveen was able to conjure up thousands of people who were curious about hypnosis and hundreds who actually wanted to experience what it was like to be hypnotized; in more than six months, I had managed to find only three.

And then the obvious struck me: *It's because of his advertising bombardment! Maybe,* I thought, *all I need to do is advertise for hypnosis subjects to practice on!*

After a few hours of investigation I discovered that advertising on billboards, in the major newspapers and on radio stations was far beyond my budget. I calculated that Reveen had spent over $50,000 (1970's money) in advertising, but I also calculated that he must have brought in as much as $150,000 in revenues. *That's not a bad return on one's investment, especially considering that he did it by having six days of fun,* I thought.

However, quite by happenstance I found an advertising medium that I *could* afford—a weekly circular called the *Little Nickel:* Five dollars a week for a one-inch advertisement.

The only downside was that the ads in the *Little Nickel* were *not* classified, so the reader had to go through all five hundred or so notices if they were to, for sure, find mine:

SELF-IMPROVEMENT
Hypnosis can help you break bad habits
And give you the confidence to be successful.
Call 123-4567

Four weeks went by and $20 went down the drain without a single call.

The sales rep "guaranteed" that if I would run the ad for another four weeks I'd get *some* response. "It just takes longevity for an ad to get the attention of our readers," she said.

I reasoned with myself. *I know that there are people out there, thousands of them, who are interested in hypnosis. Why am I not getting any calls? What if I go for another four weeks and end up spending $40 and still find no one to practice on? That's one month's car payment! But then, if I don't advertise, I'll for sure find nobody.* "All right," I told her, "I'll try it for one more month."

Back then there was no voice mail or, for that matter, telephone answering machines that I could afford, but there were telephone answering services.

These were companies that employed a room full of operators who would answer an exclusive number for each of their customers. When that line would ring, one of the operators would physically answer the phone and take a message along with the caller's phone number. I was subscribing to such a service for my industrial supply sales and Ecology II, so I used the same phone number in my *Little Nickel* ad.

A few times a day I would call the answering service and retrieve my messages. So far, the only messages I had received were regarding industrial supply sales or Ecology II.

Then one day, as the operator was passing on my calls, she hesitated for a moment as she came to the "I want to be hypnotized to get over my fear of bugs" message.

She asked, "What in the world is this all about?" (I had neglected to inform them that I was also advertising for hypnosis subjects.)

"I have hypnotized a few people (I could now honestly say a few!) and have been advertising to find individuals who are interested in using hypnosis to break bad habits, improve their self-confidence and get over their 'fear of bugs' (I improvised) ... and stuff like that," I told her.

She came back with, "I went to see Reveen. Twice! I sat in the front few rows both times and still couldn't tell if what I was seeing was real or if he had just hired a bunch of shills to act like they were hypnotized." Without hesitation she asked, "Can you *make* me stop smoking with hypnosis?"

I told her that I had hypnotized *some* people who had successfully stopped smoking (again I fudged the truth a little—one for sure and maybe another one).

And, catching me off guard, she asked, "How much do you charge?"

Up until then I hadn't even thought about charging money for the chance to hypnotize people. I was only advertising to find a few people to practice on—until I got good enough at it so I *could* charge for my service. So, after thinking about it, I stammered, "$10... I think."

Art Baker had been hypnotizing people for many years and charged $20 a session, so $10 seemed to be a fair price for someone who was just getting started.

Again catching me off guard, she asked, "How long does it take to get an appointment—how long is your waiting list? How soon can I come and see you?"

I again stammered (anxious to get a client as soon as I could, without sounding like I was anxious to get a client as soon as I could), "I can probably work you in tomorrow... I suppose."

Sue made an appointment for the next evening, and added, "You had better call your 'bug person.'" So I did.

"Hello," said the tiny juvenile voice that answered the telephone.

"My name is Lindsay Brady. I'm a hypnotist (I had never before called myself a "hypnotist" and it seemed a little strange). Someone at this number called about getting over her fear of bugs. Do you know who it was that called?" I asked, thinking I was talking to a twelve-year-old.

"Oh, that was me," she said.

Still thinking I was talking to a child, I asked in kind of a childish (almost baby talk) voice of my own, "What kind of bugs are you frightened of?"

The miniature voice on the other end of the line said, "Crickets."

I waited for an explanation about why she was afraid of crickets, but none was given. So I said, "Why did you think of hypnosis as a way to get over your fear of crickets?"

"I didn't," she said in her adolescent voice.

Again I waited for a moment and she finally said, "My son saw an advertisement in a newspaper; he told me that hypnosis could make me get over my phobia. He gave me your telephone number, so I called."

It seems that lately, every time I turn around I'm getting caught off guard—how can a twelve-year-old have a son old enough to read a newspaper? I thought.

After recovering my senses and feeling embarrassed about having just used baby talk to a grown-up, I asked (stupidly), "How old is your son?"

With a "little" chuckle she said, "Oh, he's twenty-one and I'm forty-one; I just *sound* like I'm in my pre-teens. But that's okay, I'm used to it."

For several seconds this time *I* paused. After collecting my wits again I asked, "Why do you want to get over the fear of crickets?"

"Because I really love being outdoors in the cool air in the early evenings, but every time the crickets start chirping I have to go into the house. I can still hear them singing when I'm inside, and I'm fine with that, but if I'm outside and they start chirping, I get this wet clammy feeling all over my body. It's not the crickets—it's their chirping! I've had this irrational behavior for as long as I can remember.

"Can hypnosis cure me of this phobia?" she asked.

"What do you think happened that gives you these feelings?" I (again stupidly) asked.

"If I knew, I wouldn't have the feelings, would I? That's what you're supposed to do—find out what *causes* these clammy feelings when I hear the sound of crickets...isn't it?

"Don't you hypnotize me, and while hypnotized, ask me why I have my phobia, and then I remember, and when I remember what caused it I'm over it? Isn't that how it works? Do you think you can help me?" She asked again.

I went through my, "I'm not sure, but I've hypnotized several people (stretching the truth again) who, as a result of having been hypnotized, made some significant changes in their behavior," routine.

I said to her, "If you would like to try it I'd be happy to work with you. I charge $10 a session and I have some time open tomorrow afternoon."

She said, "That would be a perfect time to come in. My son will be home from school by then and he can watch my two-year-old grandson."

We agreed to meet at one o'clock the next day, and we hung up.

Two appointments in one day... and getting paid! That'll pay for half of my advertising bill, I thought with gleeful excitement.

All of a sudden I was thinking in terms of earning money by hypnotizing people, not just finding people to practice on. *Besides, if I can keep the session to an hour and a half (like Art said I should) that's $6.60 an hour! Not as much as I can earn selling industrial supplies, but still, $6.50 an hour is a good wage for most working people.* I thought "working people" because doing hypnosis was not work at all. Challenging (as with Sonnie), but certainly not work.

I was not only curious to find out what had caused a juvenile-sounding forty-one-year-old grandmother to be afraid of the sound of crickets, but even more, I could hardly wait to see what she looked like!

When she arrived I was surprised to meet a trim, very well-dressed, sophisticated, confident, society-type woman who *looked* like she was about forty years old...but when she spoke, out of her mouth came this little tiny soft voice that distracted my attention from her natural physical attractiveness. I may not have recalled this session in such vivid detail had it not been for her child-like voice.

I introduced myself and invited her to sit down on a chair at my newly re-finished desk.

Before sitting down she extended her hand and with a firm handshake said, "My name is Mrs. Wilma Smith, but most people just call me Willy and I'd prefer that you do the same," without a hint of impertinence.

My lack of planning, un-preparedness, and un-professionalism smacked me right in the face when she asked, "Don't I need to do some paperwork before we get started?"

Caught off guard again! I thought. *Recently, it seems, all I have been doing is a lot of stammering and engaging in trivial deceptions, but this time I'm really stretching the truth:* "Right now I'm out of forms," I explained (which was true), "but if you will just write down your name, address and phone number on this yellow pad, I'll transfer the information to one of my forms when I get them back from the printer." *Which I will do as soon as I get some,* I quickly rationalized.

I doubt that she believed me but she wrote down the information anyway.

After Willy slid the notepad back to me she said, "I've never been hypnotized before so I'm really quite apprehensive about the whole thing." (To me, however, she didn't look or act apprehensive at all; she seemed confident and straightforward.) "Can you tell me what to expect during the session?"

"Sure," I said. And then I went into my practiced speech about never being unconscious and that she would do nothing that would violate her standards nor do anything that would cause her harm.

I told her that in a few minutes I would have her move to my recliner and go through my "hypnosis induction" process, and that all she needed to do was listen. "And after you are hypnotized I'll be asking you a few questions about why you are afraid of crickets," I explained.

Immediately she corrected me, "I am not afraid of crickets; I just don't like their chirping sound when I'm outside, just like I told you on the telephone. Don't you remember?

"Being out of doors while the crickets chirp gives me this clammy feeling, not the crickets themselves. As a matter of fact, I think crickets are cute little things. It's just when I'm outside and they're singing is what I don't like. Actually, right now, just talking about being outside when the crickets are chirping is making my skin crawl!"

Another early lesson learned from a client: Listen to what they say and how they say it, and don't make assumptions about what they mean based on my own preconceived notions. Although she had very specifically explained her fear the day before on the phone, I had still erroneously made the assumption that what she *really* meant was that she had a fear of crickets—not the sound of their singing. As a result, I had to suffer her tart reproval as she recounted exactly what she had told me the day before.

Another thing that struck me: *How can such a little voice have such an air of authority and confident assertiveness?*

When I had recovered (again) I told her that I *did* remember what she said on the telephone and that I should have listened more closely.

I asked her to move over to my recliner, where "we'll do some hypnotizing."

Hearing that comment slip out of my mouth, not to mention the way I had said it, I thought, *Now, that was a really professional and classy way to start a session with a person of her sophistication; and a really great way to engender her confidence in me as being a polished expert in my field!*

I vowed at that moment to work on developing, if nothing else, an "appearance" of being professional when working with clients.

After she sat down in my recliner I asked her to make herself comfortable and to look at the ring I was holding....

After going through the "induction" I asked her if she was comfortable, and in her "pre-teen voice," but so very softly that I could barely hear her, she said, "Yes."

I asked, *"What about the sound of crickets chirping makes you feel uneasy and fearful, and causes a feeling of clamminess?"*

As was the case with Sonnie, I waited for a long time for her to answer, while she just sat there perfectly still, except for a few facial expressions that gave me reason to believe that she was recalling some experience.

Bracing myself for an emotional explosion, I cautiously asked, *"What are you thinking about? What is going on in your mind?"*

With a gentle smile she said (speaking in the present tense, as though it was happening at this moment), "I hear a chirping sound, kind of like crickets chirping. I like the sound crickets make when they sing. The sound makes me feel good.

"I'm sitting in a little wagon being pulled up the street by my brother. The chirping sound is coming from the wheels of the wagon.... It reminds me of the sounds made by crickets when they are singing. I wonder if there are crickets in the wheels.

"The wagon handle just slipped out of my brother's hand and we (the wagon and me) are starting to roll down the street backwards. The wheel chirping is getting louder and louder and the wagon is going faster and faster. I am holding on for dear life. Oops! We (me and the wagon) just plunged into a big bush. I'm unharmed and none the worse for wear—except for a fine mist of water that is spraying on me. I think it's coming from a sprinkler head we just hit inside the bush."

I waited for the tale to continue, or for an explanation of why the experience had created her fear (while she was telling it she seemed to be enjoying the telling), but she just sat there seemingly amused about what was going on in her head.

I prepared myself again for some kind of an emotional response as I asked, *"What does this experience have to do with your fear of the sound of crickets? As you tell of the event it doesn't seem to be a frightening experience at all."*

With her eyes still closed, Willy slipped out of being *in* the experience to telling me *about* it, and said, "Oh, that part wasn't frightening. As a matter of fact I thought it was quite fun and that my brother had intentionally let go of the wagon handle. It was what happened after we (the wagon and me) ended up inside the bush and had knocked loose the sprinkler head that I didn't like."

She opened her eyes, looked at me pleasantly, and began explaining. "While I was sitting there being drenched by the mist, I heard my brother screaming at the top of his voice as he ran down the hill, closely followed by my mother. 'I've killed her! She's dead in the bush!' And then I heard my mother at the top of her voice criticizing my brother for being a clumsy, worthless idiot who had just killed his little sister! All this happened in just a few seconds but by the time they got to me it wasn't fun anymore. And when my mom reached inside the bush and felt the mist on my body she thought it was blood and she fainted. My brother finally dragged my 'dead body' out of the bush and also fainted when I sat up and cried, 'I'm not *really* dead!'

"You would have to understand the wimpiness of my mother and brother to relate to their fainting," she explained. "But *I* felt like I was responsible for their fainting and when they finally came to, all they could do was sob and criticize me for having made them think I was dead, for having made them faint and for having gotten my clothes all clammy and dirty."

By this time Willy was sitting up in the recliner and conversing in her ordinary, everyday little voice. So I asked her, "*What does this scenario have to do with your phobia of the sound of crickets when out of doors and not feeling the clamminess when indoors?*"

"Oh that's simple," she said. "Wagons and mists are not allowed indoors! When I'm indoors, I'm safe. I won't be criticized because there will never be 'squeaky-chirpy' wagon wheel sounds and mist soaking up my clothes, if I'm inside."

"*So how do you feel now when you think about being outside when the crickets are chirping?*" I asked.

"That's really queer! Not only can I think about it now, but I can even talk about it and it doesn't make me feel clammy like it used to. I like it. I think I'm cured!" she exclaimed.

Since the "sale was made," and since she had already given me ten of her dollars (and because both of us felt good about it), I shut up and sent her out the door.

And then *I* sat down in my recliner, closed my eyes and began to methodically analyze what I had just experienced:

1. *Where were all of the emotions that were supposed to be vented? Willy just told her story in her child-like voice (with a little prodding from me), but related the whole event matter-of-factly.*

2. *Why, halfway through her account, did she open her eyes, sit up and finish telling it in everyday conversation?*

3. *Since I didn't tell her to "wake-up," I wonder if she is still hypnotized?*

4. *I don't understand it: Why does a squeaky wagon wheel, that just <u>sounds</u> like a cricket, cause a person to feel clammy when crickets start chirping? It is obvious that the clammy feeling was associated with the broken sprinkler mist and that her fearful feelings were associated with how her brother and mom reacted to her "being dead," but why did it cause her to feel clammy when out of doors and the crickets started to sing?* (At that time in my life I had no knowledge of classical conditioning.)

5. *Why, with my unprofessional beginning, did she still go under hypnosis, and seem to regard me as some sort of an expert who knew what he was doing?*

6. *Why did she have such seemingly good results without me having to give her any suggestions whatsoever about her phobia being removed as the result of chucking all of the garbage, and a little red wagon, into the drink? Maybe Furst and the other authors were right: All the subject needs is to find out what the experience was that caused the fear and the fear just disappears–once they know the event that caused it.*

7. *Why, when a person is hypnotized, do they speak so softly?*

8. *Why does it take so long for them to respond when asked questions?*

9. *This session lasted less than fifty minutes: Wow! More than ten bucks an hour, and it was fun! Maybe I'll stick with clinical-type hypnosis and give up any notions of that stage-show stuff.*

10. *Either I'm really good at this–four clients now and all appear to have been successful in making the change they came in to change–or maybe hypnosis is really simple and anyone can do it.... I think it must be the latter.*

After an hour or more of introspection and self-questioning, I came up with no answers. Only when I began rehashing the same questions did I open my eyes, sit up and set about preparing myself for my appointment with "Answering Service Sue"–which turned out to be an experience of an entirely different variety!

Just as a side note: Although Willy never called back, her son made an appointment with me several months later and immediately after introducing himself said, "You totally 'cured' my mom. She's the one with the tiny voice who didn't like the sound of crickets. Do you remember her?"

I said "Yes I do." But then I quickly added, "But I didn't do any curing, she did it."

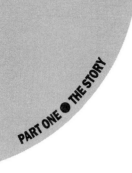

CHAPTER 9

The Sage

Figuring that I ought to be better prepared, and wanting to appear more professional for "Answering Service Sue's" appointment later on that evening, I picked up a copy of a patient information intake sheet from a nearby psychiatrist's office. I took it back to my office, made a label with stick-on lettering and covered up the psychiatrist's name with: *Lindsay A. Brady, Hypnotist*, and under it in smaller letters *Confidential Information Sheet*.

I took *my* intake sheet to the no-longer-imposing SLC Public Library, went in without hesitation, and as I walked by the volunteer sitting beneath the "HELP" sign, I gave her a wink and proceeded to *her* "copy machine."

I put "copy machine" in quotes because in those days copy machines were nothing at all like they are now. The copies came out on a slightly brownish wax-like paper. They were very susceptible to smearing if they got wet and the fidelity was severely compromised, by today's standards. But I now had an intake form for my appointment with Sue and a few extras just in case I had more appointments someday.

I got back to my office a few minutes before Sue's appointment time and I waited. Twenty minutes later I was still waiting. Disappointed, I began wondering what could have kept her from arriving on time. *Maybe she got here early and, because I wasn't here, left. Or maybe she lost her nerve because she thought I'd make her cluck like a chicken. Or maybe she changed her mind about stopping smoking. Or maybe she got lost and can't find my office. Or maybe she is unreliable or just one of those people who is always late. I'll give her another fifteen minutes and if she doesn't show up I'll go home.*

Fifteen minutes passed, and as I was getting ready to leave, there was a brash rapping on my office door and my disappointment about not having another client to practice on disappeared.

From the moment Sue walked into my office, in grubby-looking garb that was meant for a person two sizes smaller, we were on different frequencies.

I introduced myself, offered her my hand and said, "You must be Sue." She hesitated and looked at me suspiciously with glassy eyes. She looked at my extended hand and then back at me.

She reeked of cigarette smoke, and had the odor of alcohol on her breath. After a slight teeter, she reluctantly placed a sweaty, fish-like hand in mine and slurred, "Don't ever call me Sue! I hate that name. I go by Sue only at the answering service because there was already a Suzy there when I started. And for sure don't ever call me Susan, either; I hate that name more than Sue! My name is Suzy."

As politely as I could, I asked her to sit down at my desk. I slid a pen and my newly acquired intake sheet in front of her and asked if she wouldn't mind filling it out.

Grudgingly, she picked up the pen and looked at the intake sheet for a long time. Then she started penning in the requested information, starting with an over-sized "SUZY," leaving smudges as she moved her sweaty hand from question to question.

When she had answered only about half a dozen of the thirty questions, she stopped and said, "Why do you want to know all of this stuff about me? I mean my parents' names, my siblings' mental state and who should be contacted in the event of an emergency? This is ridiculous!" She slammed the pen down on the paper, leaving a splotchy handprint.

Because I had been in a hurry to get some "paperwork" for my appointment with "SUZY" I had just glanced at the content of the psychiatrist's form and had assumed that the questions would be relevant. *There I go assuming again. When am I ever going to learn not to assume things—just because I think that things and people are as I think them to be?*

I was straightforward and completely honest with her when I said, "I just picked up an information sheet from a psychiatrist's office today and made copies of it after sticking a label with my name on it. All I really need is your name, address and phone number."

She seemed to be okay with this since she had already filled in that much of the information. As she slid the sheet back to me she spluttered out, "You *are* really new at this, aren't you?"

I again honestly responded, "Yes."

In spite of my resentment over how she had sneered at my inexperience, I asked her to move to my recliner.

While struggling to get her body from chair to recliner she mumbled, with hardly understandable, run-together words, "Well, make me stop smoking now. I hope I get my ten bucks' worth!"

After she had plopped into the recliner, I went through my pre-hypnotic talk (wondering the whole time if she was grasping a word of it) and then asked her to look at the ring I was holding.

When I was three or four minutes into my "induction" dialogue, Suzy opened her eyes and slurred out, "This is nothing like I saw at Reveen's stage-show. I can hear every word you are saying. This is not how you are supposed to hypnotize a person. You are supposed to snap your fingers and say 'Sleep.' Then I go unconscious and don't remember or hear anything until you snap your fingers again." And with that she hoisted herself out of the recliner, staggered to the door and slammed it, after stumbling out.

I sat there dumbfounded. My ego was crushed, and I was dejected and angry. My euphoria of just a few hours before, after my session with Willy, had in just a few minutes been shattered and transformed into misery. *What did I do wrong?* I wondered.

In an attempt to calm myself down, and to rid myself of the yucky feeling down in my belly, I sat down in my recliner and went through my self-hypnosis "ceremony." When I had gotten myself relaxed, and the negative emotions had subsided considerably, I began to evaluate what I had just experienced.

I wasn't aware of when it began (I just kind of slid into it), but I found myself engaged in an imaginary conversation with what seemed like another person.

Only twice before (once, when I had discovered that my brain understands mental images, not words; and again, when I *didn't* drive off the cliff) had I experienced talking to my alter ego (if that's what it was). I don't know how long it lasted, but it was as if I was talking with a wise old sage who was not only answering some of my questions, but was scolding me, as well.

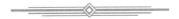

Me: What did I do wrong when working with Suzy?

Sage: Well, you could have shown a little more compassion for her! Obviously she was apprehensive about being hypnotized in the first place and probably spent a good deal of time at a pub trying to conjure up the courage to come here at all. That's why she was late. Besides that, she was probably afraid she was going to "spill her guts" and tell a stranger about all of those hidden secrets that she has been trying to keep from everyone.... Now doesn't that sound familiar?

From the moment she walked through the door you were judgmental of her appearance and the aromas that exuded from her presence.

The first thing you must do if you want to be successful in the business of helping people to improve their circumstance in life is to develop a totally nonjudgmental attitude and accept each person just as they are, even if at first they seem repulsive. You don't have to like them or agree with them, but you must have compassion for them and understand that most folks who are abrupt, defensive and critical are very insecure people and probably don't like themselves very much.

Me: Except for not being understanding and compassionate, what else could I have done that might have made her feel more at ease?

Sage: That form you pilfered from the psychiatrist's office....

Me: I didn't pilfer it! I asked the receptionist if she had a spare copy of their information intake sheet that I could take home with me.

Sage: You gave her the impression that you wanted it for their purpose, not yours, and that you would be bringing it back when you had filled it out. You didn't take it home, you didn't fill it out, and you didn't take it back. You marched right to the library after having covered up their name with your name. So you pilfered it. And besides that, you plagiarized it.

Me: What do you mean I plagiarized it?

Sage: You used someone else's creative work, you used it for your own gain without their permission, you didn't compensate them for it, and you didn't give them recognition for having created it. That's plagiarism!

You often stretch the truth, and recently even engaged in outright deceitful covert lying. It is time for you to start practicing complete honesty.

Me: Okay, you're right, but most of my deceitfulness "until recently" was *not* to protect or bolster my ego, it was to protect others from experiencing ill feelings and anxieties. So what do I do now?

Sage: You can start by creating your own client information sheet. One that gives you just enough information so you can get *some* insight into the client's circumstances: Their name; their address; what kind of work they do, if any; their marital status; how they heard about you and the reason they have engaged your service. Make it short and easy for them to fill out. Didn't you notice how Suzy recoiled when you slipped that pilfered psychiatrist's form in front of her? It may as well have been a rattlesnake.

Some people just don't like filling out forms, others don't like giving out information about themselves, and for some, writing anything is a challenge because of ineptness in their writing skills. You should understand the latter reason better than most people: Don't you know one of the reasons you didn't like making sales calls was that if someone bought something it meant you were going to have to fill out a form—a contract or the order? And when you did make a sale, half of the stuff you wrote down was spelled wrong. Don't you remember?

Me: Yes, I remember. At times, even now, I still struggle with writing and spelling. I don't know why, but sometimes I just can't think of how a word should be spelled, even simple ones that I have spelled many times before. Do you think there is something wrong with my brain?

Sage: I don't know if there is or if there isn't, but even if there is it shouldn't get in the way of you creating a simple intake form for your clients to fill out—one that is so simple that even you would feel good about filling it out.

Me: Why did the session with Willy go so well, although she was critical of me for being a little on the short end of professional?

Sage: Because Willy is confident and comfortable with herself, has high self-esteem, and is compassionate and non-judgmental. Besides that, she didn't *criticize* you for not having some paperwork for her to fill out; she just *asked* if you did. It was you who took it as criticism.

She knew from the beginning that you were new at hypnotizing people and that her tiny voice amused you, but she has the self-esteem that allows her to rise above all that, so she was free to listen to what you had to say.

Me: But why didn't Willy have to go back and re-experience all of the emotions—like Sonnie did—in order to get rid of the clammy feeling she experienced when being out of doors and hearing crickets chirping—or even when she thought about it, for that matter?

And in addition to that, although she *said* she was "cured," I'm not *sure* that she is.

Sage: It seems that some people don't have to re-experience the emotions in order to get rid of them, and maybe *nobody* does, but this is something you will figure out with experience.

Whether Willy is "cured" or is not "cured" is not up to you. You are not responsible for another person's behavior. You can't choose for Richard or Rob to start smoking again or to not smoke. If they choose to pick up a cigarette and start smoking again it is their choice, not yours. Once a client leaves your office it is out of your hands.

Me: Why don't people call me back, tell me how great a hypnotist I am and rave about how if it hadn't been for me hypnotizing them they would still be trying to get over their unwanted maladies?

Sage: You not only need to work on your compassion, honesty and acceptance of other people, but developing a little humility wouldn't hurt either.

It was not you who changed them—it was they who changed themselves. You didn't do it; they did. You didn't hypnotize them; they hypnotized themselves. Sure, you talked to them and gave them a little insight into making changes in their lives, but all you did was talk and because they saw you as an authority figure, what you said had credibility. Your words changed how they thought of themselves, but the power within *them* is what made the change.

Listen closely: The power that causes the change in each person's behavior through hypnosis has very little to do with the hypnotist; it all comes from an innate power within the subject. It isn't the hypnotist who causes the subjects to change their behavior; the process that causes the change is in them.

It's like a doctor: The doctor doesn't heal the patient; all of the healing is done by the natural healing processes in the patients, themselves. Sure, a doctor performs surgical procedures and prescribes and administers drugs, radiation and chemotherapy, but it is still the patient who does the healing. True, some doctors are better than others at advising their patients about what to do to get well, but that comes from study, experience and a sincere desire to help their patients heal themselves.

During the hypnotic session, all the hypnotist does is talk—he or she just uses words to convey ideas. And if the client accepts your words as being true, the idea that it is true invokes a natural process in their brain that causes them to behave consistent with what *they* believe. The hypnotist does not choose for the subject what to believe; the subject does.

Me: But isn't it up to the hypnotist to create the belief by using words?

Sage: Yes, that is true. With more practice, learning the right words to use, developing convincing logic and rational arguments, you will get better at helping them to believe. But still, the images that are created by your words are the messages, not the words.

It may be a very long time before you fully grasp and understand the power imbedded in what I just said.

So, whenever you happen upon someone that you have worked with and they attribute the change in their behavior to you, thank them for the compliment but then rave about how great they are for having used the powers that they possess that caused it to happen!

As with Richard and Rob, you helped them to see themselves as being non-smokers; but they were the ones who did the quitting, not you. So why do you think you should take the credit?"

Me: Well, you are right. It's just that I haven't been thinking of it from that perspective!

But what was the difference between Sonnie and Willy? They both seemed to get the results they wanted, but Sonnie burst out with all of those emotions and Willy didn't.

Sage: The difference between Sonnie and Willy was that Willy *knew* what triggered her clamminess (the sound of crickets when out of doors) and Sonnie *didn't know* why the word "assertive" triggered her fear of *being* assertive.

Sonnie knew on a conscious level the experience that created her phobia and had even talked about it with her friends. Willy knew it was the sound of crickets that triggered her clammy feelings, but she had forgotten about the experience associated with the phobia until you asked her to go back to it. All you did was to help them change how they thought about the experience that triggered the emotions—the word "assertive" and the sound of crickets.

In that respect you helped them to change their view of how they now respond to the stimuli, but it is not *you* who is causing them to respond differently when triggers occur—it is not you who is keeping them from having those negative feelings now.

Me: Well, I hadn't thought about it that way, either. So what do I do next? And how do I find people to practice on?

Sage: Start by creating your own information sheet and keep on doing what you did to find Willy and Suzy: Advertise! And for sure, work on your honesty, compassionate acceptance of others and humility…. Oh yes, and stop *assuming* that people and things are as you think them to be, because that doesn't mean that is how they necessarily are.

Me: I can create a form easily enough, but it's going to be tough learning to be compassionate and humble…. And it's going to be really hard to be completely honest, especially when being bare-facedly honest—when I express what I really think—it is going to make other people uneasy and even resentful. How do I get around that?

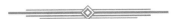

I got no answer. Suddenly I was wide awake, sitting up in my recliner, wringing wet with perspiration and feeling like I had just been reproached and counseled by God Himself. I knew I hadn't been, but I *felt* as though I had.

So the next day I followed "His" advice: I designed an intake information sheet:

Name: _____

Address: _____

Phone Number: _____

Date: _____

Age: _____

Occupation: _____

Marital Status: _____

How did you hear of me? _____

Have you been hypnotized before? _____

For what reason do you want to be hypnotized now? _____

_____

I figured that would give me enough information to at least get a "feel" for the client's status in life and disclose the behavior they wanted to change. I thought to myself, *This is simple enough that even I could fill it out without feeling threatened or challenged.*

Note: I have used this basic information sheet for 38 years and only twice did it threaten or challenge a client.

One time, many years ago, a young woman (about 30 years old) came in and when I asked her to fill out the information sheet she told me that she could neither read nor write so would I mind filling it out for her. She didn't lack intelligence or the ability to engage in rational dialogue, but had been raised in a very backward family and had been forbidden to go to school when she was growing up and had learned to get along fairly well being illiterate.

The second time happened today (the very day I am writing this). A fellow filled in only his first name (I suspect even that was fictitious), the date, his age and paid me in cash.

He wanted to make sure the session would be completely confidential (which it would have been anyway) because of his embarrassment about his issue: Taking longer to urinate than other men when using public restrooms!

Although to *almost* all of us, this would seem to be an insignificant problem; to *him* it was a major issue.... So I was compassionate and accepted the condition as being a valid matter to resolve... which it was.

Not only did I *create* a simple intake information sheet but I took it to a printer, had it typeset and ordered 500 copies. I figured that 500 copies (for as many clients I had been seeing) would probably last me a lifetime.

I called the *Little Nickel* rep and extended my ad for an additional six months and I began thinking about being honest, compassionate and humble.... Then I called my answering service to pick up my messages, and who should answer but Suzy!

The moment that I identified myself she said, "Hi Lindsay, I've been hoping that I'd be the one who answered when you called in for your messages. I want to apologize for my behavior last night. I had been out drinking because I needed to muster up the courage to be hypnotized and the thought of giving up smoking made me all the more anxious. I was a mess!

"I really feel bad about how I acted and treated you. Will you forgive me? I don't think I am ready to give up smoking right now, but will you give me another chance when I am? I put a check in the mail this morning for $10. Is that okay?"

I was more flabbergasted than I had been the night before. After (again) gathering my composure, I said, "There is no need to apologize. I didn't handle last night's situation any better than you did, and besides that, I learned some wonderful lessons from the experience and I want to thank you for that. If it hadn't been for you I would have missed out on an unusually insightful experience. So yes, I accept your apology, but any forgiveness will have to come from some source other than me, because I don't think I ever condemned you. Thanks for sending the check and I will just consider it as payment in advance for when you are ready to stop smoking. Now, do I have any messages?" I didn't.

When I hung up I contemplated, *This hypnosis business is really emotionally unpredictable—one moment I'm ecstatic about doing it, the next moment I'm questioning if it's something I even want to be involved in, and the next moment I'm excited about pursuing it further. I wonder if hypnosis will be a significant part of my future?*

It wouldn't be long until I found out!

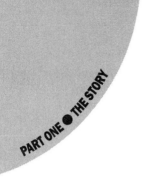

CHAPTER 10

Eric

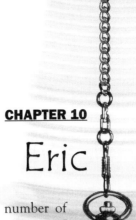

The *Little Nickel* ad produced a moderate number of sessions over the next ten months and from time to time I had additional appointments with clients who had been referred to me by (apparently satisfied) previous clients. I scarcely made enough money to cover my advertising expense and overhead but, still (I rationalized), I was getting valuable experience.

Many of my clients were successful in achieving the change they were seeking, but some of them weren't. *But at least I'm doing as well as Art Baker, who has been hypnotizing people for many years,* I reasoned.

However, I was not satisfied with my success rate and thought, *I wonder if there is, as yet, some undiscovered approach that could improve the effectiveness of hypnosis, or do I just have to accept that some people can't be hypnotized and consequently are excluded from experiencing the benefits of the process? Or if, in fact, everyone can be hypnotized and the only reason some people don't successfully achieve the change they're hoping for is that they really didn't want to change anyway?* Remembering Art's viewpoint.

But I was not content with that philosophy. So after each session (regardless of whether *they* felt the session was successful or not) I explained to my client that I was in the process of refining my approach in an attempt to increase my effectiveness and asked, "What do you think would have made the session more successful? What were you expecting me to do or say that I didn't do or say? Is there anything that I said that was unclear or seemed abrasive or offensive and distracted your attention from what I was saying?"

I realized that asking such questions might, at least for some people, lessen the client's confidence in me as a hypnotist but I was willing to take that chance. I figured that if I could gain some fresh insight from other people it might give me some fresh ideas that I would not have otherwise come up with—which it did.

(In a later chapter I will recap how the opinions of my clients profoundly influenced *my* thinking about hypnosis, and how that led to the development of a unique approach and, consequently, a higher level of effectiveness.)

Except for Richard, who from time to time referred a client to me, I had given little thought to those early clients. And then one morning when I picked up my messages, one of them was marked urgent! It was from Sonnie. I wondered what could possibly warrant the "urgent" status and hoped that she hadn't had a cataclysmic relapse and was in a fit of desperation waiting for me to rescue her from despair. So my first call was to her.

But when she answered she sounded bubbly, enthusiastic and seemed pleased that I had returned her call. So I asked, "Well, how are you doing and what can I help you with? I was a little alarmed when your call was marked 'urgent.'"

"Oh that," she said. "It wasn't an emergency 'urgent' but rather an exciting 'urgent.' It is something I thought that you might want to follow up on.

"A fellow came into my office wanting to find work with a painting contractor. He told me that he has all of the equipment (compressor, spray guns, scaffolding, brushes, rollers, etc.) and he has just arrived in town and is ready to go to work. He advised me that he is the 'world's best' house painter but just needs to find a painting contractor who needs his skills until he can get back on his feet."

I interrupted her before she could continue and asked, "What in the world is so exciting about meeting the 'world's best' house painter? I don't know any painting contractors that need help and I don't think that my house needs any more paint."

"Oh, that's not what's exciting about him," she said. "It's been a long time since I was in your office, but I think you told me that you were interested in learning stage hypnosis but didn't know how you would ever find someone who could teach you how to do it. Am I right? Are you still interested?"

"Well, I don't know," I answered. "It has been almost a year and I haven't thought much about doing stage-show hypnosis since you were in. But what does this have to do with the 'world's best' house painter?"

"Well, he said that he is an even better stage hypnotist than he is a painter—the 'world's greatest.' He told me that he just needs to earn enough money painting houses so he can advertise and book some hypnosis stage-show performances.

"I told him that *I* had been hypnotized to do better at work and in my personal life and that it has really made a big difference.

"He said he hoped that whoever had hypnotized me was certified, very good and had had a lot of experience, because if he hadn't he could have messed up my psyche for the rest of my life. I told him that you must have been a very good hypnotist because of the positive influence our sessions had on me... but I *didn't* tell him that I was only your third client!

"By the way, I don't think I ever thanked you for your help. If it hadn't been for you, I'd still be wallowing around in my self-imposed limitations."

I said, "You're welcome, but it wasn't me who made the change in you, it was you who changed you, so I think *you* should get all of the credit. I just said a few words that changed how you thought about being assertive and the change just happened. It wasn't me who did it; it was you. True?"

"Yes, that's true, but if it hadn't been for you I wouldn't have changed how I thought about it. True?"

"Well, what does this guy being the 'world's greatest' stage hypnotist have to do with me?" I asked, intentionally changing the topic.

"He told me that he teaches hypnotists how to do stage hypnosis and that he trains people so they can be certified hypnotists! He gave me his phone number and said he would like to meet you and if *he* thought you had the 'right stuff' he *might* be interested in letting you be his apprentice."

I thought about how she had said it, and commented, "It sounds to me like he is a little arrogant and self-centered. If being arrogant and self-centered is what it takes to be a stage hypnotist I'm not sure I want to be one. I have been strongly advised that I need to acquire some humility. I don't know that I have made much progress in that area but I've been trying. But give me his name and phone number and I'll think it over."

"His name is Eric and his phone number is…"

I found myself in a real dilemma. *What do I want to do with the rest of my life? I enjoy hypnotizing people in a clinical setting and over the last year I've made considerable progress in being confident about hypnotizing people and I'm getting better results as time goes on, but maybe I could expand my knowledge and improve my effectiveness sooner if I had a teacher who, although arrogant, seemed to have enough confidence and experience to be arrogant. Would I have to give up selling industrial supplies and doing clinical hypnosis to be a stage hypnotist? Would it mean traveling from city to city, living in hotel rooms and being away from my family for weeks at a time? I'm not sure that I would like that kind of a lifestyle…. Well, it won't hurt to at least call the guy.*

So I called Eric and after a brief introduction arranged to meet him at the downtown Walgreen's lunch counter.

I recognized him from the description he had given me over the phone. Eric was a man who looked fortyish and was about my height, with a reddish complexion, a receding hairline and a large round head and—as I was to discover—an ego to fill it. He was wearing a gray pullover sweater. He looked like he had made an attempt at neatness but still looked rather disheveled. *I guess he just climbed down from his scaffolding,* I thought.

I motioned him to the booth where I was sitting and when he sat down, without any attempt to introduce himself, he said, "So you want to be a stage hypnotist. I've been doing hypnosis stage-shows for over fifteen years; I studied under The Baron Von Brennon, who, when in Germany, hypnotized Hitler. But when Hitler found out that he had Jewish blood Hitler wanted to kill him, so he came to America back in 1938 and that's how he found me. The Baron was the finest stage hypnotist in the world. He taught me everything he knew and then he died, and I am better than he ever was. What makes you think you can be a stage hypnotist, anyway?"

"I don't know that I can or even if I want to be a stage-show hypnotist if it requires being a braggart," I answered, without caring if what I said was offensive to him.

My frankness took him aback a little, but then he said, "Oh, by the way, I'm Dr. Eric. That lady over at the employment agency said you had hypnotized her. Are you certified to do that?"

"I didn't know that I was breaking the law by hypnotizing people or that I need to be certified to not break the law," I said.

"Well, technically you aren't breaking any laws, but if you are not certified it leaves you open to lawsuits if someone complains about your ethical conduct," he asserted.

"Well then, I should have nothing to worry about since I have no intention of engaging in unethical conduct," I asserted back.

"You really are a feisty little guy, aren't you?" he said.

I thought to myself, *Yes I am feisty, and I like being this way with you since I think that you are full of crap anyway. And besides that you can't be more than a fraction of an inch taller than me so what do you mean calling me little?*

He went on. "Well, whether or not you plan to do unethical things with hypnosis you still need to be certified to, at least, give the appearance of being legitimate. I can certify you if you go through my certification training program. You will not only learn how to hypnotize people the "right way," but for the small fee of $2,000 in advance, I'll also teach you how to do stage hypnosis. And if you prove to be competent enough, as part of your training I'll let you be my assistant when I perform on stage."

My brain was churning. *I probably would have more credibility if I had a certificate hanging on my wall and I think I want to learn how to do stage hypnosis, but do I want to do it with this shady oddball?*

Without saying a word, Eric reached in his pocket, pulled out a book of matches, lit one, closed his eyes for a moment, opened them with a little jerk of his head, stretched out his arm, and placed the palm of his hand right into the flame and held it there for several seconds. After shaking out the flame and giving another little jerk of his head, he showed me the soot that had accumulated on his palm. "And I can teach you how to do *that* by using instant self-hypnosis," he stated smugly.

Well, I was impressed, but I still had my doubts about hooking up with this character. So I said, "I'll have to think about it. $2,000 may be a small amount to you, but to me that is a lot of money to come up with right now."

"Well then, for you, I'll make an exception. I'll let you pay me in installments of $200 a week for ten weeks."

"That's still $2,000 and a lot of money. I'm not trying to talk you down, but I don't have that kind of cash flow and I'm not willing to go into debt to get it."

In an attempt to show me some compassion and understanding he placed his soot-stained hand on the back of mine and said, "I like your straightforward honesty, so I will compromise even more.

"The woman at the employment agency said you have an office where you hypnotize people. I need a place where I can do private clinical sessions. So, if you would let me use your office ten hours a week, I'd be willing to teach you the *right* way to do clinical hypnosis, teach you stage hypnosis and present you with a *Master of Hypnosis* certificate, all for just $500—$100 now and the balance paid at a rate of $100 a week over following four weeks. How does that sound?"

"That sounds a lot better, but it seems to me that I have very little evidence that you can do all of that. I mean, all I have to go on is what you told Sonnie at the employment agency about you and what you have told me about you, which is the same thing you told *her* about you. So all I have to rely on is what *you* think of *you*. I don't even know if you can hypnotize anyone. For me to make a decision based only on what you tell me about yourself may be a little naive and irresponsible. Do you have any credentials that verify that you are qualified to teach hypnosis and that you have the authority to certify me as a Master Hypnotist?" I asked.

"Are you suggesting that I am a fraud and a con artist?" he said with an angry voice.

Getting a little irritated myself, I responded, "If you can't back up your egotistical claims, then yes!"

"Well, if you need proof I'll give it to you. Just tell me where to meet you and I'll show you my credentials," he said in a huff.

"Even if you have verification that you are qualified, I'll still have to think about it. I'll call you tomorrow and let you know my decision," I said, just before he got up and stomped out without a word.

I will have to admit that in spite of his questionable character he is a quick thinker and is able to flex his position when push comes to shove. And he at least attempted to show some compassion before I questioned his authenticity. But even if he can deliver his claims, could I tolerate his arrogance? I really do need to consider his proposal closely.

When I returned to my office I sat down in my recliner, took in a deep breath and went through my self-hypnosis process. Without intentionally conjuring him up, I found myself in another conversation with "The Sage."

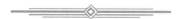

Me: Am I ready to make hypnosis my primary source of income? I'm doing very well with my industrial supply selling, and even making a little money doing clinical hypnosis. If I start learning stage hypnosis won't that distract me from selling and hypnotizing people in my office? And then there is Eric's arrogant sleaziness. Do I want to get mixed up with someone like that?

Sage: Lindsay, don't you remember that you are supposed to be practicing compassion and acceptance of other people? You have regressed into your judgmental attitude, and it has clouded your thinking.

Me: What do you mean judgmental attitude and clouded thinking?

Sage: You called him arrogant, self-centered and sleazy, and that's clouded your thinking. If your thinking had not been clouded then why are we in this dialogue? Whenever you are critical and judgmental of another person, it not only fogs up your brain, but it also lowers your self-esteem. Did it *really* make you feel good about yourself when you were critical and judgmental of Eric? Have you so soon forgotten that the only reason a person (including you) is boastful, arrogant, and critical is because of their own insecurities? And that they feel they must degrade others, thinking by doing so it elevates themselves, when in reality it does exactly the opposite? That's why your thinking is foggy and you are reluctant to make rational decisions.

If you want to elevate yourself, then speak to and treat others in ways that cause them to feel good about themselves. Just try it. It always works. I'm not talking about flattery; that always backfires. I'm talking about genuine compliments about another person's qualities. You can always find something good to say about someone else.

Me: Okay, but what about getting mixed up with this... oops, what I meant to say was: Based on Eric's personality, and what little I know about him, would entering into an arrangement with him to learn stage hypnosis and become certified be a good idea?

Sage: You will surely have to keep it strictly on a business level and be sure that every agreement is written down and clearly spelled out from the beginning. On the other hand, remember what Napoleon Hill said: "When a desire or need is conceived in the mind of man the means whereby to fulfill the need or desire will surely appear." If you don't act on opportunities as they appear, the need or desire will surely go unfulfilled.

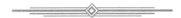

Two days later Eric was in my office working out an equitable arrangement that would be acceptable to both of us.

I could tell that Eric was doing his best to be congenial and that he was trying to suppress his habitual bragging as he sat down on the other side of my desk. He said, "You have a splendid office here. It must be nice to have such a pleasant setting in which to hypnotize people."

I politely replied, "It has worked out well for me but you should have seen it a year ago. It was nothing more than a place to store stuff, until I started doing hypnosis. My first two sessions were conducted sitting on a couple of folding chairs surrounded by stacks of inventory, but it didn't seem to matter to my clients; as far as I know, neither of them has smoked since.

"I've hypnotized about fifty people in the last year, and with fairly good success, but I would like to improve my effectiveness. That's why I am entertaining the idea of entering into some kind of an arrangement with you—so I can get better," I told him.

His attempt at modesty was short-lived when he said, "In that case it is very fortunate that you stumbled onto me, because I know more about hypnosis than anyone alive. My teacher, The Baron Von Brennon, whom I told you about the other day, knew more about hypnosis than any other person, until he died a few years ago. He taught me everything he knew and I've continued to learn more so I have become more knowledgeable than he was.

"You asked for my credentials and to verify that I can hypnotize people and teach you how to be a better hypnotist. Is that right?" he asked with contempt.

"Well, here are my certificates, which were issued to me by The Baron Von Brennon. They certify me as a *Master of Hypnosis* and a *Certified Hypnosis Trainer*. The Most Reverend St John, who is not only an ordained minister but a very fine hypnotist, as well, issued my Doctor of Divinity certificate. I am also an ordained minister, so my DD certificate allows me to legitimately call myself 'Doctor.'

"And here are newspaper articles reporting several stage-shows I have performed in various cities around the country and some clippings from interviews with reporters about my clinical hypnosis work."

Well, again I was impressed. I still questioned the validity of the "*Doctor of Divinity*" title, but the rest of his evidence was undoubtedly valid.

Eric went on, "If we come to some kind of an agreement would it be okay if I hang my certificates on the wall of your office? I've never had an office where I could display them. Until now all of my clinical hypnosis has been conducted in hotel rooms or at a client's home or office, as I traveled from city to city. I've never stayed in one place long enough to open an office of my own."

I said, "I suppose so, but let's get very specific about an agreement. I have written a list of the items we talked about the other day and I've tried to make it simple. Is this close to what you had in mind?"

I handed him my typed proposal:

1. You will teach me how to do stage-show hypnosis and as part of that training allow me to assist you during some of your stage-show performances.

2. You will instruct me in clinical hypnosis and grant me a *Master of Hypnosis* certificate when I meet your requirements for certification.

3. In return for these services I will pay you $100 a week over the next five weeks.

4. I will give you access to my office for your clinical practice up to ten hours a week.

5. After five weeks, this agreement will be null and void. And at that time another arrangement can be entered into if we choose to continue a business relationship.

"Yes, that is pretty much what we talked about, except for letting me hang my certificates on the wall of the office."

He went on, "I've been seriously thinking about our conversation the other day and, although you challenged my integrity, I was impressed with your straightforward frankness and candor. I like those qualities in a person because then I know exactly where I stand. I don't very often come across someone who has the courage to stand up to me like that. I'm looking for someone with those qualities to assist me in establishing an *Institute of Hypnosis*.

"If you prove to be trustworthy and reliable after our five week trial period, I will invite you to be a part of my plan to create a corporation for the purpose of raising money to promote 'mega' stage-shows and to establish an organization for the certification of *all* hypnotists. I plan to lobby for legislation that would require all hypnotists nationally to be certified by this organization. What do you think of that?"

I was not sure that I fully comprehended what he proposed and questioned whether what he said was reasonable, so I answered, "Let's follow through with the five week agreement and make no commitments beyond that. We can talk about your future plans at that time.... And yes, you can hang your certificates on the wall of my office. Here is my check for $100. When do we start with my training?"

"Get out your note pad and we'll start right now," he said.

CHAPTER 11

The Teaching

"What I am going to teach you, you will find no place on this earth except from me or maybe a few others I have taught. None of my former students, however, pursued their learning beyond what I taught them, so none of them have ever become more knowledgeable about the workings of hypnosis than I am," Eric told me.

I was not at all impressed with his egotism but was willing to sift out as much information as I could from his self-important dialogue. But even as he spoke I wondered how *he* knew that he knew more than anyone else unless somehow he had talked to *all* of them to find out what *they* knew—my innate skepticism at work.

He went on, "My teacher, The Baron Von Brennon, learned about hypnosis from Sigmund Freud when he was in Germany. But Freud gave up on hypnosis because he was part of the medical and academic community and his colleagues frowned on even the mention of Mesmerism or hypnotism—they viewed discussion on such topics as mysticism. Besides that, Freud didn't have the temperament for hypnotizing his patients. Even if he did get them hypnotized, if they didn't respond well to his suggestions he would spontaneously go into a rage. But The Baron could see how powerful hypnosis was, and he took what little he had learned from Freud and set out on his own."

This is interesting history, I thought, *but I question the validity of his story.*

He continued, "In Germany in the early thirties, hypnosis was very popular at theaters and in cabarets; that is where The Baron started practicing stage-show hypnosis, and he became very good at it. He even *almost* hypnotized Adolf Hitler at one of his shows but when Hitler began going under hypnosis he abruptly opened his eyes and shouted, 'No one will ever control my mind!' and then stormed out."

Now I was even more skeptical of his tale. But if not factual, at least it was entertaining.

He went on, "When Hitler started his ethnic cleansing in earnest, The Baron, like many other people with Jewish blood, immigrated to America, and after mastering the English language began doing stage-show hypnosis here. And that's how I met him.

"Over his thirty-year career he hypnotized more than 500,000 people in Germany, the United States and Canada. By hypnotizing more people than any other person alive, he not only learned a great deal about the practice of hypnosis but also uncovered some anomalies that *could* happen when a person goes under hypnosis—obscure characteristics that could have been discovered only by hypnotizing hundreds of thousands of people.... And before he died he taught me everything he knew. So, what I am about to teach you now you will find no place on earth except from me."

The more he talked the more I became doubtful of the legitimacy of what he was saying. *If someone had hypnotized half a million people it would seem that he would be famous, and his name recognition as common as Mesmer, Freud and Houdini. And how can a person teach another person "everything" he knows? It would take as long to teach someone everything a person knows as it took to learn it in the first place—a lifetime. I knew he didn't mean it literally, but I did think that the things he was telling me were boastful exaggerations.* But I was curious about the obscure anomalies he had made reference to, so I began listening with greater interest.

He continued in all seriousness. "The first thing I will teach you is to recognize and become competent in dealing with the *five hypnotic fits*. I want you to write their names on five separate sheets and then I will go back and explain each fit. I want you to write down everything I say, just as I tell it."

So I picked up my pen and wrote on the top of five pages the name of each "fit" as he recited it:

1. Pent Emotions
2. Cataleptic Fit
3. Needles Hypnosis
4. Somnambulistic Sleep
5. Somnambulistic Fit

I had not an inkling of what the name of each "fit" meant, and wondered why he called them "fits."

Eric began: "*Pent Emotions* is when a person for no apparent reason, or as the result of being asked a sensitive question, breaks out into an uncontrolled state of emotional hysteria. It is the release of emotions that have been pent up inside a person and when a person goes into hypnosis they all come gushing out. This happens about once in 25 subjects when doing clinical hypnosis and less often during stage-shows, so it is relatively common.

"The way you handle this condition, if it is in a clinical setting, is to just let them vent their emotions until they get it all out of their system. Just wait, and occasionally encourage them to let it all out and explain that when all of it has been vented they will feel a great sense of relief and whatever caused the emotion will be gone—because it has been vented. I've had some people sob for more than an hour before they got it all out," he said.

He paused to give me time to write it all down, and then he said, "When you are doing stage-shows and this happens, immediately wake up the subject and assure them that they are fine, and that you will visit with them after the show. You do it as a matter-of-fact—as though it happens all the time—because you don't want to contaminate the other subjects. After all, a stage-show is supposed to be entertaining and hilarious, not therapeutic."

What he just said has some validity, I thought. I've hypnotized only fifty people and have already had one. This must have been the condition that Sonnie experienced and, thanks to Art Baker, it appears that I handled it right.

"Next page," Eric said. "A *Cataleptic Fit* is a condition that occurs once in about 5,000 subjects. No one knows why it happens, but rather than relaxing when the suggestion is given to relax, the subject becomes more and more rigid and tense. You will recognize this condition by their white-knuckled, clenched fists and when you try to pick up their arm it feels as though their body is a granite statue—their whole body moves with their arm."

Well I'm glad I haven't had that happen yet, but then I haven't hypnotized 5,000 people, either, I thought.

"You deal with this condition by giving a loud clap of your hands close to one ear and in the other ear shouting, 'WAKE UP NOW.'"

I could feel the shock it had on my psyche when he demonstrated exactly how to do it.

He explained, "This is a very effective way to break any trance, whether you are doing clinical hypnosis or stage hypnosis. With a little practice, when on stage, you can make it look like it is just part of the show.

"Next page," he said. "*Needles Hypnosis* is a situation that takes care of itself. When a subject goes into hypnosis spontaneously it feels to them like their whole body is being pricked with needles—kind of like when you hit your crazy bone or your foot goes to sleep. When this happens, the subject automatically wakes up but the sensation remains for twenty or thirty seconds and the subject usually complains about the severity of the discomfort before it goes away. Needles hypnosis also happens once in maybe 5,000 subjects."

He then said, "Now things get a little more difficult. Not that there is anything dangerous about the condition itself, but how to handle it is a little tricky.

"A *Somnambulistic Sleep* may occur once in about 20,000 subjects. This state arises when a person has been deprived of sleep for a long period of time or is facing a stressful situation they want to avoid. You will recognize this condition when your subject doesn't *want* to wake up when you suggest to them to wake up—it isn't that they can't wake up, it is just that they don't want to.

"This is different from when a subject just falls asleep during a session. Just falling asleep may happen once in twenty-five or thirty subjects when doing clinical hypnosis. If that happens during a session just shake the chair they are sitting in and tell them to wake up. Just falling asleep seldom happens during stage-shows.

"A Somnambulistic Sleep is quite different—you can't get them to wake up no matter what you do. You can even throw water on them or vigorously shake them and they still won't wake up."

"Well, what do I do if this happens?" I asked.

"You just let them sleep. They will eventually wake up on their own although it may take a good deal of time—many hours or even a day—but they *will* eventually wake up. Obviously this could create some problems because just letting them sleep for a day is seldom feasible—like during a stage-show."

"You are right," I interjected. "Or even during a private session; I'm sure *someone* would be worried about them when they didn't show up for supper."

"That's right," Eric said as he gave a little chuckle. "However, since a hypnotized person is never unaware of the hypnotist's voice you can still give them suggestions.

"Should this happen to you, the most effective way to deal with the situation is to suggest to them: *In a moment I'm going to count up from one to five and if you do not wake up when I reach the number five I'll give you suggestions that will never allow you to enter back into this peaceful state again.* And then count up and when you say 'five,' simultaneously clap your hands and shout 'WAKE UP NOW!' I've used this method several times and so far it has worked."

And then he elaborated: "The Baron explained that a person who is in a Somnambulistic Sleep is experiencing a state of euphoria and doesn't want to be deprived of experiencing it again sometime in the future, so they just wake up. He never told me what to do if they didn't wake up or the suggestions to give them so they would never experience the euphoric state again. I guess it was because this method always worked for him, too, so he didn't need to think about an alternative."

Eric said, "Now it gets serious: The *Somnambulistic Fit.*

"Once in about 100,000 people," Eric said, "you will come across a person who is a 'hyper-natural somnambulist'—they take every suggestion so literally that they follow every suggestion precisely as they are given—without any logic or reasoning whatsoever.

"A hyper-natural somnambulist is quite different than a natural somnambulist. A natural somnambulist is a person who is an excellent hypnotic subject and they, too, take suggestions literally but a hyper-natural somnambulist takes it to the extreme.

"When the suggestion is given to a hyper-natural somnambulist to relax every muscle of their body they do; including the muscles used for breathing, their heart muscles and all other vital organs, and they start to die!

"This happened to The Baron three times during his career and it happened to me twice... both within two weeks. And it happened to my uncle, who was also a hypnotist, once.

"The problem with statistics is that you don't know if the one in 100,000 is going to be this one or the two hundred thousandth one. Statistically I am due for another one any moment, but then, again, I may never have it happen again in my lifetime."

"Now, this sounds very frightening," I said. "How do you deal with it? You don't just sit there and let them die, do you?"

"No," Eric said, "you inflict some kind of physical pain: Slap them, kick them, pinch them, yank on their hair... anything that will cause them to feel pain and at the same time keep shouting, 'WAKE UP NOW!' Give no heed to the reaction of the people who are observing the situation. You'll probably be criticized for treating a person with such cruelty and the person or their family may even sue you; but that's better than having them die. My uncle *was* sued and I think that is the reason he doesn't do stage hypnosis any more. But both times it happened to me the person and their family thanked me for saving their lives, once they understood what the consequences would have been if I had not taken the action.

"The way you recognize this condition," he went on to explain, "is the subject's skin will start turning gray and you will hear a 'death rattle' coming from deep in their throat through an open mouth. This is one reason you want to have an assistant (or at least a designated person in the audience keep a close watch on the subjects) when doing stage-shows—while your attention is directed on one subject sometimes you lose track of the other ten or fifteen."

Eric told me to memorize what he had just passed on, and at the beginning of our next training lesson he would expect me to explain the five fits and demonstrate what to do if (or when) they happen.

With that advice we set a time for the following day's training session.

After he was gone I spent the rest of the morning memorizing the "five fits" and practiced what to do if they ever occurred.

And then I began my habitual wondering. *Does Eric really know what he's talking about? Maybe he was just making this stuff up to give me the impression that I am getting my $500 worth of knowledge that I can get nowhere on earth except from him. Or had he just taken a few rumors and imagined them into fact? I can relate to the Pent Emotions condition because I experienced something similar to that with Sonnie, but the other "fits" seem a little too far-fetched and bizarre to hold much legitimacy. However, I guess I should keep an open mind about it just in case what he told me holds some truth.*

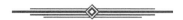

Well, over the next thirty years of my profession it was confirmed that all five "fits" *could* occur—some with greater frequency than others.

In the early years of my hypnosis career, Pent Emotions seldom materialized during stage-shows but quite often popped up during hypnotherapy sessions. It happened maybe once in ten or fifteen subjects—a big box of tissues worth every month. But as my approach changed it happened less frequently, and now sitting at my desk is a half-empty box of Kleenex that was purchased more than a year ago; and most of that was used for someone to get rid of their chewing gum so they wouldn't choke on it during the session.

A Cataleptic Fit has happened only once so far. A young woman came in to get over her fear of flying and as I began going through my "induction" process, I noticed that her hands started curling up into clenched fists, and the more I suggested relaxation the more rigid and tense she became. I took hold of her wrist and when I tried to pick up her arm it was like picking up one of King Tut's mummified arms—her whole body moved with my tug. So I got close to her ear and shouted, "WAKE UP NOW" as I clapped my hands next to her other ear. With that, she opened her eyes and her whole body went limp.

"That was really weird," she said. "It felt like my whole body was stiff as a board and I couldn't move. The more I tried to relax everything just got stiffer. What happened?"

I explained to her that this condition rarely occurs and that no one knows why it does. "During my training I was instructed how to handle it if it ever happened, but this is my first experience with the situation. I'm curious to learn how you would explain what happened? What do *you* think caused it?"

She thought for a very long time and then said, "I think it started during your pre-hypnotic talk when you made it sound as though being rid of my fear of flying was going to be easy. I know it is irrational to have the fear at all, but if it was all that easy to get rid of, why hadn't I been able to get rid of it on my own? Once I started thinking that way I felt myself resisting all the more and I don't think I heard half of what you said during your pre-hypnotic talk.

"I am very independent and strong-minded so when you made it sound so easy I felt like you were telling me I was a weak person. It sounds crazy I know, but I did exactly the opposite of what you suggested. I didn't do it intentionally, it was just my rebellious nature that kicked in, I guess."

She didn't say any of this critically. She just answered my question in a relaxed yet analytical way as though she was as curious about the event as I was. So I asked her, "What would have been a better approach for you? Would you have responded better had I made it sound like it was going to be a hard, long, drawn-out process?"

She thought again for a long time and then said, "No, I want it to be easy.... Can we go back and start from the beginning?"

I said, "Yes."

So I started over and from time to time I asked her if what I was saying was acceptable to her or if she was feeling any resistance to it. As it turned out, this time she made an excellent hypnotic subject.

A couple of weeks later I received a post card from her that was postmarked Italy, telling me how much she had enjoyed her flight.

Needles Hypnosis has occurred three or four times, but never with the severe discomfort that Eric told me the subject would experience. In each case the subjects *did* wake up by themselves, but none complained of prolonged pain. "It was like a tingling feeling all over my body so I opened my eyes to see what was causing it and when you asked why I had opened my eyes, it just went away," was their response in general. In every case when I went through the hypnosis induction process a second time, the condition did not happen again.

Somnambulistic Sleep has never happened to any of my hypnotherapy clients or stage-show subjects; however, I did have an experience that confirmed that it could happen.

One New Year's morning at about 2:00 a.m., my phone rang and the voice on the other end of the line said, "Are you a hypnotist?"

I answered, "Yes I am, how can I help you?"

He said, "We have been playing around with hypnosis at our New Year's Eve party and now we can't get one of the guests to wake up. We've tried everything. We have tried shaking her awake, we've tried scaring her awake, we've even tried throwing a pail of ice water on her and she still won't wake up. We're really worried. Can you come and help us wake her up? We'll pay you any amount you want if you can just get her to wake up!"

I explained that there was nothing to worry about and if they would just let her sleep she'd eventually wake up on her own and ended with, "It might take several hours or maybe even a day but she *will*, sooner or later, wake up."

"Well, we kind of can't wait that long," he said.

"Why not?" I asked.

"Well it's like this. She is married and her husband doesn't know that she came to our party and he will be getting home from his night-shift job in three hours. Do you understand our problem?" he asked.

I answered, "Yes, I do. Give me half an hour and I'll be there. It's going to cost you $200 whether I can wake her up or not."

"We'll have the money ready for you. It's worth the chance, if you know what I mean," he said before hanging up.

Thirty minutes later I was at the door of a home in a fashionable part of town. When I entered I saw twenty or so anxious people milling around and one on a sofa in a bright green water-drenched dress, seemingly asleep. The fellow who appeared to be the host of the party greeted me, pointed to her limp body and said, "Well, there she is."

"What is her name?" I asked.

"Sharon. And my name is Tom," he said.

I went to the couch and felt her arm just to make sure she was warm and alive—she was. So I leaned down close to her ear and said, "*Sharon, my name is Lindsay Brady; I'm a professional hypnotist. Your friends have asked me to come and see if you are ready to wake up yet. If you can hear my voice move your right pointing finger; it doesn't have to be very much, just enough so I will know you are aware of what I am saying.*"

I had my doubts that she had heard me, but momentarily her right pointing finger gave an almost imperceptible little twitch. So I went on, "*I know that you are enjoying this state of euphoria and that you feel that you need to sleep, or maybe there is something that you would rather not face when you wake up, but you have had plenty of sleep now and I will promise you that when you wake up whatever it is that is distressing you, if anything, no longer will.*"

And then I said to her, "*In a moment I'm going to count up from one to five, and when I reach the number five just open your eyes and you will be wide awake, feeling like you have had a whole night's sleep and if there is something that has been bothering you, it no longer will.*

"*One, two, three, four, five, open your eyes and WIDE AWAKE,*" I said with a clap of my hands near one of her ears. And she just continued to lie there in her soggy green dress with her eyes closed.

"*Sharon, I'm going to count up once again from one to five and this time if you do not open your eyes and awaken when I reach the number five, I will give you a suggestion that will never again allow you to return to this state of peace and tranquility. When you open your eyes you will be wide-awake, still feeling as peaceful and tranquil as you are right now.... And, you will remember everything that has been going on.*"

I added the remembering part hoping that I could gain some insight into what had produced the condition and what she had been experiencing while it was happening.

"*One, two, three, four and five, open your eyes now and WIDE AWAKE!*" I said with an accompanied loud clap of my hands.

This time her eyes snapped open, and she smiled and said, "That was a very nice nap, but I'd better head for home now before my husband gets off work. I think that he knows I came to the party anyway, although he asked me not to come by myself, but I don't want him to get home and find me missing—he would be worried."

Just before she walked out the door, I pulled her to one side for a moment and asked, "Why didn't you want to wake up?"

She answered, "Even though I was enjoying a very pleasant state of mind and body—kind of like floating weightlessly in space—I *couldn't* wake up.... Well, that's not exactly right, in the *beginning* I didn't want to wake up because it was so peaceful—nothing seemed to matter. Even later when they dumped ice water on me, I didn't mind. But when I heard Tom say that he *couldn't* wake me up I *thought* I couldn't. And then I heard *everyone* saying that I couldn't wake up so I just laid there enjoyed the pleasant relaxing sleep while I waited for someone to tell me that I could. Does that make any sense?" she asked.

"Yes it does, but why didn't you wake up the first time I asked you to?" I inquired.

She answered, "Because I didn't want to go back to feeling lousy. Before Tom hypnotized me I was really feeling guilty about coming to the party because I told my husband that I wouldn't. But I didn't want to miss out on the fun of a New Year's Eve party just because he had to work, so I came anyway. I don't lie very often so I wasn't enjoying being here because I was feeling so guilty. Then when you told me that I'd still feel good when I woke up, which I still do, I felt that it was okay to wake up."

I thanked her for sharing her experience with me and said, "You had better be getting on home."

After she left I visited with the remaining guests and explained to them that she was a very good hypnotic subject and at first she *didn't* want to wake up because she was enjoying the peacefulness, so she didn't wake up. But when she heard Tom say that he couldn't wake her up that became a hypnotic suggestion and the more she heard everyone else saying that she couldn't wake up it reinforced the suggestion all the more.

I advised them to, in the future, be aware that some people are "natural somnambulists" and once hypnotized take every suggestion literally, whether the suggestion is intended or just a slip of the tongue.

Tom handed me my $200 and said thanks, and I went home to enjoy what was left of my New Year's Eve sleep—which was not much.

I have never personally had a client go into a Somnambulistic Fit, however, a colleague of mine did... or, at least something like it.

In the early 1980's I was still performing an occasional stage-show, mostly for company parties, private parties and high school fundraisers.

Leo Gagnon, who was the president of the Arizona Society for Professional Hypnosis (ASPH) at that time, wanted to get into stage-show hypnosis, and he asked me if I would give him some tips on how to do it. I told him, "Sure, I'd be happy to," since I was no longer interested in becoming the world's most famous stage-show hypnotist.

As a part of telling him what I had learned from doing stage-shows, I explained the five hypnotic fits just as Eric had taught me. Actually, I dug out the notes I still had from Eric's tutoring and read them to Leo verbatim. He was (and still is) a very accomplished clinical hypnotist and he viewed my recitation with as much skepticism as I had when Eric first explained them to me—except for Pent Emotions, something that he had encountered many times himself.

One day about a year later, my phone rang. It was Leo. "I just got one of those! I don't remember what you called it but one of those people who start to die when they get hypnotized!"

"You mean a Somnambulistic Fit," I helped him.

"Yeah, that's what you called it, I remember now," he said. And went on to explain, "I was conducting a group session of eight clients when my wife Donna, who was assisting me, tugged on my sleeve and pointed to one of the subjects who was slumped over in his chair with these gurgling sounds coming from his open mouth. I thought at first that he was just snoring until I noticed that his skin was kind of grayish and he wasn't breathing. I didn't remember what you called it but I did remember what you said I should do. So I went over to him, slapped him on the cheek and shouted, 'WAKE UP!'"

I asked Leo how the client responded to his actions and what the after-effects were on that client as well as the others.

Leo said, "Oh, after I slapped him he took in a deep breath, opened his eyes and asked me why his cheek was smarting. I told him I had slapped him on the cheek because he looked like he was dying and that was the only way I knew how to wake him up. I escorted him out of the office and advised him to never consider being hypnotized again, and especially by me.

"The other clients just about jumped out of their skin when I slapped him (it must have sounded like a loud clap of my hands) and when I shouted, 'Wake up,' they thought I was talking to them. They didn't know what had happened, except for what they gleaned from the conversation I had with the survivor as I pushed him out the door."

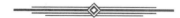

That said, when Eric left my office I still questioned the validity of the five fits and wondered if there would be any other surprises in the offing. As it turned out, there were.

CHAPTER 12

The Corporation

The next day Eric came through my door an hour and a half late, looking unkempt and red-eyed. I couldn't tell if he had spent my hundred dollars for booze; had been in a fight with his ex-wife, whom he had followed to Salt Lake City; or had been sniffing too many paint fumes. Whatever the reason he really didn't look all that sharp.

After I had demonstrated my prowess in dealing with the five hypnotic fits, he instructed me to write down word for word the "correct" language for inducing the hypnotic state when doing stage-show hypnosis. It was simple and repetitious but he insisted that I write down each word as he spoke it. And then he said, "After you have written it all down I want you to recite it back to me phrase by phrase, exactly as I have dictated it."

"Look into my eyes.... Place your hands on your lap not touching each other.... Now take in a very deep breath and hold it in while I count down, five, four, three, two, one.... And now through pursed lips exhale.

"And now take in another deep breath.... Hold it in while I count down, five, four, three, two, one.... And through pursed lips exhale.

"And now just once more. Take in a deep breath.... Hold it in while I count down, five, four, three, two, one.... And through pursed lips exhale.

"Still looking into my eyes, I'm going to count down once again. Each number I count you will feel yourself relax deeper and deeper, and as I count down your eyelids will get heavier and heavier and by the time I reach the number one your eyelids will be so heavy that you will be unable to keep them open and you will just let them close. When you close your eyes you will go into a deep hypnotic sleep.

"Five, your eyes are getting very tired and sleepy.

"Four, your eyelids are getting very heavy.

"Three, you are very tired and sleepy.

"Two, your eyes are so very heavy that you can no longer keep them open.

"One, just close your eyes and SLEEP NOW!

"And now your arms are getting very, very heavy.

"And now your legs are getting very, very heavy.

"And now your entire body is getting very, very heavy.... SLEEP NOW!

"Now your arms are very, very heavy.

"Your legs are very, very heavy.

"Your entire body is very, very heavy.... SLEEP NOW!

"I am going to pick up your arms at the wrist. When I do, notice how heavy your arms are and when I let go of your wrist your arm will drop back down into your lap and you will go into an even deeper hypnotic sleep."

Using me as a subject he demonstrated how to pick up the person's arm and said, "You want to pick up an arm of each person who has volunteered to be hypnotized. When you do this you are testing to see how well the subject has relaxed, to see if anyone has gone into a cataleptic fit and to deepen the trance.

"If a subject helps you lift his or her arm up, or if their arm doesn't "plop" down into their lap when you let go of it, then send them back down to the audience because they have not followed your suggestions exactly. If they can't follow this simple suggestion they are not going to carry out more complex ones."

Once I had mastered this "induction" and the "arm pick-up/drop test" to his satisfaction, Eric engaged himself in a monologue about how he was going to revolutionize the hypnosis social order (with himself at the top), and create an institute with the purpose of establishing laws and setting rules that would govern all hypnotists and spell out the standards by which hypnosis is to be conducted—his way.

He told me all he needed was $35,000 to make it all happen but then grumbled, "It would take me forever to earn and save up that much money painting houses, even if they paid me as much as I am worth. And doing clinical hypnosis sessions would take just as long. I only charge $50 a half hour, but it's tough to find clients who are willing to pay that much—as much as *I* am worth. So my only hope is to create a corporation and put together a business plan that will entice investors to fund an advertising scheme for putting on 'mega' stage-shows. I mean stage-shows that will fill up a concert hall—3,000 people at each performance.... And that's where you come in. I need you to do the 'leg work' for creating a corporation that will handle all of our business transactions and to come up with a business plan to present to potential investors."

I was puzzled as to why he thought I could create a business plan that would attract investors who would part with their money, and why he thought I would know how to create a corporation. I knew nothing about fundraising and even less (if that is possible) about creating a corporation. So I asked, "Why do you think I would know how to do all of this and why are you asking *me* to do it when *you* could do it just as well yourself?"

He answered, "Because it is apparent that you are successful in your present businesses, you have credibility in the community and you probably have connections with people who have money who would like to make a handsome return on a sure thing."

Little did he know that I was still in the process of overcoming a lifetime of mediocrity and financial devastation. *I guess I am still very good at putting on a good act,* I thought.

But then I considered, *Of the three points he made, the first two were probably just for flattery and the third was the real reason; he thinks I have connections with people who have money to invest. I probably do know a few such people but I think they would be leery about investing in a "sure thing."*

"And why would *I* want to do all of this for *you*, even if I knew how?" I asked.

Eric answered, "Because by helping *me*, you can make more money than you could ever dream of earning by selling your stinking little industrial supplies and drain pipes. And, you would be a major player in a revolution that will shape the domain of hypnosis for centuries to come—*I* will make *you* famous."

I replied, "I'm not sure I want to be a part of it. And I don't think that it's even realistic, for that matter. I'm not talking about the 'mega stage-show' part because Reveen was able to do it with his advertising blitz. When I say unrealistic, I'm referring to changing the worldview of hypnosis and creating some kind of an institute to legislate laws that would require hypnosis to be conducted in accordance with how you think it should be done.

"Why don't we just stick to our original agreement of *you* teaching *me* how to do stage hypnosis for $500?"

And as an afterthought I asked, "And how do you know that it will take $35,000 if you haven't already worked up a business plan?"

Apparently he had no answer, because rather than responding to my question he said, "Okay, I just thought you would be as excited about my plan as I am. But in the meantime I'm going to teach you how to book stage-shows on a mini scale so you will have had real-life experience assisting me when the big things happen. And we can put a few bucks in our pockets while we are getting all of the other stuff put together."

He didn't say it directly but I knew that "the other stuff" was fleecing people out of their money while creating a corporation to change the worldview of hypnosis.

For the rest of the week my "training" took the form of traveling around the greater Salt Lake City area and stopping at every nightclub and bar we could find in an attempt to secure a stage-show booking.

As we were driving back to my office after four days of fruitless endeavor Eric said (for at least the tenth time), "All it takes is one booking and we'll be on our way. I'll have more bookings than we will have time to perform. Once we have a track record in this city, and I can show other nightclub owners how my shows will quadruple their business, I can write my own ticket. They will be clamoring for me and then I can demand more money."

It is interesting how he is able to so easily weave "I" and "we" into his scenario, I thought.

He was probably trying to convince himself more than me when he said, "Just think about it. When nightclub owners see how much additional money I bring in they will be willing to pay more money just to keep me from taking their patrons to some other club. Just wait and see. I've seen it happen many times."

While he continued his prattling (and since I had heard it all before anyway) I was free to engage in my own thoughts on the matter. *Yeah, we've traveled all over the Salt Lake Valley and out of the fifty nightclub owners we've visited only one showed any interest whatsoever until she found out it would cost her "only $2,000 a week" and she pointed us in the direction of the door.*

It appears to me that booking a stage-show is a hundred times less likely than finding people for clinical hypnosis. If this approach is all that you have cracked it up to be, why aren't you still in Las Vegas, rolling in cash, with more business than you can handle? I think I should give up this stage-show hypnosis stuff and just stick to doing it clinically one-on-one.... Or maybe I should give up on hypnosis altogether and focus my energies on industrial supply and Ecology II selling.

I was so lost in my thoughts that if Eric was still talking I wasn't aware of it as I continued thinking. *We have spent four days and two tanks of <u>my</u> gas and* *haven't made a cent. I could have earned two or three hundred dollars if I'd been out there selling bolts and drainage pipe. In addition to that, next Monday Eric is going to want his second $100 installment and I've learned almost nothing from him about doing stage hypnosis. I really am discouraged. I think hooking up with Eric was a very bad idea. And as I think about it, I don't like this nightclub environment and most of the unsavory people who are associated with it. And I'm sick and tired of being in Eric's presence with his non-stop bragging and repetitive jabbering. Maybe I should just tell him I'm going to go back on our agreement so he can go his way and I can get back to a lifestyle with which I am familiar.*

All of these negative thoughts, and the bad feelings associated with them, vanished into the ether when we got back to my office and I called my answering service. "Hi, Lindsay," Suzy said (I don't know if she had a choice but it seemed that she was the only operator who delivered my messages anymore). "I have just one message for you. It's a call from David at *David's Nightclub*. He says he wants to talk to you again about doing a stage-show at his place. I know about *David's*, that's where I got drunk the night I came to see you. I'm still embarrassed about that. *David's* is just a block from your office. If you do a stage-show there let me know, I'd love to come see you perform."

I just left it at that, since I didn't want to bother explaining that *I* wouldn't be hypnotizing anyone; I'd only be assisting Eric and he would be doing all of the hypnosis.

Of all the nightclub owners we had called on, David, although having shown little interest, was the only one who had any class and seemed to have a good business sense. While Eric was going through his "sales pitch," David just sat there writing down a few notes and asking a few relevant questions. He said that he would consider our proposal, but that $2,000 a week seemed far too much and he doubted that we would draw in enough new business to cover the cost, let alone earn any additional money from the venture.

The next day we called on David and after some negotiating agreed to (as I recall) a contract for two performances a night on Thursdays, Fridays and Saturdays over the next four weeks. He would pay us $1,000 a week and forty percent of any increase in profits, as compared to an average of the four previous weeks. In addition he would commit $1,000 up front for advertising the show and we would pay back half of the advertising amount with the first $500 of our 40% override.

"You will just have to trust me on the override. I don't open my books to anyone except the IRS," he said as we left with a signed contract in hand.

"We have a lot of training to do if we're going to be ready by next Thursday night. That gives us only four days to get you trained so plan on spending a solid five hours each day, starting on Monday," Eric said.

On Monday and each of the following four days (though always late), Eric brought with him a different "friend" to pose as a stage-show subject so I could have a real live person with whom to practice as he taught me how to assist him. Except for his friend Linda, they were rather "seedy-looking" males. I didn't know where he came up with them on such short notice since I had assumed this was his first visit to Salt Lake City. *Maybe he found them at the boarding house where he is staying*, I thought.

For the next four days Eric grilled me over and over until I could recite his introduction exactly as *he* wanted to be introduced at the beginning of each show. He expected my delivery to sound like a prizefight announcer, or like Ed McMahon introducing Johnny Carson. I had had little experience speaking to an audience from a stage, and certainly none announcing prizefights, so it was a very arduous process.

I was also instructed that while the show was going on I should keep a sharp lookout just in case any of the five hypnotic fits occurred in the audience or on stage. "And if anyone in the audience spontaneously goes under hypnosis, go down and wake them up," he said.

Using the people he brought in for the purpose, we systematically practiced some of the hypnotic routines he planned to use during his performances and how I was to participate in their execution. Eric explained, "The routines we are practicing are just the foundation of the performance—we will probably use these in every show. I have more than a hundred other routines in my repertoire of tricks but I am not sure which ones I'll be using on any given night, so you need to be prepared to assist me in carrying them out. I am 'freewheeling' when I perform, so if something happens that sparks my creative genius I may just, on impulse, create a new routine that I've never used before. So be alert!"

Contrary to the agreement I thought we had come to the week before, from time to time Eric interjected into my training conversations about his "mega plan." I was willing to consider the "mega stage-show" part and we even came up with a name for the corporation: *Positive Suggestion Institute* (PSI).

I was relieved to discover that one of Eric's "friends," John, was a fledgling attorney who had just graduated with his law degree, so I didn't have to do the "leg work" to form the corporation. John certainly didn't look like any attorney I'd ever seen (I think he was a left-over from the bohemian era and had not yet moved up to being a hippie) and I wondered if he knew how to create a legitimate corporation. As it turned out, he did—and he did it in less than a week for the right price: No money up front (except for filing fees which were paid for out of my pocket) and five percent of PSI's annual net income for the life of the corporation.

For reasons that I was not aware of at the time, I was chosen to be the president of PSI; John, the attorney, was the vice president; Terry, another one of Eric's "friends," was secretary and Eric was treasurer. Eric choosing to be treasurer should have tipped me off as to why *I* was president!

We agreed that any money (above actual expenses) that came in from stage-show performances and any income from clinical sessions that were a spin-off from doing stage-shows would be placed in the corporation's checking account, as would (of course) any money that came in from outside funding. We also agreed that we would let the funds accumulate until there was sufficient money to launch an advertising campaign for putting on "mega stage-shows." "All we need now is to come up with a business plan and find some investors," Eric said.

I remember the week of our premier performance at *David's* as being a hectic one for me: A rock flipped up while driving down the dirt lane to my home and punched a hole in the oil pan of my Fiat Spider (the car that I didn't drive off of the cliff) so Darlene and I were down to sharing one car. Dick Baker, my partner in Ecology II, had just made a giant acquisition of plastic drainpipe that ended up sitting in an alfalfa field on my parents' property. And I was also involved in the creation of "the corporation" (like opening a PSI checking account with money from *my* personal bank account). And I was sick and tired of announcing prizefights and trying to speak and sound like Ed McMahon. But Thursday night came anyway, ready or not.

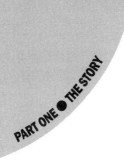

CHAPTER 13

The Stage

I arrived twenty minutes before show time thinking Eric would be there making final preparations and getting psyched up for his premier performance at *David's*.

Fifteen minutes passed and I began to worry that Eric's promptness for his stage-show performances would be the same as it was for my training sessions—an hour late.

I spied David at his office door shifting from foot to foot with his eyes fixed on the entrance—probably thinking the same thing I was.

I walked up to him and asked, "Have you seen or heard from Eric?"

With more than a hint of irritation he said, "When I booked you guys I assumed I was dealing with reliable professionals. I expected that your friend would be here well before show time to take care of any preliminaries. Is he always late for his performances?"

"I'm just as mystified as you are," I said. "This is the first time I've worked with him on stage so I don't know if he is or if he isn't dependable when it comes to his performances. For the short time I have known him, however, punctuality has not proven to be one of his finest qualities."

David said, "He called me earlier today and asked me to have ten chairs set up close together in a semicircle near the back of the stage, to leave the microphone hot when the DJ takes his break and, for some reason that he didn't explain, to have a wet bar towel on stage. All of which I've taken care of. So where is he?

"I've spent a lot of money promoting this show," he continued, "with newspaper ads and even a couple of radio spots. Look how packed the place is, and especially for a Thursday. And that's good. But if he doesn't get here soon and deliver an entertaining show, future promotions will suffer, to say nothing of the money lost on advertising and the ill consequences it will have on my reputation as a reasonable businessman. And that's bad."

My stomach leaped up into my esophagus at his next words. "I hope that you are ready to step in if he doesn't show!"

At that moment (7:29 pm on the dot) Eric walked through the door and all of my doubts about his professionalism as a stage-show hypnotist vanished.

He was dressed in a spotless, freshly-pressed black tuxedo; a lace-front white silk shirt; a black bow tie; a bright red cummerbund and black shoes that reflected the overhead lights as he strolled up carrying an over-sized briefcase.

He walked up to David and said, "Is the mic hot?"

David was probably as stunned with Eric's flashy appearance as I was and answered with only a nod.

Eric turned to me and said, "Are you ready? I hope you remember what you are supposed to do. It's not all that hard but I'm depending on you to look and be sharp. Let's go do it!"

Briefcase in hand, he stopped at the foot of the stairs that led to the stage and said, "Take my briefcase up and place it where it will be handy and then introduce the world's greatest stage-show hypnotist."

I continued up the stairs, grabbed the microphone from its stand, tapped it a couple of times and then barked into it, "*Ladies and Gentlemen, may I have your attention . . . please!*"

As I had been coached by Eric, I waited for a moment until the bar sounds quieted down, and then repeated, "*Ladies and Gentlemen, your attention please.*

"*It is my pleasure to introduce DR. ERIC, the world's greatest hypnotist to have ever performed on stage. In his illustrious career, <u>Dr. Eric</u> has astonished audiences internationally with his performances. And now, having just arrived from his sell-out engagements in Las Vegas, Nevada, he is here at David's to entertain <u>you</u>!*"

I don't think many people in the audience believed the part about Eric being the "greatest hypnotist to have ever performed on stage," because I didn't believe it either. But as it turned out I was wrong—maybe not the world's greatest stage-show hypnotist but certainly a highly accomplished one.

I continued, "*Acclaimed by the newsprint media as 'The Master of Mesmerism,' Dr. Eric will to take you on a journey into the mystical realm of the subconscious mind. And now . . . heeeeere's DR. ERIC!*"

Eric leaped up on stage, I handed him the microphone and the show began.

"Ladies and Gentlemen, I am *Dr. Eric,* the world's greatest stage-show hypnotist! Tonight I will be taking you on an adventure into your subconscious mind. I am assisted by Lindsay Brady, an accomplished hypnotist in his own right.

"The subconscious mind is powerful and wondrous. Let me demonstrate how *my* subconscious mind can eliminate all feelings of discomfort and pain."

With that he reached into his "magic briefcase" and pulled out a six-inch-long ice pick. Then with a quick jerk of his head (to give the appearance of entering into a trance), he leaned his head back and inserted the shank of the ice pick into his right nostril, all the way to its hilt. Leaving it in place, he stretched out his arms, turned from side to side so the audience could see that it was indeed inside his head, waited a moment or two and then in one easy motion extracted the ice pick and spiked it into the stage floor three feet in front of himself.

The crowd went silent.

Without a word he reached back into his case and took out a pure white six-inch-long candle. He took a cigarette lighter from his pocket and lit the candle. He turned sideways and stretched out his right arm palm down, placed the flame right under it and held it there for five seconds. He removed the candle, blew it out and turned his hand outwards to show the audience the soot that had accumulated on his palm.

With another jerk of his head (to give the appearance of coming out of a trance), Eric said, "That demonstrates how the subconscious mind can control the human body. Medical records tell of major surgery being performed without the patient feeling any pain whatsoever while under hypnosis!

"Hypnosis is used every day to help people stop smoking, lose weight and get over phobias. But that is not what I will be doing tonight. Tonight I will be entertaining you and taking you on an adventure into the realm of your subconscious mind.

"In a few moments I will be asking for volunteers to come up to the stage to be hypnotized. When you volunteer, come up with the intention of being hypnotized and following my every command. Prepare yourself to come up and participate in an adventure using powers of *your* subconscious mind. I will treat you with total respect and cause you to do nothing that will harm you or embarrass you.

"I am calling now for volunteers. Come up now and enjoy the experience of being hypnotized and discover the power of *your* subconscious mind. Come up now."

At least twenty-five people walked to the base of the stairs that led up to the stage. One by one Eric beckoned the volunteers to come up and stand facing him so they were about two feet apart. He asked each person their name, waited for an answer, and then calling them by their name said, "*Look into my eye,*" as he pointed with his right finger to his right "eyebrow-raised" eye.

"*As you gaze into my eye you feel yourself starting to fall backwards. You are leaning further and further backwards. My assistant is stationed right behind you to catch you as you are starting to fall backwards now.*"

As I had been instructed, I had positioned myself behind the person who was looking into Eric's eye so I could catch them when they fell backwards.

He moved his hand from pointing to his eye and together with his other hand (with all of his fingers slightly bent and pointing in the direction of the subject's face in typical hypnotic fashion—as if some mystical force was emanating from each fingertip) said, *"Fall back NOW!"*

If they fell backwards into my arms Eric invited them to sit on one of the ten chairs. If the person didn't fall backwards, he or she was "invited" to return to the audience. After all ten chairs were occupied Eric asked the remaining volunteers to return to their seats with the suggestion, *"I will be performing another show at 9:30. So stick around, and enjoy a few extra drinks—along with everyone else* (he emphasized)—*and volunteer again later."*

During my training Eric had instructed me, "When working a nightclub, from time to time suggest to the audience that they 'enjoy a few extra drinks,' or that 'it's time for another round,' especially when you are getting an override on an increase in the nightclub's profits. With a little practice you can make it so subtle no one will know that you just gave them a "hypnotic suggestion" to buy more drinks. If you will closely observe, you will see the cocktail waitresses and bartenders getting busier right after the suggestion."

I had no difficulty performing my task except for the last guy—Bert was a foot taller than me and outweighed me by at least a hundred and fifty pounds. When he started to fall backwards Eric helped me by grabbing him by his shirt collar to keep him from hitting the floor.

While the unused volunteers were returning to their chairs Eric reminded me, "Keep an eye on the audience and if any of them start acting out my suggestions or if anyone slumps over in their chair, go down and wake them up."

During my training sessions he had tutored me, "Often times a person or two in the audience will get hypnotized without realizing it. Any suggestion I give on stage they take as a suggestion to *them* and they act out the suggestion. There is nothing serious about this, unless of course they go into a somnambulistic fit—and you know what to do if that happens—but it creates an aura of mystery when the assistant needs to go down and wake someone up."

Once all of the selected volunteers were seated shoulder-to-shoulder in the tightly positioned chairs (as Eric had instructed David to have them placed), Eric faced them and said, *"Place your hands on your lap, not touching each other, and look into my eyes... And take in a deep breath and hold it in while I count down, five, four, three, two, one, and now through pursed lips, exhale... "* He continued to recite word for word his "induction" precisely as he had trained *me* to do.

As the subjects' eyes began closing and their heads began to droop, Eric leaned each person against the person seated next to them, positioning a few so that their heads rested on their neighbors' shoulders, creating an amusing sight all by itself.

After the chuckles in the audience had subsided, Eric suggested to the subjects, "*In a moment I am going to ask you to open your eyes. When you open your eyes, sit upright in your chair and fix your gaze only on me. When you open your eyes you will go even deeper into hypnosis.*

"*Open your eyes now. Sit upright in your chair, looking only at me and drifting into a deep hypnotic sleep.*"

Showing them with his own hands what he wanted them to do he said, "*Clasp your hands together like this, with your fingers entwined* (which they all did) *and follow these suggestions exactly: Whenever you have your eyes open, until I instruct you to do otherwise, your gaze will be only on me. Now close your eyes.*"

He went down the line and with a squeeze of each subject's clasped hands suggested, "*Your hands are locked tight together, you cannot take them apart. The harder you try to get them apart the more they just stick tighter and tighter together, and only by* my *next touch will you be able to take them apart. Now try to take your hands apart, but they will just stick tighter and tighter.*"

Although it was impressive to witness ten people trying to get their hands apart, it wasn't all that humorous—very little laughter came from the audience.

Eric began at one end of the subjects and one after the other grasped their clasped hands and very easily pulled them apart, except for one fellow who defiantly refused to let his hands separate. The more Eric struggled to get his hands apart the more the young man resisted. Eric let go and with a loud clap of his hands right next to the chap's ear shouted, "*Freddie, WAKE UP NOW!*" Freddie opened his eyes, and looked at the audience with a smirk on his face. Eric said, "Freddie, you can go back down to the audience now."

He turned to the remaining nine subjects, whose eyes were all fixed on him, and then one by one, he grasped each person's arm, pulled on it to make it straight, and placed each arm out in different directions—some straight up in the air, some right out in front, some to the side of the subject—with the suggestion, "*Your arm is stiff, like a bar of steel; you cannot bend it.*" After everyone's arms were sticking out every which way Eric suggested, "*Try to bend your arms now. The more you try to bend your arms, they just get stiffer and stiffer, but the moment I snap my fingers your arms will float comfortably back to your lap and you will go even deeper into hypnosis.*"

The audience was a little more amused at the peculiar site of nine people with their arms sticking out in every direction and trying to get them to bend, but failing.

Eric waited for a moment and suggested, "*When I snap my fingers your arms will no longer be stiff and they will gently float down to your lap.*" [Snap!]

Like balloons having lost their buoyancy, each person's arms drifted down to their lap.

Next, Eric pulled a cigar box out of his briefcase, walked over to Patty, gently touched her forehead and said, "*Patty, in a moment I will ask you to open your eyes. When you do I will hand you a magical box. Take it and sit down on the floor to the left side of the stage and open its lid. When you do, look into it and you will witness some strange things going on inside this magical box...you will see a bunch of tiny people having a party. Your job is to keep all of the partiers in the box so none of them get stepped on. From time to time one of them will escape so you must capture the runaway and return him or her to the party. Open your eyes now, Patty. Take this box and sit down on the floor over there, open the lid, look inside and tell us what you see.*"

After Patty seated herself cross-legged on the floor, Eric asked, "*Patty, what is going on in that magical box?*" He placed the microphone close to her mouth and waited for her to answer.

Patty placed the box up to eye level, gingerly lifted the lid and peeked in for a few seconds then slammed it closed and said, "There's a party going on in there! These little people are in there having a party! I don't know how they got to be so tiny or how they got into this box but it looks like they're sure having fun—boogying around and just having a good old time."

Eric suggested, "*With all of that partying going on I think they need some fresh air. Open the lid wide so they can breathe. Look at them more closely because they are miniature versions of people you know. Tell us what they are doing.*"

She opened the lid wide, set the box on the floor, stuck her nose down close and began giggling as she said, "I see my grade school principal, Mr. Sanders, dancing with Miss Hildebrand, my sixth grade teacher. I always knew they had this thing going for each other. Hey, *all* of them are my old school teachers. They're having some kind of a reunion. I think they are celebrating because I graduated and they don't have to put up with any more of my fooling around. Whoops, Miss Nelson just jumped out of the box. I'll save her before someone steps on her... Maybe not, I never liked her anyway, after she gave me that 'D.' But it *would* make an awful mess if she got squashed. I guess I'd better save her."

She reached out her hand and with a gentle motion swooped up Miss Nelson and returned to her party. She placed her ear down right next to the box, as though listening to Miss Nelson, and said, "You can't use *that one*, it's much too large for you and if you could get up to the seat you might fall in and drown. I think there's a little one right over there," pointing to one corner of the box . . . and said, "You're welcome."

The crowd went wild with laughter.

Eric told her to keep a close watch on the partygoers and that he'd check back with her from time to time.

He then reached into his briefcase again and took out a pair of heavy-rimmed glasses, touched George's head and said, "*George, in a moment when you open your eyes I will hand you a pair of magical glasses. When you place them on you will look out at the audience and make some snide remarks about what you see. When you look through these magic glasses you will see that the people out there are wearing no clothes—they are stark naked—and you will probably discover a few things about them that you were not expecting. But then, when I ask you to take a closer look you will see that they have their clothes back on but they all have animal heads. Although they look like animals you will still recognize who they are and make a few clever remarks about their appearance.*

"*Open your eyes, slip on this pair of magical glasses and tell us what you see.*"

"Hey, everyone out there's naked! Why aren't they wearing their clothes when out in public like this? Don't they know that it is immoral? Gee, Mary, you've just been putting up a false front for all these years, haven't you? You're really not all that well stacked after all. Hey Peter, you are so skinny you look like a scarecrow. You really ought to put your clothes back on. Wow, Audrey you look great without your glasses and no clothes."

Eric said, "*Hey George, you'd better look more closely; I think something has changed.*"

The bespectacled George took a closer look, removed the glasses, gave them a good rubbing, put them back on and said, "Peter you look much better with your clothes on, but you look like an ass—I mean a donkey. Jenny, until now I always thought you were a cute chick, not an old biddy hen... By the way, who's the Dumbo with his arm around your shoulder? Ho, it's you, Mac!"

And then George turned to Eric and said, "Why do all of these people have animal heads? I'm getting a little freaked-out about all this."

At that instant Eric snapped his fingers in front of George's face and said, "George, *WIDE AWAKE!*" George jerked, blinked his eyes, took off the glasses and handed them back to Eric.

Eric said, "*You can return back to your seat now, George, and make sure you buy a few extra drinks for those people you have been insulting.*"

As George walked off the stage Eric whispered to me, "Bring a small table up and put it at center stage, while I send a few of these other folks back to the audience."

While I was running my errand I heard Eric call six of the remaining volunteers by name and say to each of them, "*Open your eyes, and wide awake. Return to your table and have a drink or two.*"

This left Bert, Maggie and Patty still on stage.

Patty had been watching the party in the cigar box the whole time, but from time to time she scurried around the stage rescuing an escapee.

Eric went over to Patty and asked, "How's the party going?"

Patty said, "At first everything was fine, but I think they're getting really drunk. Mr. Woods just punched Mr. Stryker in the nose because he was kissing Mrs. Woods, his wife. And when Miss Michaels saw all of those people out there in the audience with no clothes on, she fainted."

Leaving Patty to her party, Eric touched Bert on the head and said, "*I know your name is Bert, but I'm going to call you "Brute," because of the task I'm going to ask you to attempt. Open your eyes now, 'Brute.'*" And the six foot four, two hundred seventy-five pounder opened his eyes and looked at Eric. "*Now take your chair and lumber over to that little table and sit down facing its center.*"

Brute picked up his chair and lumbered to the table and sat down facing its center.

Eric walked over to the petite, one hundred twenty-five pound, five foot four Maggie, touched her head and said, "*Maggie, open your eyes and take your chair to the other side of that little table and sit down facing Brute.*"

"Don't step on Miss Killian! She's right over there hiding behind the table leg," Patty shouted as she slammed the lid of the party box closed. "Mr. Stryker is after *her*, too." On all fours, she scrambled over to the table, reached down, rescued Miss Killian from her impending dilemma, jumped up and stomped on Mr. Stryker. "That'll show you, you . . . you . . . womanizing creep!" The audience went crazy with laughter as Patty was going through her spontaneous routine.

Eric looked at Patty, and with a snap of his fingers said, "*Patty, open your eyes and WIDE AWAKE!*" Patty opened her eyes, rubbed them with one hand, looked at the cigar box in her other hand and said, "Where did this cigar box come from?"

Eric said, "*Give me the box.*" And then suggested, "*Go back to your seat and get your friends and have an extra drink or two to celebrate your fine performance.... The one of which you have no memory.*"

Eric turned to Brute, who was sitting at the table looking glary-eyed at Maggie, and said to him, "*You look like a pretty strong fellow. Am I right?*"

Brute responded (sounding like you would think a 'Brute' should sound—with a mouth full of mush), "Yeah."

"*Do you like to arm wrestle?*" Eric asked.

"Yeah."

"*Are you good at it?*"

"Yeah, I never lost an arm wrestle to nobody," he said in his brutish voice.

"*Do you think that you can beat Maggie here in an arm wrestling contest?*"

Brute looked at Maggie with disapproval and said, "Yeah, I'd bet that anyone—even my grandmother—could beat that little 'pipsqueak' in an arm wrestle."

"*So it sounds like you like to bet, do you?*"

"Yeah."

"Do you have any cash money in your pocket that you would bet on you beating Maggie in an arm wrestle?"

"Yeah, I have a hundred and I'll bet it all on whipping that little pipsqueak in an arm wrestle."

"You took the words right out of my mouth," Eric said, as he stripped a crisp $100 bill off of his money clip and held it up for everyone to see.

"Well, where's yours?" Eric asked Brute.

Brute stood up, pulled out his wallet and withdrew some twenties, a couple of tens and the rest in fives, ones and some change from his pocket.

Eric motioned to David, who was still standing next to his office door looking like he was in a much better mood than he had been in fifteen minutes earlier.

"We'll have David keep the purse until after the contest is over."

No one thought of it as a hypnotic suggestion when Eric said, *"If you can beat 'pipsqueak' in an arm wrestle, then you get your money back plus my hundred bucks. When you lose to "Pipsqueak," then David gives me back my hundred dollars and uses your money for drinks on the house until it is used up–after you lose the contest.*

"Do you agree with this wager?"

"Yeah."

"Shall I call you Maggie or 'Pipsqueak'?" Eric asked Maggie.

"I want Pipsqueak because it makes me fighting mad when people call me that."

"Have you ever arm wrestled before?"

"Yes, I have . . . with my dad many times. I always win, but I think that he lets me."

"Do you think you can beat Brute, here, in an arm wrestle?"

"I don't know, but I think I can give him a good run for his money."

"If you were going to bet on the outcome, who would you bet on?"

Without hesitation, she said, "Brute."

"How much money do you have to bet on Brute?"

"Twenty bucks," said Pipsqueak, as she slid her hand into the back pocket of her jeans and handed a twenty-dollar bill to David.

Eric peeled off a twenty from his clip and handed it to David, too.

He asked her, *"Same deal?"*

Again as a suggestion he said, *"If Brute wins, you get my twenty. When you win . . . your twenty-dollar bill goes into the pot and pays for additional drinks on the house. Is that an acceptable wager?"*

"Yes."

"Will you still try hard to pin Brute's arm to the table and win the match, even though you'll lose the bet?"

"Yes, it would be worth twenty bucks just to say I whipped this guy for calling me 'Pipsqueak'!"

"Okay, take your positions, but first, before you clasp hands, Brute, you probably don't know that I had your last drink laced with a tonic that makes your right arm very weak, do you? It turns the muscles in your right arm to jelly. And did you know that I had Pipsqueak's last drink laced with a potion that will suck all of the strength out of your arm and put it into her arm the moment you grasp her hand? It makes her arm a hundred times stronger than ever before and yours a hundred times weaker, the moment you grasp each other's hand. You didn't know that, did you, Brute?"

Brute just sat there looking dumbfounded.

"I need some help from the audience," Eric said. "When I say get ready, get set, I want everyone in David's place to shout GO!

"Brute and Pipsqueak, clasp each other's hand now and when you hear everyone say 'GO,' with all of your might try to pin your opponent's hand to the table. It will be a good contest, but we all know the outcome because of the tonic and the potion I had put into your drinks.

"Get ready, get set . . ." David's place erupted with a resounding GO, and the contest began.

The scene was a comical sight all by itself. An enormous 'Brute' and an elf-sized 'pipsqueak' facing off on either side of a two-person bar table competing in arm wrestle—Pipsqueak's arm straight up and Brute's on a forty-five degree angle so both could have their elbows on the table.

The frustration on Brute's face was apparent as he felt his arm begin to move in the direction of being pinned—his teeth clenched tight and the veins on his neck bulged, but to no avail.... His arm just continued to sink closer to the table. The crowd cheered, most of them for Pipsqueak, who had a determined sneer of satisfaction on her face. The instant that Brute's hand hit the table, the patrons at David's burst into an uproar of cheering.

Eric snapped his fingers and shouted, "Everyone, WIDE AWAKE." The show was over.

Eric grabbed my elbow and pulled me close so I could hear him over the noise of the crowd and said, "I'll meet you out in my truck, but first I'm going to get my hundred and twenty bucks back from David."

CHAPTER 14

Stage-Show
Lesson One

Eric had an old truck that he used for his painting business—maybe ten years old—but everything was neatly stowed and kept spotless. I was waiting for him and after he crawled into the driver's side and pulled up the passenger side lock, I slid in.

"Well, that went fairly well," he said. "But it could have been a little more polished. Luckily we had a few breaks so it came off okay anyway."

"It seemed to me that it couldn't have been any better," I said, "but I do have a lot of questions to ask. And what do you mean 'lucky breaks'?"

Eric answered, "I knew you would have a few questions about the performance. That's why we are sitting out here in the cold talking.

"The lucky breaks started with the large number of people who volunteered. Sometimes it's difficult to find two or three people who are willing to volunteer. It's harder to orchestrate an entertaining show if you don't have a good number of people to pick and choose from. Another lucky break was when I was close enough to help you catch Bert before he hit the floor and broke something—he really was a "Brute," wasn't he?

"Most people don't give any consideration to the potential hazards involved in a good hypnosis stage-show. Occasionally a volunteer will sustain an injury when carrying out a suggestion or just by accident, and that can spoil the whole show. But if you are going to be a stage-show hypnotist it's a risk you are going to have to take...especially if you want the show to be exciting.

"I've had people fall off the stage, fall off chairs, get stepped on, tripped over, get kicked by another volunteer who overreacted, break an arm as they missed the bottom step when leaving the stage, and one time a fellow sustained a concussion when he went back to the audience and sat down on a chair that wasn't there.

"No one has ever brought legal action as a result of the injuries, but someone getting hurt—even if it's just an accident—can mess up an otherwise successful performance.

"When we get enough funds in PSI's account we should take out a liability policy. It will cover both of us if it's in the corporation's name and it's not all that expensive."

(Note: Remember, this was back in the 70's and liability insurance was *not* all that expensive, nor were people suing other people at the drop of a hat.)

"By the way, you did a very good job assisting me. Tomorrow night we'll do an ESP demonstration—you and me—to give the crowd a little something different to think about."

After recovering from what seemed to be a genuine compliment (the first I had heard him bestow on anyone) I protested. "What do you mean 'do an ESP demonstration'? I don't have any ESP powers."

"You're right. You don't and neither do I, but the people in the audience don't know that. We'll just make it look like we do." And then he said, "Well, fire away!"

"First, why were you so late getting here?" I asked. "David and I were at our wits' end until you came through the door at the very last minute."

"I wasn't late; I was right on time," he said with a glint in his eye—obviously knowing that would be one of my questions. "I was sitting out here in my truck getting mentally prepared for the show.

"Never be early for a show and never be late for a show and always walk on stage or into the nightclub right on queue. Did you ever see Frank Sinatra or Wayne Newton meandering around, setting things up or mingling with the crowd before or after a performance? I know that I am not all that punctual when it comes to other things in my life, but when it comes to stage-shows I am a professional. I'm never late, I'm never early; I'm always right on time."

"That makes a lot of sense. I'll always remember that lesson," I said. "It is obvious to me *now* why you asked David to place volunteers' chairs so close together—so you could lean people on one another and keep them from falling over when they got so relaxed. But why did you ask David to have a wet bar towel on stage? You didn't use it for anything."

"And it is a good thing I didn't have to use it," he said. "I always have a wet bar towel handy so I can use it to slap a subject on the face if one of them happens to go into a somnambulistic fit. Once you have had that happen you become very sensitive to the possibility of it happening again. If it ever happens to you—it probably never will, but you need to be prepared if it does—use a wet bar towel to inflict pain by slapping the subject on the face until they open their eyes and start breathing again. It looks much more professional to be slapping someone with a wet bar towel than just slapping them with your hand. I think that is what made the difference between my uncle getting sued and me not—by using a towel, it was apparent that I knew it could happen and that I had made preparations just in case it did."

"Well, that makes good sense and I'll remember that too," I said. "But why did you send that first guy off the stage when he couldn't get his hands apart? He appeared to be a very good subject."

"He wasn't a good subject; he was a phony," Eric said in an angry tone. "I suggested to the volunteers that they could take their hands apart only upon my touch and that when they did their gaze would be only on me. Each of the other subjects opened their eyes first (to see if it was indeed me who was tugging on their hands) and the instant they saw it was me their hands fell apart with no resistance and they continued to look at me.

"Freddie, on the other hand, did neither. He didn't open his eyes to see if it was me touching his hands, nor did he look at me when he did; instead, he looked out into the audience, probably at his cronies, and had that silly smirk on his face. This is a good way to weed out the pretenders. A subject just faking a routine can mess up a show as much as someone getting hurt.

"There will always be people who will try to sabotage your stage-shows just to prove a point. I don't know why they do it, they just do, and you'd better be prepared for when they do it to you."

"That rigid arm routine didn't seem to get much of a reaction from the audience and it appeared to me that you didn't expect it to. So why did you do it?" I asked.

"That was a test as much as the falling backwards and hand clasp suggestions were tests. I was not testing to discover if they were hypnotized—I already knew they were. I was testing to see how well they could follow and carry out my suggestions while hypnotized. I was also deepening the hypnotic trance. You probably noticed that after each of those first routines, I gave the additional suggestion that when they had completed the task they would go deeper into hypnosis.

"Something else to remember: just because a person doesn't make a good hypnotic subject on stage doesn't mean that they wouldn't make an excellent subject for clinical hypnosis. Being up on stage in front of a bunch of people doing silly things while hypnotized is quite a different ballgame than being in the privacy of a clinical setting for the purpose of changing one's behavior."

He continued, "With the stiff arm suggestion, if any one of them would have bent their arm so much as a fraction I'd have sent them down to be part of the audience—as I would have had their arms not *floated* down into their lap. If a subject does not have the ability to comprehend, understand and respond to those first few simple suggestions, they will never be able to carry out the more complex ones.

"For example, I gave George several suggestions at the same time: I suggested that the people would have no clothes on and that he would make snide remarks about what he would see when he looked through the magical glasses. And then I suggested that when he looked more closely they'd be wearing people clothes but have animal heads and he would make comments about their appearance. Those were relatively simple multiple suggestions, but at times you may want to string as many as seven or eight suggestions together. With a little experience you will be able to determine which subjects have the ability to keep them straight.

"Another thing, if you want the show to be entertaining, you *don't* want a routine to over-run the audience's interest, nor do you want a subject to out-run their ability to keep focused. Patty was a side-show as she busily kept the little people in the cigar box—she was the perfect subject for that because she didn't get tired of chasing the little people around the stage nor did the audience get tired of watching her doing it.

"With experience, you will also learn when the routine has run its course, like with George. That routine might have played out better had I chosen a different volunteer, because George soon lost interest in following my suggestions and started to analyze. The moment he said, 'I'm anxious about this,' I immediately woke him up and sent him down to the audience because his usefulness had run its course. If I would have let him carry on feeling anxious he could have blown the whole show. So I sent him down to buy an extra drink and put a few extra bucks in David's till.

"By the way, did you notice how packed the place was, and especially for a Thursday? David did a good job of promoting us."

I agreed. "Yes, I did notice and so did he." But I had more questions for Eric. "How did you remember everyone's name? That was impressive all by itself. I couldn't keep everyone's names straight, and I wasn't doing anything but watching."

"Practice," he said. "After having given the same suggestions over and over again as many times as *I* have, saying the words of the suggestion become habitual and I don't have to even think about what I am saying. That gives me plenty of time to make an association with something about the subject and their name. Once the association has been established the name is easy to recall.

"For example: Freddie looked like the person who played the fiddler in *Fiddler on the Roof*. I know this is a stretch of one's imagination, but *Freddie* is close enough to *fiddler* for me to make a snap association. It is essential to know the name of each volunteer so you can address a suggestion directly to that particular subject. If I had not called Freddie by name when I clapped my hands and commanded him to wake up, the other subjects would have thought I was telling them to wake up.

"Also, now that suggestions become habitual, it gives me plenty of time to plan ahead and decide which subject will fit into upcoming routines. It also gives me time to improvise if the opportunity arises."

"Why didn't you use *all* of the volunteers and why did you decide to use 'Brute' and 'Pipsqueak' for the arm wrestling routine?" I asked.

"I sent the other people down from the stage because I didn't need them, and because they weren't buying drinks while they were sitting on stage. Remember this: The reason a nightclub owner hires you is to make more money by selling more drinks. While those people were sitting on stage they were not making David—or us—any money. We are not doing stage-shows just to have fun, but to earn money *while* we are having fun—you can't beat that for a profession, can you?

"But the main reason I sent the other volunteers off the stage was that I knew the time was getting short—we agreed with David that each show would be about forty-five minutes—and I had a pretty good idea how long the arm wrestling would take. It is as important to stop a show on time as it is to start it on time.

"And as for the arm wrestling.... I decided to exploit 'Brute' and 'Pipsqueak' for that routine while doing the rigid arm test—he was so burly and she was so fragile-looking—the contrast was perfect."

"How did you know that 'Brute' would want to bet? Does that always happen?" I asked.

Eric answered, "That is the first time I have ever used the betting part of that routine, and it just came to me when Bert said, 'I'll bet anyone could beat that little pipsqueak in an arm wrestle, even my grandmother.'

"I don't think that *you* ought to try anything like that yet... until *you* get as good as *I* am. You could have easily lost 120 bucks. I'm the only stage-show hypnotist in the world who could have pulled it off so smoothly."

Until this point the conversation had been tutorial and he had treated me as an intelligent equal. For forty-five minutes I had been enlightened by a skilled professional and the conversation had been rewarding and enjoyable, rather than being lectured to by someone trying to convince me that he was the greatest thing that had ever happened in the history of mankind. But once he got started bragging it seemed that he couldn't stop:

"No other hypnotist in the world would have thought of that on the fly. And even if they would have they wouldn't have been able to incorporate it into the routine as well as I did; nor could anyone else have explained the conditions of the wager as well as I did. I'll bet that David was really impressed by me putting an extra $120 into his till.... I am a genius!"

And on he went. "No one else was, is or will ever be as good, or as great, a hypnotist as I am."

He reminded me of Cassius Clay before he became Muhammad Ali—"I am the greatest! I am the greatest!"

Eric continued his boasting for another twenty minutes and then finally said, "We need to get prepared for the next show. Go in and get everything ready for the best stage-show hypnotist in the world. I hope you remember how you are going to introduce me for this second show.... And, if you think that first performance was good, just wait until you see this one. I'm going to knock their socks off!"

CHAPTER 15

The Second Performance

When I walked back into *David's*, David motioned me over and asked, "Where have you guys been? That was a fantastic performance! All kinds of people have been looking for you or Eric. Most of them probably just want to talk about hypnosis but one gal wants to make an appointment to lose some weight.

"Eric is a real entertainer. I think you guys might cover your part of the advertising in a single weekend. I have never had that kind of sales volume in that short of a time, especially on a Thursday. Of course, those extra hundred and twenty bucks didn't hurt. It was particularly good for my help; some of the people who got free drinks triple tipped the bartenders and cocktail waitresses. And happy employees make for better sales. What do you have planned for this second show?"

"I have no idea whatsoever. I am as curious as you are but I'm sure Eric will have something spectacular," I said before going up to the stage to announce the second show.

With a great deal more conviction than earlier, I articulated: "La—dies and Gentle—men, it is my pleasure once again to introduce the world's greatest hypnotist.... *the renowned* DR. ERIC! Having just finished his spellbinding sell-out premiere performance here at *David's*, the most popular nightclub in the Salt Lake Valley, and booked exclusively at *David's* for the next four weeks, Dr. Eric will again take you into another adventure into the realm of the subconscious mind. And now . . . heeeeere's DR. ERIC!"

It appeared that not a person had left *David's*. Not only was every seat occupied, but people were standing around the walls with drink in hand. It was probably a good thing that the local fire marshal was not among them—the place was packed.

When Eric charged out of the foyer and jumped up on the stage he was greeted with resounding applause. He grabbed the microphone and said,

"Ladies and gentlemen, I am *Dr. Eric,* the world's greatest hypnotist, and I am here to entertain you with another spellbinding adventure into the subconscious mind. In a moment I will be asking for volunteers to come up to the stage to experience the powers of your subconscious mind. I promise that I will do nothing that will embarrass or harm you in any way... unless it is financial pain and embarrassment for making a foolish bet on what seemed to be a sure thing."

He looked out into the audience, found "Brute," nodded to him, and said, "Brute, did anyone thank you for those free drinks?"

The place burst out in a chorus of "Thank you, Brute! Thank you, Brute!" amid peals of laughter.

Brute stood up and motioned with his arms for everyone to quiet down so they could hear what he had to say. "If I had another hundred bucks with me I'd challenge Pipsqueak to another try, but this time without the laced drinks.... Or maybe I should just hire her to work on my construction crew—I'll bet that she could out-lift the lot of them!"

"How much are you willing to bet on *that?*" Eric retorted, and the place again exploded in laughter. He was a master at getting audiences to participate in his shows and at knitting an assortment of groups and individuals into a single coherent body.

The thing that struck me most about the exchange between Eric and Brute was that Brute seemed to be convinced that it was the stuff in his drink that had made his arm weak, not the hypnotic suggestion. *Here's something else to ponder when I get a chance,* I thought.

"I am now calling for volunteers to come up to the stage with the intention of being hypnotized and to experience an exciting adventure into your subconscious mind."

This time there were *far* too many volunteers and Eric said into the mic, "I can use only the fifteen volunteers who are closest to the stage. We will be back tomorrow and Saturday nights, so if I don't select you tonight, come back and volunteer then.... And bring a few friends and buy lots of drinks!"

Eric went through his selection process and obtained the name of each participant, and I did my "catch them if they fall" thing. When each of the ten chairs had someone sitting on it, and Eric had recited his hypnosis induction and testing suggestions, he walked over to a well-dressed, professional-looking woman, touched her head and said, *"Rose, you look like a very intelligent woman. What kind of work do you do?"*

"I'm here from out of town and I am in advertising," she explained.

"Are you here by yourself or do you have an escort?"

"I am here with a date."

"Is he the jealous type?"

"I don't know. This is our first date, and a blind one at that."

"Well, in that case I had better have you return to your seat so you can become better-acquainted with him."

He suggested, *"When I snap my fingers, return to your seat and enjoy a drink. It's a special drink... one that has been mixed with a magical love potion. Upon drinking the potion, if your date is receptive to your advances, you will be so enamored with him that nothing else matters. You will gently brush back his hair, gaze lovingly into his eyes, whisper sweet nothings into his ear and gently kiss his face... but nothing beyond that. If he is not receptive, then look around until you find someone who is.*

"The effects of the love potion last for only five minutes, however, so you need to make every moment count. After five minutes have passed you will snap out of your enchanted state, wondering why you are being so friendly with a blind date. Your degree of interest in the gentleman will return back to the very level of friendliness you had before coming up on stage."

Eric snapped his fingers and said, *"Rose, you can return to your seat now and take pleasure in being with your date. And enjoy the effects of your drink!"*

Rose, stood up, looked over the audience and gave a little wave of her hand to a professional-looking gentleman sitting next to an empty chair.

Eric placed his touch on another subject, who looked like she was too young to be in a bar, and said to her, *"Judy, open your eyes and look at me."* Judy opened her eyes and then Eric asked, *"Does your mother know you're out? And how old are you, anyway?"*

"I just turned twenty-one, and my mother doesn't know I am out because she died," she replied, then burst into tears and began sobbing.

Eric calmly placed his hand on her shoulder and said, *"I'm sorry to hear that your mom has passed away. My mom is dead, too, so I can understand the sorrow you are feeling."*

The sobbing became a whimper and Eric continued, *"Just close your eyes again; everything is fine."* Eric waited for a moment and then said, *"I am going to count up from one to five, when I say 'five,' open your eyes and you will be wide awake and feeling fine. You will return to your seat and enjoy the rest of the evening being with your friends. After the show we can visit and we'll see if I can help you with your sorrow."*

"One, two, three, four and five, open your eyes Judy, and wide awake feeling fine."

Just as Judy was stepping off of the stage, there was a commotion coming from the vicinity of Rose's table. Rose was sensually leaning toward her date, gently stroking his hair back with her fingers and gazing into his eyes.

She and her date were obviously the center of interest and he seemed to be enjoying the attention he was getting from her, although he had a little extra color in his cheeks as he giggled when Rose put her mouth up to his ear and began to whisper.

Almost every eye in *David's* was turned toward the loving couple and amid the chuckles came many "oohs and aahs" when she began gently kissing his face.

All of a sudden she drew back, looked at her date and said, "Gee, what am I doing?! I don't do things like that on the *first date*. Did I do anything that embarrassed you?"

"No, not at all," said her date. "I just wish he would have told you that the potion lasted for a lifetime!"

(By the way, they got along very well for the rest of the evening, and maybe even beyond that.)

Back on stage, Eric asked a scholastic-looking girl to open her eyes, stand up and look into his eyes. *"Angela,"* he said, *"you look like a very intelligent young woman. What kind of work do you do?"*

I thought to myself, *That is the same question he asked Rose. I wonder if he had just improvised when Rose said she was out of town and here on a blind date. I'll have to ask him if that was the case.*

"Well, I don't work. I'm a graduate accounting student at the U of U," she answered.

"Then you are probably good with numbers. Is that correct?"

"Yes."

"Are you good with spelling?"

"Yes, Business English is my minor."

"What is your grade point average?"

"I have straight A's."

"So you have a pretty good memory, too. Is that right?"

"Yes."

"Then you are just what the doctor ordered," Eric said.

"In a moment when I snap my fingers you will no longer be able to remember or say your last name, nor will you be able to add, subtract or spell correctly."

He snapped his fingers and asked, *"What is your full name, Angela?"*

"My name is Angela Ann.... uhhh.... My last name is.... Mmmmm. Gee, I remembered it just a minute ago."

"How much is two plus three, Angela?"

"Two plus three is ... i-i-i-s... four?"

Mingled with the laughter coming from the audience I could hear a few shouts of, "Five."

"*Angela, if I had three apples and took two of them away, how many would I have left?*"

The crowd tried to coach her again but she seemed oblivious to everything except what Eric was saying.

"... Twooo?"

"*And attempt to spell cat.*"

"K... a... t, I think."

"*When I snap my fingers, Angela, you will be able to remember your whole name and be able to add, subtract and spell better than you ever have, and you will be wide awake feeling wonderfully well but wondering what has been going on.*"

Eric snapped his fingers. Angela gave a little jump and Eric asked, "What is your full name?"

"Angela Ann Johnson."

"What is two plus three?"

"Five."

"If I had three apples and took two of them away, how many would I have left?"

"One."

"And spell cat for me."

"C–a–t."

"You did very well and I thank you for such a fine job. You can go down to your seat now... and have your friends *buy you a few extra drinks. I think you probably got behind while you were up here demonstrating your skills in higher math, spelling and memory.*"

As I watched Angela return to her seat, I noticed a young heavy-set blond, with her head on the table and her hands loosely dangling toward the floor, in what looked like a deep sleep. I thought, *She looks like she has just had too much to drink but I had better go down and check her out anyway.*

When I got to her table I asked her companions, "Is she okay? Or has she just had too much to drink?"

The gal sitting next to her said, "I *think* she's okay. She hasn't had a single alcoholic drink the whole night, but she's been awake since early this morning, so I think she just got tired and fell asleep while sitting there. She was fine until the last show started, but then she just leaned over, laid her head down on the table and went to sleep.... Do *you* think she's okay?"

"I am sure she is but she may have just become hypnotized without knowing it. What is her name?"

"Jeanie."

I leaned down to Jeanie and said in her ear, "*Jeanie, when I clap my hands just open your eyes and you will be wide awake feeling refreshed, just like you have had a nice, long nap.*"

I clapped my hands and said, "*WIDE AWAKE!*" Jeanie's eyes popped open; she sat up in her chair and said, "I wasn't asleep. I've heard everything that has been going on. I just felt like laying my head down on the table. I guess I must have been resting, though, because I feel really refreshed, but I wasn't asleep."

I told her to enjoy the rest of the show and returned to the stage. Eric was standing in front of Mike, a slender, wiry fellow of medium height, who was standing as rigid as a board, arms pressed tightly against the sides of his body. I knew what Eric was up to because this was the only routine we had practiced during my training sessions, except for the falling backwards test.

Eric motioned to me and I snatched a couple of chairs, set them up about five feet apart and stationed myself behind Mike. Eric gave him a gentle push with a single finger and Mike's rigid body fell into my arms. I took him by his neck as Eric picked him up by the feet and set his rigid body between the back of each of the chairs—the back of his neck on one chair and his heels on the other, stiff as a board.

Eric let him balance there for ten seconds and then placed another chair right under Mike and sat on it so when Mike relaxed he would fall right into his lap.

"*Mike, the next time I say 'relax now' all of the muscles in your body will relax and you will comfortably fall right on my lap and be wide awake. When you open your eyes you will be surprised to find yourself sitting on the lap of a strange man. You will jump up and return to your chair in the audience, wondering why you have been sitting in the lap of a total stranger.... When you get back to your table you'll probably need a drink or two while you try to sort it all out.*"

Eric waited for a moment or two longer, positioned himself under Mike, and then sharply said, "*Mike, RELAX NOW!*" Mike's body went limp and fell right onto Eric's lap; he opened his eyes, looked at Eric indignantly, jumped off of his lap and walked off of the stage shaking his head in disgust.

Eric touched his hand to the head of a rather plain-looking young woman (not unattractive physically, but her hair style was old-fashioned and her figure was hidden under a dowdy dress) and said, "*Sara, open your eyes and look at me.*

"*When I snap my fingers you will feel and act like a high-fashion model. You will stroll up and down the stage as though you are on a runway at a fashion show. You will enjoy showing off the latest style in high-society fashion clothes with grace, confidence and poise...and you will charm the audience with your radiant smile.*"

SNAP! Sara straightened up her posture, looked out over the audience, put on a smile and gracefully, with swinging hips, strolled back and forth on the stage as though it were a runway. The transformation was astounding. Her smile, graceful manner and confident charm caused her wardrobe and her hairstyle to go unnoticed. There were whistles, cheers and applause from the audience (no jeers, just genuine recognition of the transformation that they had just witnessed).

Eric let her glory in her fame for a few minutes and then said, *"Sara, when I snap my fingers you will be wide awake feeling wonderfully well, and will return to your chair and continue to feel as good about yourself as you do right now. And this feeling will continue on with you as you go on with your life."*

Eric snapped his fingers and Sara gracefully descended the stairs, modestly showing off her natural poise and enchanting smile.

Eric touched the heads of three of the remaining volunteers, called them by name in succession and said, *"Alan, Victoria and Beth, when I snap my fingers you will return to your chairs, but when you sit down you will immediately jump up and impersonate a vendor who is selling 'plaid fish.' You will act like you have a strap around your neck that is attached to a tray on which you are carrying your wares and shout, 'Plaid fish for sale, anyone for some nice, fresh, plaid fish?' You will continue until I clap my hands and say, 'Wide awake.' When I do, the tray and the plaid fish will be gone and you will return to your chair, order a drink and wonder why you have been trying to sell plaid fish."*

Eric touched the heads of Mike and Nina and said, *"When I snap my fingers you will open your eyes and return to your chair and order a drink. But while you are waiting for it you will notice a dribble of water coming out of one of the far walls. Your attention will be focused on the leak and as you look it becomes a trickle and then it becomes a little squirt. You will jump up and go over to the spot and realize that the wall is a dike and you are the little Dutch Boy and you must do something to keep the dike from breaking. You start by trying to stop the leak with your finger but the hole just gets bigger, so you use your hand but it still gets bigger. You begin asking people for towels or buckets or anything else you can think of that would keep the dike from breaking, and warning the people here in David's of the impending disaster that they will experience if they don't do something to help. You will continue until I clap my hands and say, 'Wide awake.' When I do, the water will disappear and you will go back to your table and enjoy the drink that you just ordered.*

"And Peter, when I snap my fingers you will open your eyes and return to your chair but when you sit on it, it will feel very hot; you will jump up, rub your hind side and express the discomfort you have just experienced. You will look around for another chair or stool. You will test it with your hand and it will feel cool to your touch but

when you sit on it, it will feel very hot and you will jump up and continue looking for a cool seat to sit on. But when I clap my hands and say, 'Wide awake,' you will be able to comfortably sit on any chair in the house."

Eric snapped his fingers. The volunteers opened their eyes, stood up, walked off of the stage and returned to their chairs.

Almost at once, there were three people out in the audience shouting, "Plaid fish for sale, plaid fish for sale! Anyone for some nice, fresh, plaid fish?" At the same time, two more people were shouting for towels, mops, buckets, sandbags and bulldozers, while warning people around them that the dike was about to burst and they were in imminent danger of being washed out *David's* door. And Peter was running around *David's* rubbing his hind side and cursing that he couldn't find a seat in the whole place that didn't burn his butt when he sat on it.

For a few minutes it seemed that the whole place was in a state of pandemonium until Eric clapped his hands together and shouted, *"Everyone, WIDE AWAKE!"*

The place went silent for a moment or two, and then burst into applause, cheers and whistles as Eric left the stage. He stopped at Judy's table, said a few words, gave her one of his calling cards and slipped out the door.

As I was trying to do the same, Jeanie caught my arm and said, "Do you help people lose weight? I need to lose at least eighty-five pounds but I just can't stick to a diet. Can you help me?"

I gave her one of my just-off-of-the-printing-press "Stage-Show Hypnotist" calling cards and told her that *I* had lost seventy-five pounds myself with hypnosis and that I was sure that she could, too. "Give me a call tomorrow and we can talk about it," I said, before sneaking out the door.

When I got out to the parking lot neither Eric nor his truck were anywhere to be found, so I figured I'd just have to wait until the next day to get my next batch of questions answered. *He did say that tomorrow he was going to teach me how to create the illusion of having some kind of psychic powers, didn't he?* I thought to myself.

Little did I know that there was another surprise anomaly I'd be exposed to. Maybe not for the metaphysical oriented person but for my rational, analytical, reasoning, logical, right-brained, scientific oriented mind, it seemed even more bizarre than feigning psychic powers.... Past life regression!

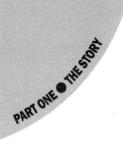
Lesson Two

The next day I arrived at my office at twelve o'clock sharp. Eric immediately said, "Where have you been? I've been waiting for you."

I replied, "Our meeting time is twelve noon and I'm a professional when it comes to keeping my appointments. A great teacher once enlightened me, 'Always on time... never early or late!'"

After a brief smile he said, "We've got a lot of work to do before tonight's performance. So let's get started."

And with no more explanation, he said, "Get out your note pad and write this down:

"The number 'one' is represented by the letter 'o'—as in 'once, oh or over'— because the word 'one' starts with the letter 'o.' First, I'll ask you, 'Are you ready?' and you'll respond, 'Yes.' Now when the first word of the next sentence I speak begins with the letter 'o,' you will respond back, 'One.'

"So if I say, 'Are you ready?' and you answer, 'Yes' and then I say, 'Oh, you should have no problem with this number,' you will know that you are to say back to me, 'One.'

"We'll each have our own microphone. I'll be out in the audience and you'll be up on stage and I'll announce to the crowd, 'We will now demonstrate the physic and telepathic powers of the subconscious mind. My associate Lindsay Brady and I have established a mental link and we will demonstrate it now.'

"I'll ask someone for a dollar bill and then gather a few people around me so they can see the serial number on the bill to confirm that you respond with the correct number. We'll take each number one by one. Do you get it?"

"I think so," I said.

"Okay, write down the rest of the code letters and the number each represents."

I picked up my pad and wrote:

> One is "o" because the word "one" starts with the letter "o"
> Two is "t" because it starts with "t"

Three is "e" because it has two of them and "t" is already used
Four is "f" because it starts with "f"
Five is "v" because it has a "v" in it and "f" is already used
Six is "i" because "s" is seven and few words start with "x"
Seven is "s" because it starts with "s"
Eight is "g" because it looks like an "8"
Nine is "n" because it starts with "n"
Zero is "r" because very few words start with "z" and the other
letters have already been used

After going over the list for ten minutes, I said, "Okay, try me out."
Eric took a bill from his clip and said, "Are you ready?"
"Yes," I said.
"Good, this is an easy number to start with."
I said, "Eight."
"Are you ready?"
"Yes."
"Now this number has magical powers. Have you received it yet?"
"Nine," I said.
"Are you ready?"....

We continued to finish that bill's serial number, and practiced on five more.

"Well, you caught on very quickly to that, but now we need to add another wrinkle. Someone will probably challenge us by saying, 'What about the letters in the serial numbers?' When I say, 'So you want the letters, too?' it will signal you that the rest of the serial number will be letters. At that point, I will probably get into a conversation with the audience to give me some time to think of a word that will represent the letter. When I've done that, you'll hear me say, 'Are you ready?' and you'll reply, 'Yes.' Then when you hear me say, 'Okay,' the first letter of the *second* word I speak after 'okay' will be the letter to repeat. Most often the first word after I say 'okay' will be 'now,' and then the first letter of the next word will be the key word. Is that clear?"

"I think so," I answered.

"Almost always, one of the on-lookers will ask about the letters in the serial number (thinking that they can trip us up) and that is good. If *they* bring it up then it gives the routine more credibility and makes it look like we really do have telepathic powers; but even if no one asks about the letters I'll make it *sound* like someone in the group did. Either way, when you hear me say, 'So you want the letters, too?' you will know that the rest of the serial number will be letters.

"For example, if I say, 'Okay. Now do you think you can get this one?' you will respond, 'D.' Or if I say, 'Okay, what then is this letter?' you will respond, 'T.'"

After we practiced the letters a dozen times, Eric continued. "We need to make it look like there is really something telepathic going on between us so take your time before answering—you can even put your fingers to your forehead as if in deep concentration, and I will do the same before giving you your clue. I will even get the onlookers to think of the number or letter and then have them confirm it's right by exclaiming, 'YES!'"

It was surprising how easy it was to make the association between the first letter of the first word and the number it represented, as well as catching on to the letter of the second word that represented the letter.

Eric seemed pleased when we had finished and said, "That didn't take nearly as long as I thought it would. Now let's talk about last night's performance."

He took a small note pad out of his shirt pocket. As he leafed through it, he said, "First of all, you did a good job assisting me and waking up that gal in the audience, but ALWAYS let me know when you leave the stage. Mike was standing there like a statue for two or three minutes while I was waiting for you to get back, so I had to do a dog and pony act to keep the audience's attention until you returned to the stage.

"Whenever you do the rigid body demonstration, don't let the person stay in that state for more than four or five minutes; it may cause muscle damage, and the subject's muscles are almost always sore the next day. And before giving a person a suggestion of that kind, always ask the subject if they have, or have ever had, back problems. If they have, never use them for that demonstration... and always choose a subject that is thin and wiry—it never works with a fat person.

"Always look like you are having fun while doing stage shows. And the show goes a lot better if you interact and joke with the audience... like I did with Brute. When he voluntarily responded with some humor, I knew I had the audience in my hands.

"If you are going to use only one person for a routine, ask them a few questions to determine which of your routines would best fit that person. I had intended to use Rose for the 'you can't remember your name, add, subtract or spell' routine because she looked smart and educated, but when she said she was there on a blind date I switched gears and used the love potion suggestion instead. Usually I use the love potion routine with two people who are on stage, but I spontaneously used it for an entirely different circumstance.... That's why I am the greatest stage hypnotist in the world—because I can think on my feet and improvise!

"Once in a while I do make a mistake. I really misread Judy. If she would have been under 21, which is the drinking age limit in Utah, as you know, I would have sent her off of the stage. I figured that if she was over 21, asking 'Does your mother know you're out?' would have some humor to it because she looked like she was in her early teens. But as it turned out it was the wrong question to ask and it triggered that emotional outburst. But did you notice how I handled it? That kind of calmness when handling unexpected responses only comes from many years of experience, like I have had."

I had a few questions of my own for Eric. "It appeared that Brute thought that you really *had* laced his drink and that is why his right arm turned to mush. How long after a person has been hypnotized does the idea of a suggestion last? Will Brute spend the rest of his life thinking that there is a magical brew out there that will turn only one's right arm to mush?"

"Yes he will; that is, until I (the hypnotist that gave the initial suggestion) undo the suggestion by telling him to forget about it, or until someone else convinces him through pure reason and logic that he was just tricked into *thinking* such a potion exists," Eric said.

Because of my innate curiosity about the process of hypnosis and how it works I wondered, *What he just said, or maybe how he said it, doesn't seem to quite fit the stereotype of a hypnotist. If someone using logic and reason can undo a suggestion, isn't that person as much of a hypnotist as the hypnotist?*

I was shocked back into the topic at hand—stage-show hypnosis, not how hypnosis works—when Eric went on, "It is good showmanship when doing stage shows to make it as mysterious as you can and to create the impression that there is a subconscious mind—a second mind—that operates below the level of our conscious awareness. People really like that kind of stuff. Many of the spectators at the show last night thought that *I* had a mystical power and that *I* could make anyone do anything I chose just by talking to their subconscious mind. I do have an unusual talent to convince people to do what I ask them or tell them to do, but it is not a mystical power—it just *seems* that way because I'm so good at it.

"You want to give hypnosis the appearance of being mystical and make it look like the volunteer's conscious mind was oblivious to what was being said and to what he or she did while hypnotized. To do that, when you bring a person out of hypnosis suggest to them that they will wake up 'wondering what has been going on' or that they'll 'remember nothing that has happened.' It's like Angela not remembering her last name. If you don't give that kind of a suggestion, almost every subject, when they return to their chair, will say 'I wasn't hypnotized because I heard everything that the hypnotist said and I remember everything I did. I just went along with the suggestions so it wouldn't embarrass the hypnotist.'

"On the other hand, if the suggestion *is* given that the subject won't remember what happened, when the subject returns to their seat most of them (not all, however) will have no recollection of the suggestions or remember what they did while on stage. Even when their friends tell them what they did, they still won't remember and will think that their friends are just making it up. People really like mysterious and mystical things.

"Did you notice how surprised Mike was when he found himself sitting on my lap and how Rose asked her date if she did anything that embarrassed him? Neither of them remembered what they had been doing after they woke up. That's what makes hypnosis mysterious and that's what will pack the house every night for the next four weeks."

I said, "Jeanie, the gal in the audience that I woke up, said she would call for an appointment to lose weight. The self-hypnotic suggestions that I gave to myself when I lost seventy-five pounds worked well for me, but the effectiveness for my clients seems to drop off for weight loss as compared to getting people to stop smoking or to get over fears and anxiety. What kind of suggestions should I give to her if she comes in for a session?"

I was shocked to the core when Eric retorted, "You won't be giving Jeanie any suggestions. Jeanie is my client, not yours. Any clients that are generated at *my* stage shows are *my* clients. It is *me* that produced them so it will be *me* that will hypnotize them and it will be *me* that will earn the money for doing it. Is that clear?"

Instantly my dander was up and I said, "Yes, what you said is clear, but not acceptable if you are thinking about putting money from private sessions generated from stage-shows into your own pocket. We agreed that we are partners in accumulating money to advertise for a mega stage-show.

"When I agreed to participate in creating *Positive Suggestion Institute* and when I opened the PSI checking account yesterday—incidentally, with *my* hundred dollars—we agreed that all of the proceeds generated from stage-shows would be deposited into the account and we would let it accumulate until there was enough to advertise for your 'mega event,' except for direct expenses related to PSI business. Apparently, I wrongly assumed that meant any money we earned from private sessions that were generated from the stage shows, as well. Was not that our agreement?"

Not giving him a moment to respond, I continued. "You may have an unusual talent to manipulate people into doing what you ask them to do or what you tell them to do, but it doesn't work on me. You are dealing with a master of trickery and I can spot a fraud a mile away. And besides that, *I* have an excellent memory and expect that any agreement we make, whether verbal or written, is adhered to. Do I make *myself* clear?"

"Well, you don't have to get in a huff about it," Eric said quickly. "I thought that you were going to pocket the money yourself. Well then, let's teach you what to say when hypnotizing people to lose weight."

And the rowel was instantly defused.

He knew that what I said was exactly what we had agreed on and knew I wouldn't back down when confronted with deceptive conduct. I was amazed, however, how quickly he could switch his position and disposition when met head-on with the truth. He seemed to be genuine, but still I wondered, *Is he just feigning agreement? I wonder if he would have pocketed the money from private sessions if I had said nothing. I can see that he's a master stage-show performer, but I think I had better keep my guard up regarding personal and business matters.*

"The right way to make people lose weight is to make fattening foods smell and taste awful and make healthy foods smell and taste delicious. I'll demonstrate at tonight's show how easily that can be done—make things that smell bad smell good and make things that taste bad taste good," he said.

"The same thing goes for smoking and chewing tobacco. If you can make tobacco taste terrible and make the smell of tobacco smoke even worse, then people don't want to smoke because they don't like things that taste and smell terrible. Give them the suggestion that even the thought of smoking makes them feel sick so they don't want to even pick one up because they are afraid they will get sick.

"Another thing I have noticed," he said as he looked at his notepad. "You spend a great deal of time wondering why and how hypnosis works instead of just accepting the fact that it does. If you are analytical about it instead of just doing it, you will never become a great stage-show hypnotist.

"If you are going to be analytical you should enroll at a university and take some courses in behavioral psychology instead of trying to be a stage-show hypnotist. You can be analytical and be a good clinical hypnotist, because that is what it is all about—analyzing the client's problem and figuring out a way to get them to change—but there is no need to be analytical when doing stage-shows. Stage-show hypnosis is entertainment, not therapy or research—you've got to be an entertainer first and then use hypnosis to entertain."

I've always been analytical, but I wasn't so sure that a person couldn't have curiosity about how hypnosis works and be an entertainer, too—or at least learn how to be an entertainer once what makes it work was figured out.

The more I thought about it, though, the more I realized that what Eric had said had some legitimacy—it wasn't until I learned to sell the benefits of my products (and the benefits the customer would enjoy as the result of buying the products from me), that I excelled in sales. When I first started selling air nailing guns, I spent days trying to figure out how the piston inside the nail gun got back up to its firing position after it had driven a nail, instead of figuring out how to sell the benefits that my prospective customers would enjoy by investing in a nail gun and buying it from me. I *did* figure out the piston problem, but I didn't make any sales while doing so.

"And another thing," Eric said. "Before you make unhealthy food and cigarettes taste terrible (or deal with any other issue, for that matter) you must first regress your subject back to the event that produced their bad behavior or habits. The only reason people have bad habits and engage in self-destructive behavior is because their subconscious mind is responding to some adversity that happened in the past and is affecting their behavior now. So you must regress them back and dig up the experiences, examine them, and then have the client re-experience the emotions associated with the event, no matter how painful the experience; they need to vent all of those emotions before any permanent change can occur.

"Some of the sensitizing experiences may have happened very recently, like a recent divorce or the death of a loved one, but most likely the incident occurred many years earlier and often in a past life."

"What do you mean 'in a past life?'" I retorted. "Do you *really* believe we lived past lives and that they are influencing how we behave now? Do you expect me to believe that some event that occurred before I was born is determining how I act? To me, having lived past lives is mythical fantasy. The next thing you are going to tell me is that Zeus and Diana were *real* gods and that the position of the planets determines my future!"

"No, Zeus and Diana were not real gods and astrology is questionable at best, but we did live past lives. I have hypnotized hundreds of people who regressed and remembered experiences from other lives—multiple lives. As a matter of fact, everyone I hypnotize for clinical reasons I regress to past events— and quite often back to a past life so they can resolve their problems in this one. If you are going to get outstanding results from your clinical hypnosis, you are going to have to become very good at taking people back to the event that is causing them to engage in self-destructive behavior—whether it happened in this life or some other life."

"Well then, teach me how to do it if it is so important," I said.

"It's easy," said Eric. "After they are hypnotized just ask them to go back to an event that is causing them to feel and act like they *don't* want to feel and act— ask them to go back to the experience that is causing their unwanted behavior, whether it happened in this life or some past life."

"So what do I do if I tell them to go back to a past life experience and they open their eyes and laugh at me... or just sit there and say nothing? It has been my experience that when asking a hypnotized person questions, it takes forever for them to answer, if at all. Why do you think that happens?" I asked.

"There you go again, trying to figure it out instead of just doing it," he scolded. "True, if a person is in a deep hypnotic state it takes a long time for them to answer and often you get no answer at all, so you need to give them some help by answering for them. When you get as good at regressing people as I am you will learn to rely on your sixth sense—you will already know the answer before you ask the question—so you answer for them."

"Are you telling me that I'm supposed to rely on a sixth sense to discover what is going on in someone else's mind so they can resolve *their* problems, even if they aren't able to articulate what caused it? Now that sounds like *real* telepathy! That is as illogical as past life regression itself," I said.

"There you go again with your logic and trying to make things reasonable. It doesn't have to make sense if it works!" he reproached.

"Let me give you an example," he said. "Let's say a person comes in to you to lose weight. Ask them to go back to the experience that is causing them to eat so much. You already know that they are overweight because they overeat. They overeat *not* because they are hungry, but because they are emotional eaters; something is making them feel anxious, angry, worried or unhappy. Sometimes they even overeat because they are happy. Overeating is emotion-based, not hunger-based. The emotions that cause them to overeat are rooted in something that happened in the past; whether it happened this morning, yesterday, last year, when they were twelve years old or in a past life. So when you ask them why they overeat, and they don't answer the question, you answer it for them: 'You overeat because you are emotionally upset.' Then you ask them to go back to the experience that is making them unhappy or angry. And you had better be prepared for an emotional eruption, because most overeaters are trying to suppress bad emotions and when their defenses are removed while hypnotized, all of those pent up emotions just come gushing out.

"So when Jeanie comes in, you should regress her back to the experiences that make her unhappy or angry. After she gets it all vented out of her system suggest to her that now that all of the emotions have been resolved, healthy foods and drinks taste wonderful and fattening ones taste awful. It's that simple."

Although I was wholly unconvinced that it was necessary to regress a person back to some sensitizing event (or that past lives had anything to do with it) I resolved to give it a try and satisfy my curiosity on both counts.

Before Eric left he said, "We'll continue this discussion at some other time, but I need to go to the grocery store to buy a couple of props for tonight's show." And off he went.

CHAPTER 17

Back on Stage

At 7:30 on the dot, Eric came through the door donned in his tux and looking as sharp as the night before. With briefcase in hand he was greeted with applause from an overflow crowd. Apparently the word had gotten out about the hypnotist that was performing at *David's*. When I arrived fifteen minutes earlier the nightclub's bouncer and a fire marshal were there, keeping count of the number of people inside and an eye on another 50 people milling around outside, hoping to get in.

After giving my "the greatest hypnotist in the world" introduction I handed Eric the microphone and he announced to the audience, "Before I call for volunteers to participate in tonight's show, my colleague Lindsay Brady and I will demonstrate the telepathic and psychic powers of the subconscious mind. Only after hours of intense practice have we succeeded in establishing a communication link between our two minds. In a moment I'll come down among you while Lindsay remains here on stage and we will see if he can sort out *my* mental messages from all other thoughts that are going on in the minds of the people in this 'standing room only' performance at *David's*—now the most popular nightclub in the Salt Lake Valley!"

Eric handed me the stage mic and threaded the other one, with its extension cord attached, through the audience as he positioned himself at the far end of the bar (Back then cordless microphones were rare). He asked Rich, David's daytime manager who had stuck around to see the performance, for a dollar bill. Gathering a group of people around him he said, "I will see if I can telepathically transmit to Lindsay the serial number on Rich's dollar bill."

To give the demonstration a little more credibility he asked Rich, "Have either Lindsay or I talked to you about this demonstration of telepathy or have you divulged to either of us the serial number on this dollar bill?"

Rich self-consciously answered into the mic, "No. I didn't even know what you wanted it for and for sure I have never looked at its serial number."

Eric went on. "I need those of you who are closest to squeeze in a little tighter so you can verify that the number on the bill and the one Lindsay claims he has received are the same. I also want you to help me by thinking of each number as it comes up. There will probably be some of you who will try to send the wrong number in an attempt to trip us up, but I think Lindsay and I have established a good enough communication link that we can override the bogus thoughts—it's just that the more people who are thinking of the same number, the stronger the signal. So please help me. But I also want you to respond with a shout of 'YES!' or 'NO!' depending on the correctness of Lindsay's response."

Eric held up the bill so those close to him could see it and said into his microphone, "Are you ready?"

I answered into my mic. "Yes."

Eric placed two of his fingers on his forehead as if in deep concentration and said, "Everyone around me knows what this number is, do you have it yet?"

I closed my eyes for a moment, placed my fingertips to my forehead, opened my eyes and said, "Yes I do. The number is 'three.'"

A shout of "Yes!" went up from the observers.

"Are you ready?"

"Yes."

Eric said, "On this number we need to be really tuned in. I think other people are trying to send a different number."

I did my concentration pantomime and replied, "I think I've got it. Is it the number 'one'?"

"Yes!" And a few cheers went up from the audience.

"Are you ready?"

"Yes."

"Save some of your psychic powers for other numbers. This one should give you no trouble."

"I have received the number. It is 'seven.'"

"Yes!" And cheers and applause rose again from the audience.

"Are you ready?"

"Yes."

"Only four more numbers after you receive this number. Do you have it yet?"

"I believe that it is another 'one.'"

This time there was a louder "Yes!" mixed in with the applause and cheers.

"Are you ready?"

"Yes."

"Really, this number should give you no trouble."

"Zero," I answered.

"YES!" And still more cheers and applause rang out.

"Are you ready?"

"Yes."

"Ready for this one? So far you are doing great."

"It is another 'zero.'"

"YES!" Cheers, whistles and applause rang out.

"Are you ready?"

"Yes."

"From now on you are going to be famous for your telepathic powers. Do you have it yet?"

"Four."

"YES!" The whole place went into an uproar.

Eric said, "This is your last number. Are you ready?"

"Yes."

"On this last number, be careful. Someone is trying to send the wrong number again."

I gave a little extra time while "receiving" the message and then said, "I believe you are sending me another 'one.'"

After the pandemonium had settled down a bit I heard Eric say into his mic, "So, do you want to see if he can get the letters of the serial number, too?"

It seemed to me that everyone in *David's* shouted in unison, "Yes!"

"Do you think that you can do this too, Lindsay?"

"I think *I* can if *you* think *you* can!" I answered.

"Don't go putting all the blame on *me* if *you* mess up. I'll send it right so it is up to you to receive it right," he quipped. "Are you ready?"

"Yes."

Eric said, "Okay. Now let's see if you really *do* have telepathic powers. I am sending the letter now.... Do you have the letter yet?"

"Not yet, but give me a moment.... Yes, I think I have it now. The letter is 'L'?"

Again the nightclub went crazy with hoots, cheers and applause.

"Are you ready?"

"Yes."

"Okay. Don't just think anyone can do this," he said to the crowd. "Lindsay, if you can get this one you will be legendary... at least here at *David's*—which has overnight become the most popular nightclub in the entire Salt Lake Valley."

I waited again. There was complete silence. "Give me just one more moment.... Are you still sending it?" Eric placed his fingers to his head again, and I did too, and then said, "The letter you are sending me is... is... 'J.'"

The roar of the crowd was deafening.

Over the next four weeks this routine was the most popular of all. Almost every night someone would request, "Do that telepathic demonstration again." We had a group of loyal followers (or better put—skeptics). People pulled out note pads or used the back of napkins to write down Eric's clue statements attempting to decipher the code, or to see if he used the same statement for a given number, but for the most part the audience thought it truly was telepathy. Only once out of a hundred or more numbers did I come back with the wrong one. On that occasion, however, just by pure chance, Rich, the daytime manager with whom I had established a fairly good rapport by then, shouted "YES!" amid the disappointing "no's." "That's the letter *I* was thinking," he shouted into Eric's mic. "This stuff really works!"

After Eric made his way back to stage for the rest of the show and had completed his selection and hypnotizing process, he asked all of the volunteers to open their eyes and instructed them to keep their gaze on him and to be aware of what he was up to. *"Although I will be speaking to only one person, each of you will follow and carry out any suggestion that relates to you."* He placed his fingertips on the forehead of an attractive, well-dressed woman whom he had earlier seated on an end chair and said, *"Mary, you look like you take pride in your dress and appearance. What is the name of that perfume you are sporting? Do you always wear the same fragrance?"*

"No, I don't," she answered.

"What is your favorite?"

"Well it depends on the occasion. Right now I have on Chanel No. 5."

"That's pretty expensive stuff, isn't it?"

"Yes, it is. Forty-five dollars for a one ounce bottle."

"You probably use it sparingly then, but how much would you use if you had a free pint of Chanel No. 5?"

"If I had a free pint of Chanel No. 5 I'd drench myself in it. Well, not quite drench myself, but I wouldn't be so stingy when I put it on."

Eric went over to his over-sized briefcase and pulled out a pint of household ammonia; held it up for the audience to see what it was and returned to Mary and said, *"I have here a pint of household ammonia, but to you it has the aroma of Chanel No. 5. In a moment when I hand it to you, you will remove the cap and smell its contents; to you it will have the fragrance of Chanel No. 5, and because it is free, you will apply it to your body just as you do when getting ready to go out for a night on the town, but lavishly. You will then pass the bottle down the row of your fellow volunteers so they, too, can enjoy its fragrance, but to them it will smell like what it really is—household ammonia. After each of them takes a whiff of your perfume they will probably quizzically look at you and wonder why in the world an attractive, well-dressed woman like you ever chose this aroma as her favorite."*

Eric asked Mary to stand up and handed her the pint of "Chanel No. 5." She unscrewed the lid, lifted the bottle and passed it back and forth under her nose with no adverse physical reaction whatsoever; she even seemed to enjoy the fragrance, as she sniffed it and let out a sigh of "mmm." She dipped her finger into the ammonia and lavishly applied some behind each ear and a healthy amount to her throat, sat back down on her chair and handed her pint of perfume to Jill, who was sitting next to her.

Jill took one whiff of Mary's perfume, jerked back with a turning of her head in an attempt to catch her breath, gave Mary a critical look and said, "That is awful!" She passed the bottle to her neighbor as she shook her head in disbelief and disgust.

The audience was more amazed than entertained, as was I, wondering how Mary could have not reacted adversely to the smell of ammonia. Anyone who has ever gotten a good whiff of ammonia will understand how difficult it would be to *not* jerk back in an effort to avoid its pungent odor and to catch one's breath.

As the bottle was passed down to each of the volunteers, their reaction to the smell of the ammonia was identical, just as you would expect. None of them wanted a second sniff when Eric offered. And the crowd began finding the scenario more amusing with the similarity of each person's response.

Eric returned to Mary, who seemed confused and offended that no one else liked her choice of perfume. Eric touched her head, after handing the bottle back to her, and said, "*Mary, when I snap my fingers you will wake up and return to your seat with no recollection of what you have been doing on stage except that you have in your hand an almost full pint of Chanel No. 5. When you get back to your table you will invite your friends to take a sniff of your free Chanel No. 5.... And even pass it around to others in the audience so they, too, can enjoy its fragrance. Regardless of their response and comments you will still take pleasure in its fragrance; that is, until you hear me say "oranges." When I say the word "oranges," the ammonia will smell like ammonia; you will bring the bottle back to me and express your displeasure and accuse me of having turned a whole pint of Chanel No. 5 into ammonia. But when I look at you and snap my fingers the entire episode will be forgotten, and you will return to your table and act as if the event had never occurred.*

"*And for the rest of you volunteers, when I snap my fingers your eyes will close; you will lean your head against your neighbor and you will go into an even deeper hypnotic state.*"

[SNAP!]

Mary stood up and on her way back to her table took an occasional sniff of her free pint of Chanel No. 5. And on stage every head of the remaining volunteers leaned onto their neighbor as they closed their eyes.

After watching Mary make it to her table and observing that she was following his suggestions, Eric turned to Jill, touched her head and said, "Jill, open your eyes and look at me."

Jill did just as she was commanded and Eric said to her, "*Jill did you like Mary's Chanel No. 5?*"

159

"It was awful. It smelled just like ammonia. I can't believe that anyone could stand how it smells, let alone use it for perfume.... She's a whacko!"

Eric said, *"Jill, I noticed that you were drinking a screwdriver before coming up on stage. Do you like oranges?"*

Mary jumped up from her chair in the audience; grabbed the bottle of ammonia from a person who was about to sniff its contents; stormed back up to the stage; walked up to Eric and with her face right in his shouted, "You are a fraud and a liar. You gave me a whole pint of Chanel No. 5 and then you turned it into ammonia. You are really a spiteful person!"

Eric looked at her and snapped his fingers right in front of her face. She gave a little jerk and calmly returned to her table without saying another word, as though nothing had happened.

"I apologize for that interruption, Jill, but did you say that you liked oranges?"

"Yes I do. I eat them all the time."

"Have you eaten one today?"

"Well no... except for the screwdriver I had a little earlier."

"If I gave you a very nice, juicy orange would you eat a slice or two and also be willing to share a few pieces of it with the other volunteers?"

"Yes, I would be willing to do that."

Eric then suggested to the group, *"Volunteers who are on stage, in a moment, when I snap my fingers, you will open your eyes and look at me. I will give Jill a container of a very special citrus fruit; she will pass out a slice to each of you. At first, it will look and smell like a nice, juicy slice of orange and when I say 'EAT IT NOW' you will take a healthy bite but discover you have just bitten into what it really is... a very sour lemon. With surprise at what you have just chomped into, your face will contort, your lips will pucker, your eyes will water, your mouth will salivate, and you will express your displeasure at having been duped into thinking that a lemon is an orange and then wipe your face with a napkin that I will have Jill give you.*

"But Jill, yours will continue to have the aroma and taste of the most sweet and delicious orange you have ever eaten. You will eat it greedily and when finished comment on how delicious it is, but give no thought to the reaction of the other volunteers. There will probably be a few extra pieces and you will enjoy devouring those, too."

Eric pulled out of his briefcase a Tupperware container with a dozen or so slices of lemon (each inside a folded piece of wax paper—Baggies hadn't been invented yet) and a napkin for each person. He handed the Tupperware and the napkins to Jill. Jill distributed a napkin and a piece of "orange" to each of the other volunteers and took one for herself. The audience was silent with anticipation.

Eric said, *"Now that Jill has so graciously shared with each of you her special citrus fruit, I think that it is time for you to 'EAT IT NOW.'"*

Each of the participants unwrapped their "orange," took a healthy bite and, as you would expect, reacted as one would when biting into a tart, sour lemon. The volunteers reacted with puckers, facial contortions, and explicative comments upon discovering that what they thought was a sweet, juicy orange was actually a very sour lemon. And the audience's curiosity turned to amazement, laughter and hoots as they observed the spectacle.

But Jill gobbled hers down and wolfed down the remaining pieces apparently without a hint of a sour taste and said, "Boy, that was good. Where did you ever find such sweet, juicy oranges this time of year?"

Eric turned to me and said, "Lindsay, would you mind taking the Tupperware and gathering up the leftovers?"

He turned to the participants, snapped his fingers and said, *"Sleep now!"* Everyone's head either dropped to their chest or onto the shoulder of the person sitting next to them.

Eric walked over to Jill and said as he touched her forehead again, *"Jill, when I snap my fingers you will open your eyes and be wide awake, wondering what has been going on. You will return to your table, ask your friends to buy you another screwdriver and enjoy the rest of the show, but deny to everyone that you have ever eaten a lemon that tasted like an orange."*

[SNAP!]

Jill returned to her table, had her friends buy her a screwdriver, and argued with them that she had ever eaten a lemon that tasted like an orange.

Eric turned to the remaining volunteers, asked them to open their eyes and said, *"In a moment I will touch each of you on your forehead. I will give specific instructions that apply only to the person whose head I am touching at the time. When I snap my fingers you will follow and carry out <u>your</u> suggestions exactly as I have instructed you to do. Later on, when I clap my hands together, you will wake up immediately, feeling wonderfully well but wondering what in the world you are doing on a nightclub stage and why all of those people out there are looking and laughing at you. You will then return to your table and catch up on the drinks you've been missing out on and have no recollection of being on stage or what you did while on stage."*

Eric touched the head of a burly fellow and said, *"Tim, you are a dog, a big St. Bernard. When you hear the snap of my fingers you will drop down on all fours and look around. If you hear or see anything that acts or sounds like a cat you will, of course, bark and growl at it in your deepest bark and growl. You will stay in the vicinity of your chair, as though you are tethered to a leash, but act agitated because you can't get at the cat.*

"Molly, you're a duck. When I snap my fingers you will crouch down with your hands tucked into your armpits, flap your imaginary wings, and strut around the stage quacking and acting like a duck.

161

"Gerald, you are a cat, an old tomcat. When I snap my fingers you will also drop to the floor and begin yowling and carrying on just like a tomcat. If you happen to see or hear anything that acts like or sounds like another cat you will attempt to impress her with your yowling, and of course, if you happen to encounter anything that sounds or acts like a dog, you will hiss and spit at it."

Eric touched the forehead of a redheaded gal and said, "Carmen, you are a chicken, a Rhode Island red hen. When I snap my fingers you will climb up on your chair —I mean your nest—squat down on it, pose as a chicken and cluck just as a hen clucks who is laying an egg.

"Terry, you are also a dog... a yappy terrier. When I snap my fingers, you, too, will stay in the vicinity of your chair as though you are tied to a leash. If you see or hear anything that sounds or acts like another animal you will, of course, just as terriers do, yap at it.

"Tony, you are also a duck, a real quacker. When I snap my fingers you will also act like a duck and if you see or hear anything that sounds like another duck you will waddle behind it and attempt to out-quack it.

"Gary, you are a big barnyard rooster. When I snap my fingers you, too, will crouch on your chair, pose as a rooster and take it upon yourself to make sure that all of the farm animals wake up on this fine spring morning by flapping your wings, stretching out your neck and crowing at the top of your voice.

"Karen, you are also a cat; a soft, fluffy, well-bred female Persian. When I snap my fingers you will drop to the floor and slink around on all fours as you put forth soft meows. And if you should encounter anything that sounds or looks like a dog you will strut around just beyond the length of its leash as though taunting it. And should you encounter anything that sounds or acts like a tomcat you will ignore it."

[SNAP!]

The stage erupted into pandemonium. It took on the appearance of a psychotic farmyard: The low woofing and growling of a St. Bernard as a tomcat hissed and spat at it; the yapping of a terrier as a Persian cat strolled back and forth a foot beyond its leash; a hen sat on its nest clucking as she laid an egg; a rooster perched on another chair with outstretched neck, flapping its wings and crowing at the top of its voice; one quacking duck waddled around the stage while another one followed, trying to out-quack it; a tomcat hissed and spit at the yapping terrier while trying to impress a Persian cat that was ignoring it; and a nightclub full of people were in hysterics, crying out with laughter and applauding while marveling at the spectacle.

[CLAP!]

"Wide awake now, feeling wonderfully well and wondering what has been going on!"

The stage went silent as eight people looked out over an audience with no idea why they were on a stage or why all of those people were applauding and laughing at them.

Eric, in his fashion, placed the mic on its stand, picked up his briefcase and worked his way through the crowd and out the door with cheers and backslaps (high-fives hadn't been invented yet, either) as he exited.

As I went by David's office door on my way out, he grabbed me and said, "That was really a great show, especially that telepathic stunt. How did you guys do that—it wasn't really telepathic, was it? What do you think he will do for the next show?"

It is interesting how David has shifted his thoughts from worrying about making a profit as a result of hiring us to draw in more business to wondering what Eric is going to pull off at the next show, I thought, before saying, "I don't know what he has in mind but he says he has more than a hundred routines stored in his brain, so I don't think he'll be repeating any of them for awhile. I can't wait to see what he has up his sleeve, either."

By the time I got out to the parking lot, Eric and his truck were nowhere to be found. *I guess I'll just go back to the office until the second show time and analyze the things I have just witnessed,* I thought.

Back at my office I leaned back in my recliner, made myself comfortable and began wondering:

What is really going on in the brain of a hypnotized person?

Why do people act that way and do those things while hypnotized on stage, when most of them, in everyday life, probably would not have the courage, ability or inclination to do such things at all?

Is there truly a second, "subconscious or unconscious" mind that operates independently from our conscious awareness and that can override normal, rational behavior and thinking?

How can a person stick their nose into a bottle of ammonia and not react to its pungent odor—let alone think it is Chanel No. 5?

If there is an independent subconscious mind, that without questioning, causes a person to behave as though something is real that isn't real, just by a suggestion, then how do we tap into it and intentionally take control of our everyday life and eliminate limitations and self-defeating behavior?

Is "self-hypnosis" something different than being hypnotized by someone else? It appears to me that I am missing something. If self-hypnosis is as effective in affecting behavior as being hypnotized by someone else, why do I still have many of my old hang-ups and limitations? Maybe I don't understand the communication link between my conscious and unconscious minds.

In spite of the fact that Eric says I can't be a good stage-show hypnotist if I am analytical, I believe that, as powerful as hypnosis appears to be, a hypnotist would be a better hypnotist, whether on stage or clinically, by understanding what the driving force is that makes it work.

How is the brain involved in all of this?

I wonder how the human soul or spirit is involved in hypnosis—what was their soul or spirit doing while those people were on stage barking, crowing, hissing, and thinking a lemon was an orange and ammonia was perfume?

Maybe people who are hypnotized really are susceptible to evil forces. Maybe our conscious, rational mind is "good" (because we consciously know the difference between good and evil—what is real and what isn't real) and our subconscious mind is "evil" because it seems to lack rational restraint; it just does whatever it is told to do whether rational or irrational—good or evil.

Why do people smoke, drink, overeat and engage in other self-destructive behaviors, when on a conscious, rational level they know that it is bad for them? Why do they continue to engage in the behavior anyway? Is there an evil unconscious force that is trying to destroy human good health, happiness and goodness?

Did we really live past lives? Have we really experienced birth, growing up, having children and death, before this life!!!?

If what Eric says about past lives is true, why don't we remember them while not hypnotized and remember them when we are? And if we did live past lives how much are they affecting our behavior in this one? I think it would be interesting to investigate and see if there is some validity to what he says!

I know that I am a rational person and that I can figure things out when I need to, but I feel that locked up inside of me is an intellect that is howling to be used and a curiosity that is longing to be fulfilled. I also know that, outside of my narrow social and family traditions, I have missed out on being exposed to a broad insight into human wisdom and general knowledge. After all, I just squeaked through high school and have expanded my education very little since. And for sure, I lack an understanding of psychology and other behavioral sciences that may explain why we human beings behave as we do. I also lack the rich understanding that comes through literature, history, the arts, science, and by discovering how other people think.... My comprehension of what this world is all about is really limited—I've been living in a cave! I think Eric is right—enroll in college and get an education. I'm sure that would help me find answers to many of my questions and satisfy my curiosity!

All of a sudden I sat up in my recliner and realized that a stage-show was about to start without me and I rushed back to *David's* thinking, *I sure have more questions about hypnosis than I have answers. Maybe Eric is right again—just "do it" and stop analyzing what makes it work!* Little did I know that a bombshell was about to explode square in the center of my already challenged rational, questioning mind and traditional way of thinking.

CHAPTER 18

Bombshell Performance

I arrived back at *David's* just in time to get everything arranged before Eric made his grand entrance to another round of applause and cheers. He had developed quite a rapport with the audience in just three performances, so most of them thought of him as a compatriot rather than an arrogant, but highly skilled, stage performer—as I did.

This time around, once Eric had selected 10 responsive volunteers and had recited his hypnosis induction, he placed his hand on the head of a middle-aged woman whom he had intentionally seated in the middle of the group. He said, *"Everyone on stage, except for Tabitha, whose head I am touching now: when I snap my fingers you will wake up feeling wonderfully well and return to your place in the audience and enjoy an extra few drinks while you are enlightened by what you are about to witness on stage. Lindsay and I will be back tomorrow night so please come back and volunteer again. All of you are very fine hypnotic subjects but for this show I will need only one volunteer."*

With his hand still on Tabitha's head he snapped his fingers, and while the volunteers exited the stage he said into my ear, "Set all of the empty chairs to the back of the stage and bring me that stool over there; then go down and find a vantage point off stage where you can keep a close watch on the audience."

He then had Tabitha turn her chair so she was seated at an angle but facing the audience (so neither she nor Eric would have their back to the spectators but could still face one another) and placed the stool a couple of feet from Tabitha.

Eric turned to the audience and said, "This show will *not* be as packed with humor or fun-filled antics as earlier shows have been. Yet, it *will* be entertaining, enlightening, provocative and more mind-boggling than any of our previous adventures into the world of the subconscious mind.

"In the subconscious mind of every human being is stored a record of every significant event a person has experienced. To demonstrate the truth of this statement, I will now regress Tabitha back to a few experiences that have long since been forgotten by her conscious mind."

With that, Eric gave a little nod to *David's* DJ. The house lights dimmed and all of the stage lights went off, except for a single small blue floodlight that shown down only on Eric and Tabitha, giving the stage a dramatic, mysterious appearance. In the haze of cigarette smoke that filled the nightclub, the soft blue light gave the stage an eerie enigmatic and curious look—almost as though Eric and Tabitha were suspended in mid-air.

Eric swung around on the stool so he was facing Tabitha and said, *"Do you go by Tabitha?"*

"Yes."

"Tabitha, what is your present age?"

"I just turned forty-three."

"Then it has been a while since you were in grammar school, is that right?"

"Yes, more than thirty-five years."

"Tabitha, just close your eyes now, remaining upright in your chair; make yourself comfortable and SLEEP NOW!"

Tabitha wiggled around and closed her eyes, and her head sank down to her chest as she settled into what looked like a comfortable sleep.

"Tabitha, I want you to now return back to some significant event from your first grade classroom. It is as though you are there. You hear, see, smell, and emotionally feel the experience of the event just like you are there now.... Return back now to your first grade classroom and tell me, what is happening now?"

Eric put the microphone down close to her mouth and waited for a moment or two, but Tabitha said nothing, so he asked, *"Is your teacher there?"*

Another moment or two passed before she answered, "Yes."

"What is your teacher wearing?"

After a longer pause Tabitha finally said with a subdued, quiet voice, "She is wearing that ugly old grayish-brown, button-down-the-front dress that she almost always wears."

"What is your teacher's name?"

Another pause and then she said, "Her name is Miss Agnes Appleby."

"When Miss Appleby isn't around, what do you and your fellow students call her?"

Almost immediately a smile crept over Tabitha's face as she responded, "Promise you won't tell?"

"I promise."

"I'd be in big trouble, you know, if it got back to her and she found out it was me who told.... We call her 'Dogbreath Applenose!'"

There were a few chuckles from the audience, but then Tabitha opened her eyes, looked off into empty space and said, "Just look at it—I mean her red nose—and when she gets up close to you and talks in your face you can smell her stinky 'Dogbreath.' My friend Adam says her nose is always red like that and her breath stinks that way because she sips at her toddy all night long—just like his Uncle Joe."

There came from the audience a few more chuckles.

"What is Miss Dogbreath Applenose doing now?"

Tabitha's countenance changed to one of anxiety as she said, "She's yelling at me!"

"Why is she yelling at you and what is she saying?"

"'Your letter "S's" are all lying down on their side. Anyone can see the difference between a standing up "S" and one that is lying down on its side. You're really a stupid little girl!'

"Ouch! She just slapped my hand with her yardstick."

"Does she often slap students with her yardstick?"

"Yes, she does it all the time."

"What, then, is significant about this time? What is happening now?"

"Adam has grabbed the yardstick from her hand. He just whacked her on the rump with it! Now he's breaking it over his knee and is shouting at the top of his voice, 'Stop hitting my friend, Dogbreath Applenose!' He just threw the pieces of the yardstick at her and he is tearing out of the room shouting back at her, 'You'll never catch me, 'Dogbreath Applenose!'"

The audience broke out into a roar of laughter. Eric was as amused at the vision of the spectacle as the audience was, and he turned to them and with a big smile on his face said, "I thought this was supposed to be a serious show!"

Eric turned back to Tabitha and said, *"Tabitha, I want you to now return back even further in your life. Return back now.... You are two years old. It is your two-year-old birthday party. You can hear, smell, taste and feel the event in every detail, just as though you are there now. What is happening?"*

Tabitha just sat there again, so Eric said to her in baby talk, *"Is your mommy here, and if she is, what is she doing?"*

After a moment Tabitha answered back in her own baby-talk voice. "My mommy is lighting two candles on a tiny cake."

"Are there other people at your party?"

"Daddy is here and my big brother is here and my new little baby sister is here."

"What is happening now?"

"My daddy is scolding Mommy for using the last of the sugar to make my birthday cake!"

"What is he saying?"

"We're out of money, I can't find work, and here you are using our last ounce of sugar and flour to make this stinking little cake! What in the world were we thinking of when we had all of these kids? Maybe we can sell one of them so the rest of us don't starve!"

Eric reached over and placed his hand on Tabitha's head and said, *"Sleep now... drifting down now into a deep, peaceful, hypnotic sleep."*

Tabitha closed her eyes and her head again sank down to her chest.

"Tabitha, I want you to now return back even further. I want you to go back to a significant experience from a past life."

The instant Eric spoke those words I detected mixed reactions from the audience. Some were shaking their heads displaying complete disbelief that such a thing holds any credibility whatsoever. But the vast majority reacted with a positive conviction that past-life experiences are valid, and waited with anxious anticipation to witness firsthand someone actually regressing to a past life, to confirm their belief. After all, it *was* the seventies and the era of "What sign were *you* born under?" and the movie *On a Clear Day,* in which Barbra Streisand was "regressed" to a past life by a hypnotist.

Eric continued his suggestions to Tabitha: *"When I ask you to return back you will be able to easily articulate the experience as though you are there. You see, hear, smell, taste, touch and feel everything associated with the event–just as though you are there. Return back now, Tabitha, to a significant event from some previous life's experience."*

Again, Tabitha just sat there, although this time it was apparent that something was going on in her mind that was puzzling her.

Eric let her just sit there for a very long time. The nightclub was almost silent and I could sense the unrest in the audience in anticipation of what she might come up with. *Maybe it is the hocus-pocus setting–the eerie blue light illuminating the smoke–that is creating this uneasy feeling,* I thought.

Eric asked, *"What is happening now? Tell me, Tabitha, what is going on."*

Tabitha opened her eyes and looked beyond the audience–like she was watching something happening far away–and said, "They are after me. I've got to hide. If they find me they will kill me!"

With that she stood up and hunkered behind her chair as though it could hide her from a looming danger, and occasionally peeked over its back as if on the outlook for some imminent disaster.

Eric said to her, *"You are safe now that you have found a hiding place, but tell me who 'they' are and why they are out to get you."*

"It's the priest and his inquisitors. They think I am a witch!"

"Are you?"

"Of course I'm not. Everyone in the village knows that I am not a witch. Those evil men, under the guise of being holy men, trump up witch stories about women so they can take pleasure in probing and torturing them."

"What do they say you did that gives them reason to accuse you of being a witch?"

"You must not be from around here, are you? Everyone knows that Mr. Drummer—that cantankerous old tyrant whom no one can stand—wants to get his hands on my property. He told the priest I had placed a curse on his cow and caused it to dry up. The priest believed him and called his stooges to find me so they can torture and kill me."

"What is your name?"

With hesitation and a look of suspicion she said, "My name is Angela Grover. I am heiress to my father's estate. Why do you ask? You're not one of them, are you?"

"No I am not. But I am curious about people and their life's experiences—their history and how they live their lives."

Eric reached over the back of the chair, placed his hand on her head and said, "Tabitha, in a moment I will ask you to come back and sit on the chair. When you do, you will be able to remember your life as Angela Grover. When I ask you questions about this event in your life as Angela, it will be like viewing a movie—you are outside of your body watching what is happening. Although you know it is your own story of a past life you will answer my questions detached from the emotions of the experience. You will be peaceful and comfortable and tell your story as an observer. Come now and sit back on the chair and close your eyes."

With the absence of the terror she had displayed a few moments earlier, Tabitha did as he had asked. When she was seated and comfortable Eric asked, "In your life as Angela Grover, did the men find you, and if they did what happened afterwards?"

With her eyes still closed, Tabitha said in a matter of fact voice, devoid of any emotions, "Yes they did. They took me to the priest, who pronounced me to be a witch and told the inquisitors to extract a confession from me and to discover where on my body the evil spirit had entered when it took possession of my soul.

"They took all of my clothing off and while probing found a birth mark on my hip. They pronounced that it was the mark left by the devil when entering my body. It confirmed that I was a witch. For the next two days I was chained to a wall and was given no food or water, and every 'fourth bell' they whipped me, demanding a confession. Finally I did confess to being a witch, hoping that they would stop the beatings. But then they just whipped me all the more because I was a self-confessed witch and needed to be punished.

"On the morning of the third day the priest came and condemned my soul to hell for eternity. They took me and tied me to a pole in the middle of the square and burned me to death."

David's was silent as she told her story. For the few moments it took to tell her tale I didn't see a person order a drink or even take a sip of the drink they had.

Eric said to Tabitha, *"That was a fantastic firsthand account of a tragic part of human history and I think that everyone listening has compassion for you in your life as Angela Grover.*

"Tabitha, would remembering this experience as Angela Grover on a conscious level have, in any way, an adverse effect on your life now? Or, would you like your memory of it completely erased?"

Tabitha said without hesitation, "No, I don't want it erased. I want to remember it all. I have always felt that there was something in my past that caused me to feel guilt and shame. Now that I know why, there is no reason to continue feeling that way."

Eric said, *"Tabitha, when I ask you to wake up you will remember in every detail your experiences as Angela Grover. You will not only use the memory of the experience to better deal with* this *life but will be completely free from all feelings of guilt and shame. It is like a giant weight has been lifted from your being and allows you to confidently enjoy this life's experience.*

"Open your eyes now, Tabitha, and wide awake feeling wonderfully well."

Tabitha opened her eyes and sat up in her chair as Eric gave a nod to *David's* DJ and the lights came back on. Tabitha looked at Eric and said, "Thank you, that was a great adventure. I really feel wonderful."

"Let me ask you a few questions before you return to your seat," Eric said. "When did you last think of the experience of your first grade teacher, Miss Dogbreath Applenose, and Adam smacking her on the rump?"

"I don't think that I have thought about that since it happened. Maybe I thought of it for a few days afterwards, but not since. But the memory is crystal clear now."

"Did you ever think that you would be able to recall your second birthday? It sounded like your family was very poor."

"Until now I had no recollection of my second birthday, but I do remember being very poor when I was growing up. It was during the Great Depression— in the early thirties. My parents have told me stories about that period in their lives, but until now I had no recollection of my second birthday. I can remember the kitchen and the old wood stove and even the linoleum floor. I'm going to ask my mom and see if she remembers."

"Tell us a little more about your life as Angela Grover. Does it seem like you were just making it up or was it like remembering, say, your high school graduation?"

"Oh it was a real memory.... and terrifying! That is, until you took me out of experiencing it and had me view it like I was watching a movie.

"When I saw those men coming I wanted to run, but there was no place to run to. And the humiliation and beating, although watching from outside of my body, still brought on feelings of shame. Until now I could not understand why I have, for my whole life, had this underlying feeling of guilt and shame. I really knew I hadn't done anything bad and that I shouldn't feel guilt or disgrace, but now that I know about my life as Angela all those bad feelings are gone. I hope that they stay away."

"They will, and if you want to pursue the event further, give me a call and we can do it in the privacy of my office, but now is not the time to investigate it any further. You can return to your table now and enjoy visiting with your friends."

Eric turned to the audience and said, "That was a *real* adventure into the recesses of the subconscious mind, wasn't it? I only occasionally do past-life regression during my stage-show performance—stage-shows are supposed to be humorous and entertaining—but I just wanted to demonstrate to the skeptics (giving a little glance in my direction) that we did live past lives, and with hypnosis those past lives can be recalled.

"Tomorrow night Lindsay and I will be here at *David's*, now the most popular nightclub in the Salt Lake Valley, to take you on another adventure into the subconscious mind. So order a few more drinks, mull over the things you have witnessed and enjoy the rest of the evening."

Before exiting *David's* Eric said to me, "I'll see you tomorrow at noon," and then disappeared out the door. I watched and listened to the people who had gathered around Tabitha, as she filled in on more of the details of her life as Angela Grover.... And I just sat there and wondered!

CHAPTER 19

Lesson Three and Meeting Socrates

Eric was at my office door right on time (for the first time) and by the end of this tutorial session I felt that maybe my $100 installment payments were well worth the price—I really was learning about stage hypnosis and gaining fresh insights about doing clinical hypnosis. And although self-centered about it, Eric did have a great deal of experience and was sincere in his attempt to impart his knowledge.

He began, "If you are going to be an outstanding stage-show hypnotist you must always think ahead. The smoothness of last night's performance didn't just happen. It was the result of organization and planning. Some things were obvious—having the ammonia on hand, the lemons sliced and the napkins ready—but most of what you observed was either planned well in advance of the performance or planned while performing. Get your notepad out and take down some notes as I go through these items."

I pulled out my notepad and jotted down a few comments as he spoke.

"When doing past-life routines on stage always use lighting to create the illusion of mysticism; people really like that kind of stuff—mysticism. Yesterday when we were talking about past lives I knew then that I would be doing a regression on stage. So I planned ahead. I worked with *David's* DJ for several hours to get the lighting effect I wanted. I even placed a strip of tape on the floor to mark the position of the subject's chair, had the bar stool on stage and worked out a signal for turning the lights off and on.

"When we talked about smoking and weight loss and I told you to make bad tasting things taste good or good smelling things smell bad, I knew that I'd be doing the ammonia and lemon routines, so I went out and bought ammonia and lemons. These are examples of planning ahead for the show.

"Other examples of planning ahead during the show: Because I knew I was going to make lemons taste like oranges, I looked for a number of people in the audience who were drinking screwdrivers so I could select one of them for that routine; it wasn't on the spur of the moment that I chose Jill for that routine. Since *you* don't drink you may not know that a "screwdriver" is orange juice with vodka in it.

"I caught the aroma of perfume on a few other volunteer women but I selected Mary because she was attractive, well-dressed and looked like she was particular about her appearance. She turned out to be perfect.

"I had Mary and Jill sit on the end chairs because I wanted it to be convenient for them to pass their samples down the row of volunteers.

"I selected Tabitha because she was an older person and I figured that she would be less likely to have conscious recollection of her first grade classroom or second birthday.

"Because I knew I would be saying 'oranges' for the next routine I used that as a 'post-hypnotic key word' for Mary to discover that her perfume was really ammonia.

"Remember, when doing a stage-show routine never lie or attempt to use deception! I cringe when I hear a hypnotist on stage say to a subject 'this bottle contains perfume,' when it doesn't, or put ammonia in a perfume bottle thinking they need to trick the subject. As you saw last night I didn't need to use trickery. Hypnosis is powerful and you never need to use deception to get it to work. You no doubt noticed that I said, 'This *is* ammonia but to you it smells like Chanel No. 5. This *is* a piece of lemon but to you it tastes like a piece of orange.'

"I had you move all of the chairs to the back of the stage so Tabitha and I would be the focal point at center stage. And I had you go down to the audience for the same reason, and so that you could be near the audience to keep an eye on them should anything unusual occur.

"Fortunately, no incident occurred while doing the past-life regression routine. But many people, if past lives infringe on their religious beliefs, overreact which can disrupt the flow of the rest of the show. And sometimes people in the audience regress back to their own past-life experiences, and there's no telling what they might do or say if they are not quickly brought back to the present.

"If you ever do regressions on stage, keep each segment short. I could have had Tabitha go into greater detail about her first grade classroom, her second birthday or her past life as Angela. Sometimes it is a slow process to drag out past-life memories and people in the audience can quickly lose interest. So last night I had Tabitha view the experience of being tortured as an outside observer so she didn't get caught up in all of the emotion of the experience. As an outside observer she told her tale much more quickly than she would have had she been experiencing it. Besides that, our agreement with David was to keep the shows short. Also, when people are hypnotized they tend to speak quietly, so when on stage place the microphone close to their mouth so the audience can hear what they are saying.

"As you commented the other day, and as you observed last night, when a person is hypnotized it takes a while for them to respond to questions—especially when regressing to experiences from the past, whether in this life or past lives—so you need to be very patient and wait for their response. Sometimes it can take several minutes for them to come up with an answer. That is fine in a clinical setting, but it isn't entertaining on stage.

"When doing regressions on stage, to help move things along more quickly you must make a few assumptions: I assumed that there was a teacher in Tabitha's first grade classroom, but I didn't assume that her teacher was a woman, so I asked, 'Is your teacher there?' and it produced the response of 'Yes.' To discover whether her teacher was male or female I asked, 'What is your teacher wearing?' which triggered the memory of Miss Dogbreath Applenose's ugly dress.

"By the way, once in a while you strike it lucky; Dogbreath Applenose and Adam slapping her on the butt with a yardstick couldn't have been better for the purpose of entertaining the audience. I couldn't have scripted it any better.

"You want to make your questions non-leading when regressing a person (so you are not leading the subject and creating experiences that are not theirs) and especially when on stage, so it doesn't appear to the audience that you are creating fictitious memories.

"Also, when regressing a person back to their childhood while on stage, talk to them in baby-talk. It almost always produces answers back in baby-talk. You don't need to do this with clinical hypnosis but it makes for better showmanship on stage.

"Last night's routine was performed for you—as part of your training— to show you how easy it is to make bad tasting food *taste* good and make terrible smelling things *smell* good. You can just as easily do it the other way: make things that taste and smell good taste and smell bad ... And also I wanted to show you that there is something to past-life regression.

"All right, that's enough about last night's stage-show. I now want to teach you how to clinically hypnotize a client, *the right way*, and lead you through a process to discover what is going on in a client's subconscious mind and show you how to help a client discover their inner-self.

"There are thousands of people out there who are trying to 'find themselves,' but they are looking in the wrong places. They go to seminars, attend retreats, go into hibernation or travel the world in an attempt to discern who they are and to find *their* purpose in life.

"In reality, if people want to 'find themselves' all they need to do is look into a mirror (to find their physical self) and look into their subconscious mind to find their inner self—to discover who they really are. And a person's purpose in life is not found but chosen.

"I want to now teach you how to do this by leading *you* through the process to create an 'inner room' where you will meet *your* 'inner self'—just like you are a client who wants to 'find himself.'"

Although I had made some significant progress in my quest for self-confidence, the thought of possibly "spilling my guts" still made me apprehensive, but I bit the bullet and consented to his request anyway. *Maybe I am becoming more self-confident, since a year ago I never would have agreed,* I thought.

Eric pointed to my recliner and I moved over into it, leaned back and made myself comfortable. Eric explained, "When working on stage you want to hypnotize people quickly, and you can do this because you have a number of people to choose from—you can pick and choose the ones who respond best to the hypnotic susceptibility tests. But when doing clinical hypnosis you don't have that luxury—you just take whoever comes in. So the induction process is quite different. I am going to teach you the right way to hypnotize a person clinically by leading *you* through the process.

"After going through a pre-hypnotic talk that explains what hypnosis is and what the client will experience during the session, the next step is to get them perfectly relaxed and in a peaceful, tranquil state of mind *and* body.

"To do this you want to create in their mind a peaceful and tranquil scene. When a person is in a peaceful and tranquil scene, whether in real life or in their imagination, their natural tendency is to feel and be peaceful and tranquil—a state of mind and body in which nothing matters except the scene—and when in this state their subconscious mind is open and receptive to suggestions."

Eric pulled his chair up close to my recliner, held a pendulum about a foot in front of my eyes and said in a singsong voice, "*Look at this pendulum as it swings and when your eyes become heavy and tired just close your eyes and listen to my voice. Just make yourself comfortable. While watching the pendulum swing take in a deep breath and hold it in while I count down, 5,4,3,2,1, and exhale. Now take in another deep breath and hold it in, 5,4,3,2,1, and exhale. And now take in another deep breath and hold it in 5,4,3,2,1, and exhale.*

I closed my eyes and Eric continued, "*Imagine yourself in a hammock that is stretched between two palm trees that are swaying in the breeze on a beautiful sandy beach.*

"*As you sway back and forth you relax deeper and deeper. The cool breeze feels good on your face and engenders a feeling of being at peace. Nothing matters now except the serenity of this tranquil place and my voice.*

"*The waves are rolling in and the smell of the ocean breeze produces a sense of calmness and comfortable composure. And as you experience this scene you are drifting into a deeper and deeper sleep.*

"*Each word I speak and the scene I describe takes you into a deeper and deeper hypnotic sleep.*

"*In this serene, tranquil setting the muscles of your entire body are relaxing now... just relaxing now. Your muscles are becoming loose and limp. Your mind is focused only on my voice. My voice is relaxing you deeper and deeper.*

"*You are aware of the sound of seabirds in the distance and the breaking of the waves relaxes you even more.*

"*And now the muscles in your fingers are relaxing ...*"

Eric went through a muscle-by-muscle relaxation procedure which was very similar to the one Art Baker had used to hypnotize his clients. When he had completed the scenario he said, "*Now moving out of your hammock and imagine in your mind that you are now standing at the top of a staircase. There are ten steps leading down to a passageway. Just to the right of the bottom landing is a door. In a moment I am going to ask you to descend the staircase step by step and by the time you have reached the landing you will be in a deep hypnotic state. At that point you will follow and carry out my instructions.*

"*Standing now at the top of the staircase, imagine it in every detail...create it just as you would like it to be. This is your staircase so take a moment and craft it to your liking—see every feature in detail.*"

Eric remained silent, giving me time to create a mental image of a staircase leading down and said, "*Describe to me your staircase and the door at the bottom.*"

I described what I was seeing. "The steps are solid stone curving downward against a curved stone wall on the right—like the turret of a castle—but there is no railing or banister on the left, just a straight down drop-off. At the bottom is a broad passageway that seems to be leading nowhere. On the right side of the bottom landing is an old, stout, weathered oaken door that is hinged on the left by massive strap-hinges and secured on the right with a heavy, rusty, iron slide-bolt."

This image is as vivid in my mind now as it was the first time I conjured it up—in view of the fact that I have visited this place many times since and still do. In fact, since I began writing this memoir I find myself visiting my inner room quite often in an attempt to recall the experiences of my life that began at birth over 72 years ago.

Eric continued. *"I want you to step down each step as I ask you to and at each step I will give you instructions about going deeper into hypnosis and the purpose of your inner room. When you reach the bottom landing I will ask you to open the door and step into your 'inner room.'*

"Your inner room is a place where you will meet yourself, discern your innermost thoughts, and discover hidden secrets that relate to a better understanding of yourself, the world you live in and truths of the universe.

"When you enter your inner room you will find the means to recover memories that have been lost, uncover mysteries that have been hidden, find answers to questions that have been puzzling you and give you insight into your inner self.

"Your inner room is decorated just as you would choose it to be–lavish, barren or anything in between. In your inner room you will meet a wise and discerning person who knows everything about you. This person knows everything you have ever done, all of your thoughts, your limitations, your abilities and your potential. This person is really you but in your mind he or she takes the form of a wise old sage."

"I believe I have already met my inner self on a few occasions, but I never thought of the events as being involved with another person. It was more like a thought-voice (the Sage) going on in my head," I told Eric.

"That is fine, but to have a 'person' with whom you can talk face-to-face makes the experience conversational so you can more easily pose questions and receive answers.

"In your inner room it doesn't necessarily have to be a person you meet (although for most people it is) but you will find the means whereby you can uncover your inner thoughts and find direction in your life."

Eric continued. *"Standing now at the top of your staircase, step down to step number ten... As you do, you can feel yourself relaxing even more.*

"Now down to step nine... In your inner room you will find nothing but peace and peace of mind.

"Stepping down now to step eight... You are drifting down now into an even deeper and deeper sleep.

"Now to step seven... While in your inner room you are able to find and converse with your inner self.

"Six... You are sinking now deeper and deeper into a hypnotic sleep.

"Five... You find your inner room to be comfortable, quiet and serene.

"Four... Your mind is clear and your body is relaxed.

"Three... In your inner room you find the means to reveal yourself... like meeting a person who knows everything about you and your innermost thoughts.

"Two... *Your mind is open and your thoughts clear.*

"*And one... Now step down onto the landing. It is as though you are actually standing in front of your old oaken door.*

"*In a moment I want you to unlatch the door and step into your inner room. When you do I want you to describe to me what you see. I also want you to describe the means whereby you are able to reveal yourself and get answers to your questions. If you meet a person, he or she can be fictitious, a person you know and admire, a historical personality or a clone of yourself. If it is a person you meet, ask for his or her name. If it is some other means to discover your inner self, describe to me what it is.*

"*The purpose of this session is not to pose any questions (except for discovering a name) or to find any answers; it is just to establish a connection with your inner self. In another session I will have you ask questions and probe for answers and insights. Or you can use self-hypnosis and do it by yourself.*

"*Open the door now and enter into your inner room and describe what you see and experience.*"

I reached out and slid the bolt to the left and when I stepped into my inner room it seemed the experience was actually happening. It took what seemed to be several minutes before I could articulate what was going on in my mind and when I finally spoke my voice came out in a whisper.

"It is a small room finished with stained panels on the walls and ceiling. There is a single window through which I can see an outer well-tended garden and the walls of the room are lined with bookcases that are packed full with books. The floor is covered with lush green carpeting and there is a large, polished, dark wood desk in the center of the room. There are a couple of chairs on one side of the desk and a robed, bearded, scruffy, but wise-looking man sitting on the other side of the desk who is looking at me with kind eyes."

"*Ask him for his name.*"

It took several minutes for me to ask, and when I did, I spoke again in a whisper. "How should I address you? What is your name?"

I got no answer. It seemed in my imaginary scene that time had slowed down as he just sat there and looked at me with warm, understanding eyes— like a slow-motion scene in a movie.

Eric prompted, "*If he doesn't give you a name, choose one for him. If he has a name you can use it speeds up the dialogue later on when you next visit him.*"

Let me see, what would be a fitting name for this old sage? I thought. "*Old Sage?*" *No, that doesn't work very well. Whom do I know who is wise, kind, intelligent and understanding? How about my father? No, I'd never reveal my inner self to him and for sure he doesn't know everything about me. How about Einstein? No, that doesn't quite fit—his scruffiness fits but I don't think that's the right name for him.*

179

How about Jesus or Moses? No, those don't quite fit, either. How about Eric? I think that that is what he is hoping for... but for sure that doesn't fit! The name "Socrates" popped into my mind... Socrates? I don't know much about Socrates except that he was an ancient Greek philosopher who seemed to have a lot to say...

Eric burst into my thoughts impatiently. *"Well, it's long enough; just choose a name so we can get on with it!"*

"Socrates! Socrates is his name," I said quickly.

"Fine. Now bid Socrates farewell, open the door to your inner room, step out of your inner room and close the door behind you. Now as I ask you to ascend the staircase step by step, listen to my instructions and when you reach the top step you will be wide awake, feeling wonderfully well and remembering everything you have experienced in flawless detail.

"Stepping up to the first step now.... As you do you are beginning to wake up now.

"As you step up to step two your memory of your inner room is vivid.

"Up to step three now... You are able to easily return to your inner room at any time, either by my direction or by yourself using self-hypnosis.

"Step four... Your mind is clear and your body is refreshed.

"Five... By using your inner room you are able to become enlightened and clearly discern truths that have until now eluded you.

"Six... The time spent in your inner room, although actually almost an hour, seems to you to have been just a few minutes, yet it still has had the value of a great deal of sleep.

"Step up to step seven... In your everyday life you are getting better and better in every way.

"Eight... Your mind is clear and your body refreshed.

"Nine... You use your inner room to improve your life and to understand your inner self and the world around you.

"And up to step ten... Wide awake now, feeling wonderfully well."

When I opened my eyes I truly felt like I had had a nice long nap but I remembered everything that Eric had said and that I had imagined; in fact, it was more like a real event that I had actually experienced.

This was the first time that I felt I had truly reached a hypnotic state.

Eric asked, "Well, how do you feel?"

"I feel great," I replied.

Eric said, "Whenever you do clinical hypnosis always ask the client how they feel when you wake them up. Sometimes the subject will have a headache or still feel drowsy. If they do, have them close their eyes and count them up again but more slowly; and after each number you count suggest to them that their headache is gone and that they feel refreshed and energetic."

He went on, "I don't know why it is, but quite often people have a headache after being hypnotized. Maybe it is because they have been exercising a part of their brain that is out of condition, having not used it a whole lot lately."

With that, Eric gathered up his stuff and left—just like at the end of a stage show.

Well that was an interesting experience, I pondered. *I think that I was truly hypnotized but it was different than I thought it would be. I was always completely conscious but at the time nothing mattered except my imaginary staircase and my inner room. I know it was my imagination and that Socrates was an extension of my own thinking, but in the moment it was happening it seemed to be very real—strange! I wonder if I can get back into my inner room by myself?*

When I looked at my watch I was surprised to discover that what I thought had been five or ten minutes had actually been an hour and a half!

I don't have time to go back into my inner room now; I'm running late for my sales appointments, I thought. *But I can't wait to get back into my inner room and meet myself and discover the answers to a thousand questions. I hope I can do it by myself...*

As it turned out, returning to my inner room, and visiting with Socrates, became central to the development of my understanding of the hypnotic process and developing my unique approach for using it. In some respects, Socrates became an essential guide and confidant as I sorted through endless questions, ideas, theories and paradoxes in my quest to understand why we humans behave as we do and how to change our behavior if we choose to.

CHAPTER 20

My Premiere Performance

During the next three weeks I learned a great deal about how to perform a successful stage-show and the wording to use when giving suggestions for more than twenty-five different routines. Eric also instructed me in conducting private sessions the "right way"—his way. But then things began falling apart. I discovered a flaw in Eric's personal behavior (other than his vainglorious boasting) that was probably the reason he fell short of being a highly successful stage-show hypnotist—alcohol.

With one weekend to go on our contract with David, during one of my training sessions (which turned out to be the last), Eric said to me, "I know that you don't drink but you might consider taking a shot of brandy before doing a stage-show. It will loosen you up and remove some of the stress of the performance. I perform best if I take a shot just before the show. I had sworn off booze *again* and have been sober for the past nine months, until we got this job at *David's*. I just didn't feel that I was operating at my peak performance, consequently, starting our second week I engaged once again in my long-standing tradition so I'd feel more relaxed; just one shot before each performance and that's all, I've promised myself."

In my opinion, quite the opposite was true. His performances during those first two weeks were outstanding. He hit the stage right on cue, his tux was neatly pressed and his suggestions were crisp, clear and coherent. The routines were entertaining and humorous, and Eric treated the volunteers with the greatest respect and made a beeline for the door after each performance.

By the end of third weekend, however, if a subject did not follow a routine exactly as he thought he or she should, he became critical and at times belligerent.

On both Thursday and Friday nights of the fourth and final week he showed up late and his tux was wrinkled. During the performance his speech was often slurred, at times he used vulgarity when giving suggestions and he hung around at the bar between and after performances.

Not only that, but many of the routines had degenerated to being off-color and crude. Often the suggestions embarrassed the volunteers (and in my opinion many in the audience, as well) and when the volunteers refused to carry his out his suggestions (probably because the suggestions violated the subject's moral or ethical standards) he became confrontational and critical and then sent them off the stage mid-routine. Also, our post-performance tutorial sessions ceased, as did any further training for clinical hypnosis.

Not only did David notice a decline in the quality of the shows but he also observed the nonexistent line of people at his door wanting to get in to see them.

After the fourth Thursday night performance David asked me, "Is Eric all right?"

"I don't know," I answered. "He's not as sharp as he was in the beginning and, at times, I'm embarrassed to be on stage with him. I'll talk to him and see if there's anything I can do."

To myself I thought, *I think he must be taking more than just* _one_ *shot of brandy before each performance.*

David went on to say, "Since you guys started doing your shows, business has been booming; you paid off your share of the advertising that first weekend, in addition to the several hundred dollars I've paid you in bonuses. I was considering an extension of your contract but as things are going right now I've changed my mind. Business is still better than it was before you started, but have you noticed the shift in the class of the clientele? Last weekend we bounced at least half a dozen unruly people, whereas the first two weeks we bounced none. My reputation of running a high-class nightclub is being eroded."

The next morning (Friday) I made an attempt to talk to Eric face-to-face but he didn't "have the time," so I had to express David's concerns about his performances, as well as my own, by phone.

"There is nothing wrong with my performances. It is not your place to be telling me—'the best stage-show hypnotist in the world'—how to do my job. It isn't my fault that the shows have not gone all that well; it's the riffraff volunteers—they are all a bunch of imbeciles and jerks," he said, and slammed down the receiver.

Needless to say, that night's performances were strained. Eric and I put up a good pretense of being civil towards one another, but underneath our deteriorating regard for each other was brewing mutual contempt.

Both shows that night were second-rate at best. Eric, after the first show, slipped out before I could approach him, and after the second show he quickly found a table around which were gathered what appeared to be some rather questionable-looking characters—Hell's Angels types. Before leaving I attempted to engage him in a conversation but was brushed off with a curt, "Can't you see I'm busy talking to my friends? I'll talk to you later." It appeared to me that he was doing more drinking than talking.

The next afternoon I had just finished up my first session with Jeanie (who had finally made an appointment to lose her 85 pounds) when the phone rang. The voice on the other end said, "This is Rich over at *David's.* Eric showed up just after I opened and has been here drinking ever since; he's drunk, has been buying drinks for everyone and is now creating a big disturbance. Would you come over and get him out of here before I call in the police?"

David's was only a couple of minutes from my office and when I arrived I saw Eric sitting at a table trying to hypnotize a woman—who looked just as inebriated as he was—by jabbing his fingers at the side of her throat and commanding her to sleep! Not surprisingly, it wasn't working very well and the few people who were in the nightclub at that time of the day were pleading for him to stop.

During one of my "advanced" hypnosis training sessions Eric had shown me a few "pressure points" that when jabbed, were suppose to induce instantaneous hypnosis without having to go through an "induction." His attempts to demonstrate its effectiveness on *me* never worked. Besides that, it was painful and intrusive.

He caught my eye when I walked up to his table and he spoke before I could get a word out. "What are *you* doing here? You're supposed to be at the office hypnotizing that fat woman. I'm practicing my advanced hypnosis techniques on this 'bi_ _ _' and she's not cooperating."

I took him by the arm and said, "People are complaining about how you are acting and I think we should leave now."

He angrily shrugged off my grasp and said, "I don't have to do anything *you* tell me to do. This is a fine way to treat your mentor. I tell you what to do; you don't tell me what to do. So just bug-off and leave me alone. I can take care of myself."

I retorted, "Rich called and asked me to come and get you out of here (I fudged a bit) before the police show up."

The instant I said "police" Eric jumped up, grabbed his belongings, and scrambled out the door as best he could in his condition.

Before leaving I apologized to the woman whom he had been accosting and found Rich and likewise apologized to him. By the time I made my way outside Eric had vanished.

I returned to the office, thinking that Eric would be there, but the place was empty. So I waited.... and I waited. I finally tried to call him at his boarding house. They said he had stopped by earlier, picked up his stuff, and left without a word. So I waited.... and I waited.

At 6:30 pm I went home and dressed for that night's performance, thinking for sure Eric would be at *David's* when I got there.

I arrived fifteen minutes early to an almost packed house, set everything up and then I waited. I was still waiting at 7:45 when David came up and said, "I hear that there was a disturbance here earlier today with Eric. I've been waiting for him to come in so I can tell him if he ever stops by here again, except for doing stage-shows, I'll call the police and have him thrown in jail for disturbing the peace. Not only that, but he left today before settling up a sizeable tab that piled up from last night and today. Where is he, by the way? He's fifteen minutes late. If he doesn't get here in the next ten minutes I hope that you are ready to step in."

My stomach gave a little lurch, but it was nothing like the pure panic I had experienced four weeks earlier when David spoke the exact same words.

I had none of the props that Eric carried around in his magical briefcase so I improvised: I asked Rich, who was still there, if he had anything like a cigar box and some candles. Luckily, he knew where the candles were and was able to find a shoebox in David's office. He also agreed to put some lemons and napkins in a container and said he would be willing to come up on stage and assist me in the falling backwards test. Finally I asked him, "And would you please keep an eye on the audience during the show and if you see anyone who looks like they are going into hypnosis, alert me?" He agreed to that, too.

I had been practicing the "candle under the hand" routine and discovered that it was mostly a trick. It can be done without using self-hypnosis, and without causing any burning of flesh or blistering if it is done right—it's just that with self-hypnosis it is more comfortable, and making it appear like hypnosis is causing it makes it more entertaining. What I had learned was that if you hold the flame of the candle very close to your hand (so your hand is in the flame), then the lack of oxygen makes the flame not as hot as it would be if it had sufficient air; and if your hand is moist with perspiration (which mine certainly was for this surprise performance!) some of the heat is absorbed by warming up the moisture; and if you move the flame in a circular motion so the heat is not concentrated in one spot, then the discomfort is tolerable and doesn't create a blister. And, because there is a lack of oxygen the combustion is incomplete so the flame produces excessive soot that you can then display to the audience. (Just in case you, the reader, would like to try it someday...)

"Ladies and gentlemen, please give me your attention. My name is Lindsay Brady, not yet the 'greatest stage-show hypnotist in the world...' but I'm working on it!"

What I said produced a chuckle from the audience. Apparently there were a few people who had attended previous performances so they caught my attempt at some humor at Eric's expense.

"I have been studying to be a stage-show hypnotist under the tutelage of Dr. Eric, who *is* the world's greatest stage-show hypnotist...at least in his opinion."

There were a lot more chuckles from the audience.

I wonder if the people in the audience have arrived at the same conclusion about Eric that I have—that he is pompous and self-lauding, I thought.

"Unfortunately, Dr. Eric is unable to be here tonight so I will be presenting tonight's performance in his stead.

"Hypnosis is a powerful tool that can be used to help make positive changes in a person's daily life, like quitting the smoking habit; losing weight or enhancing performance in sports, profession or school. But tonight I will be using it to entertain you by taking you on an adventure into the realm of the subconscious mind. Tonight I will be presenting 'The Best of Dr. Eric.' I have asked David's day-time manager, whom many of you know as 'Rich' (I didn't know his last name), to assist me in Dr. Eric's absence.

"In a moment I will be calling for volunteers to come up to the stage.

"But first let me demonstrate to you how the powers of my subconscious mind can eliminate the feeling of physical pain."

The candle demonstration went well but after I had put out the candle and had shown the audience the soot on the palm of my hand, over a congenial applause I heard someone call out, "Aren't you going to do that 'ice pick-up-your-nose' demonstration?"

I retorted, "It is interesting that you ask, but the answer is 'No.' No disrespect to Dr. Eric, but I've always found that demonstration to be a little uncouth."

There seemed to be a consensus; I was relieved to hear a couple of "me, too's" from the audience.

The fact that I had generated some audience interaction put me a little more at ease.

"I am now calling for volunteers from the audience. If you volunteer, come up with the intention of being hypnotized."

To my surprise at least twenty people volunteered. I invited them one by one to come up on stage, asked them their first name, and as best as I could, made an association with the name and plugged it into my memory bank for later use. As each volunteer came up on stage I had them stand a foot in front of me and said, *"Look into my eyes,"* and as well as I could, did an eyebrow-raised, glassy-eyed impersonation of Eric that I had often observed but had never practiced.

"You are beginning to fall back now... Rich is stationed right behind you to catch you..."

Rich did a great "on the spur of the moment" job of catching each potential subject as they fell back into his arms, and then escorting them to one of the chairs when I gave him a nod. The ones that didn't fall backwards I sent back down to their tables.

When all ten chairs were occupied I said into the mic, "I appreciate the response to my request for volunteers but the necessary subjects have been selected, so would the remaining volunteers please return to your seats, enjoy the show and also enjoy a few drinks? But please stick around for tonight's second show and volunteer then to participate in the final scheduled hypnosis show here at *David's*.

"As you may suspect, I am hoping that Dr. Eric has been only briefly detained and that he will be here for tonight's second performance, but for now bear with me and enjoy my premier performance as a stage-show hypnotist."

Again to my surprise a round of applause came from the audience and a few people even stood up while applauding their encouragement. But I knew that it was out of sympathetic support and not because of my reputation as a renowned stage-show hypnotist.

I did the "clasped hand" test and the "your arms are like a bar of steel" test. Again to my surprise there was applause and a few shouts of encouragement from the audience.

Every stage-show hypnotist has to have a first performance, but most of them start with a few familiar people in a private setting and the participants are friends or friends of friends who have been invited for the purpose of being practiced on.

But here I was up on stage with almost two-hundred strangers looking at me—and a few antagonists, I was sure. Most of them had either witnessed Eric's performance firsthand, or had at least heard about "the greatest stage-show hypnotist in the world." All I was hoping for was to not fall flat on my face or present a disappointing, mediocre performance.

"Now your arms are getting very, very heavy..." When I had finished the hypnosis induction and all of the volunteers were relaxed and leaning against

one another with their eyes closed, I said to Maria as I touched her on the head (I remembered her name because she reminded me of Natalie Wood, who played Maria in *West Side Story*), "*Maria, open your eyes and fix your gaze only on my eyes.*"

She did as I asked so I went on. "*Maria, as you can see, I have in my hand a shoebox. It is a magical shoebox. In a moment when I hand it to you, you will take it over to the side of the stage, sit down on the floor and open its lid. When you do, you will be amazed at what you see. When you remove the lid you will see a bunch of little people in the box having a party. They will be singing and dancing and having a grand old time. You have two jobs: The first is to describe to the audience in detail what is going on in the party-box and your second job is, if any of the party-goers get out of the box (which from time to time they will), you will gather them up and return them to the box party so none of them get stepped on by the big people on stage. Later on, when I call you by name and snap my fingers, you will wake up immediately and return to your table wondering what has been going on.*"

I handed Maria the shoebox. She took it to the side of the stage, sat down, and as she opened the lid I put the mic down close to her mouth so everyone could hear what she had to say.

"Carumba! There are little people in this box and they are having a fiesta. There is a mariachi band and (pointing down into the box) this little guy is doing the Mexican hat dance. And over there are some children; one of them is blindfolded and is swinging at a piñata with a stick. People are standing around clapping their hands and tapping their toes in time with the music. Some of the others are just sitting around sipping on their margaritas.

"Oops, one hombre just jumped out of the box! I think that he is heading to the bar to get some more tequila... but that's such a long way for such a little fellow. No, he has a little burro tied up over there on the chair leg. Everyone stay where you are so you don't step on him! I'll grab him."

She put the lid back on the box (apparently to keep the other people from escaping) and scrambled on her knees over to the chair, scooped up the runaway in cupped hands and shouted to the bartender, "Can you send over a shot glass of tequila for this party? I think one will be plenty; they are such little people they probably won't drink much." She opened the box and said, "Pedro, you stay in the box; I've sent out for a supply of tequila."

As Maria was snatching up a few more runaways, one of the cocktail waitresses brought over a glass of tequila and handed it to Maria, who set it in the box and said as she looked down, "This is enough to keep you guys drunk for a year... You're welcome! De nada!

"Why are you guys trying to get out of the box? Don't you know there's free tequila over there?" she asked as she brushed a few other escapees back into the box.

"What is it, Pedro? What do you mean—it's vodka? Let me have it."

In the blink of an eye she grabbed the shot glass, gulped down its contents in a single swig and said, "You're right, that is vodka! Let me see if I can get you the right stuff."

How she knew it was vodka and not tequila still puzzles me—maybe she could smell the difference when she took it from the barmaid.... Or maybe the bartender had actually sent tequila but just went with the flow of the scenario; I'll never know. But whatever the cause, it made for an unexpected twist in the routine.

She glared over at the bartender and shouted, "You gave us vodka, not tequila. You send over the right stuff!"

The bartender shouted back, "I didn't think it would make any difference since they are just pretend people, anyway. You're lucky that I didn't send water!"

Maria jumped up, stomped her foot down hard on the stage floor and with her hands on her hips and leaning in his direction shouted back, in an exaggerated Spanish accent, "*You better send tequila this time. I know David and I'll have you fired and then thrown in the pokey if you don't!*"

The audience was howling throughout the act, and was engrossed in Maria, the little people in the box and her dialogue with the bartender; there was hardly a moment devoid of laughter and sniggering.

The bartender sent another glass. Maria sniffed it and said, "That's better; gracias." Then she placed the glass in the box.

Remembering what Eric said about not letting a routine run too long, I called Maria by name and snapped my fingers; Maria made the customary little jerk, looked at me, got up from the floor and headed off of the stage. But just before she got to the stage steps she stopped, turned around, went back to the box, bent down, grabbed the shot glass of tequila and gulped it down in one gulp, turned around and with a little wobble to her step teetered off the stage and returned to her table.

When she ambled to her seat there was a vigorous round of applause, but it seemed that she was oblivious to the accolade.

Wow! That went well, I thought. Emboldened by the success of Maria's suggestions I considered, *I wonder if I dare try the "forget your name, can't add, subtract or spell" routine?*

I turned to Alex, placed my hand on his head and said, "*Alex, open your eyes and look at me.*"

190

Although I still had some doubts about my prowess as a stage-show hypnotist (with only one successful routine under my belt) I daringly thought, *All I need to do is to give the suggestions exactly as I saw and heard Eric give them and then the volunteers should follow and carry out <u>my</u> instructions just as well as they would if it were Eric giving the suggestions.*

Alex did as I asked so I went on and said, "*You look to be an intelligent person, am I right?*"

"Well, I like to think am."

"*What do you do for a living?*"

My heart sank a little (and all of a sudden he didn't look quite as intelligent as I had thought) when he said, "I'm a truck driver. I haul concrete to construction sites." But I recovered in an instant when he added, "But I am going to school at night and majoring in Psychology."

"*Well, in that case, when I snap my fingers you will no longer be able to remember or say your last name. Nor will you be able to add, subtract or spell correctly. When I snap my fingers again you will be wide awake, feeling wonderful and you will be able to remember your last name and be able to add, subtract and spell better than you ever have.*"

Luckily I had once again chosen the right volunteer for these suggestions—he turned out to be perfect!

Alex was more amused than puzzled when he could not recall or say his last name, and his hearty laughter and enthusiastic animations infected everyone in *David's*. The audience broke into uncontrollable laughter—even giddiness.

When I asked him to add, subtract and spell he was even more animated. He tried using his fingers to decipher how many are left if you take two away from three, but was unable to come up with an answer. It sent him into hysterics when he was unable to figure it out and he kept shaking his head in puzzlement. Again his antics spun off into the audience—they were out of control.

And in an attempt to spell "cat" he came up with "F-e-l-i-n-e? I know what a cat is, but feline has too many letters. T-i-g-e-r? No, that's a big one of those. K-i-t-t-e-n? No, that's a little one... I've got it! If kitten starts with a "k" then it must be K-A-T!"

I remember Eric telling me that sometimes you just strike it lucky and get the right person for the routine. That was definitely the case with both Maria and Alex. *What great luck!* I thought.

Thinking that if Alex stayed in this absent-minded mode for a while he might even interact with people in the audience and make the routine more entertaining, I improvised my earlier suggestion and said to him, "*Alex, ignore my earlier suggestions about waking up and accept these new suggestions.*

"When I snap my fingers you will return to your table, but will still be in your forgetful state. When you return to your seat you will try to explain your lapse of memory to your friends and people around you. As you do, you will just find your condition to be all the more amusing. When you hear the clap of my hands and hear me say 'WIDE AWAKE' you will wake up immediately, feeling wonderfully well and wonder what has been going on. And of course, you will be able to remember your last name and be able to add, subtract and spell better than ever before."

[SNAP]

Alex shook his head with a few little jerks, like he was trying to clear out the cobwebs after awakening from a deep sleep. He then headed back to his seat, giggling to himself as he went. When he reached his table and tried to explain what he was experiencing, his animations and mirth spilled over into an already delirious audience.

I waited a few minutes for the scene in the audience to unfold on its own and then turned to the remaining volunteers and said, "When I clap my hands and say, "WIDE AWAKE" you will open your eyes and return to your table. But when you sit down you will immediately jump up and shout, 'The redcoats are coming; the redcoats are coming!' After you have shouted, 'The redcoats are coming, the redcoats are coming' you will wake up immediately, feeling wonderfully well and wondering what all of the shouting is about."

[CLAP]

"Everyone, WIDE AWAKE!"

The commotion around Alex's table abruptly ceased and the remaining volunteers stood up, stretched their arms and returned to their seats. And over an occasional shout of, "The redcoats are coming, the redcoats are coming," over the microphone I thanked Rich for assisting me and thanked the audience for their charitable attention and applause "on this, my premier performance as a stage-show hypnotist."

As Rich and I left the stage there was a standing ovation from most of the crowd. Although I was sure that the applause was as much empathy as it was recognition for the performance, I was still pleased to receive compliments from almost everyone we passed on our way to David's office, where we were headed in the hopes that there was some information about Eric's whereabouts. There was none, however. So I asked Rich if he'd assist me again at the second performance, and he agreed.

"Well in that case, let's go over to my office and we'll establish a telepathic link between our minds," I told him.

Rich exclaimed, "What do you mean? I don't have any psychic powers! Sure, I sent you that letter that one time, but that was only once out of a hundred tries and I really think it was just by chance anyway and had nothing to do with telepathy. I don't think I could do it a second time in a million years."

"Well you are right, you probably don't have any telepathic powers and neither do I, but the audience doesn't know that! And I can easily teach you how to make it appear as though we do."

When we arrived at my office there was still neither a sign of Eric nor any sign that he had been there. So I handed Rich a pad and pen and said, "We'll do it just like Eric and I did it."

"We'll each have our own microphone. I'll be out in the audience and you'll be up on stage and I'll announce to the crowd, 'We will now demonstrate the psychic and telepathic powers of the subconscious mind.'

"I'll ask someone for a dollar bill, gather a few people around me so they can see the serial number and ask them to confirm that you respond with the correct number. We'll take each number one by one.... And we will try to look and act like we are truly sending messages telepathically.

"Now, when you hear me say 'Are you ready?' and you respond 'Yes,' that is a signal that the *first* letter of the *next* word I speak is the 'key letter' that represents a number.

"To illustrate: the number '*one*' is represented by the letter '*o*'—as in '*o*nce, *o*h or *o*ver'—because the word '*one*' starts with the letter '*o*.' So when I ask, 'Are you ready?' you'll respond, 'Yes.' If the first letter of the next word I speak begins with the letter '*o*,' you will respond back, 'One.'

"So if I say, 'Are you ready?' and you answer, 'Yes' and then I say, '*O*n this first number you should have no problem,' you will know that you are to come back with '*O*ne.'

"Does that make sense?"

Rich said, "I think so."

And I went through the entire process for him. After he had finished writing each "key letter" down I asked, "Do you get the picture now?"

He answered, "Yes. That seems too simple. Why didn't I catch it when Eric and you were doing it? Give me a minute to think about it. I think I can easily establish the associations."

After a few moments, we went through a test session and it was clear that Rich had caught on perfectly.

We practiced both the letters and numbers a few times and then I said, "I think there's a hypnosis stage-show about ready to start in twenty minutes so I think we'd better be getting to it. If Eric has shown up let me thank you in advance for your time. If he doesn't show, this should be a lot of fun."

CHAPTER 21

My Second Performance

Just as we headed out the door for *David's*, Rich grabbed my arm and said, "I don't think I can do this—you don't know how terrified and self-conscious I was when you asked me to help you earlier. Up until two hours ago I had never been on a stage in front of an audience in my entire life, and now I'm going to have to talk into a microphone—which is something I'm terrified of and have never done except the other night when Eric had me say a few words. I still cringe when I think about it.

"I should have told you how frightening it is for me to just think about being on stage, let alone having to say anything into a microphone. I wish I had told you earlier before you spent all this time teaching me to do this telepathic thing. I'm afraid when I get up there I'll choke up and be unable to speak a word, let alone remember which key letters represent which numbers. That would be so embarrassing, especially when most of the people in the audience know who I am. Right now I'm really wishing I hadn't agreed to do it at all. I'm so nervous. Having to talk into a microphone is a lot different than just catching a few people when they start falling backwards...." Rich was so agitated that he could barely catch his breath between sentences.

I did my best to calm him down. "I can relate to how you are feeling; I felt exactly the same way that first night at *David's*. I'm sure you'll do fine. Besides, you've seen every show Eric and I performed, so you know exactly what to expect and probably know Eric's routines as well as I do. Maybe I should be assisting you!"

He laughed, but winced at even the thought of it and said, "That would scare me to death. I'd be petrified if I had to be in charge and in the center of what was going on!

"I make friends easily and I'm very good at managing David's nightclub but even that was getting to be a drag until you and Eric showed up a month ago. Then I started wondering if I'd ever have the courage to get up on a stage and perform. That's why I stick around after my working hours—just to watch you guys up there having fun and envying the fact that you're doing something you really love doing, and not only that but you're getting paid for doing it.

"When I'm around my close friends I can be a real 'cut-up'— I have a quick wit and can make them laugh when I choose—but when I get around strangers I just clam up, especially if there are a bunch of them. If I could only be as comfortable in front of a group of people as you and Eric, it would be a miracle. My friends tell me that I have a lot of talent and that I'm really good at playing my guitar and singing. I've even written a few little ditties that are just jokes I've put to music... And everyone thinks they are truly clever and funny. My friends tell me that I ought to join a group or start my own band, but I'd never be able to do that because it would mean I'd have to get up in front of a bunch of people and talk or sing into a microphone. Have you ever heard a recording of your own voice? Once some of my friends were fooling around with a tape recorder and my voice just happened to be on it. When I heard my voice I was horrified. How awful my voice sounds is all I can think about when I even consider performing in front of an audience."

I told him that I had the same feelings when I first heard my recorded voice. "All I can remember is that it sounded like my brother but with a clothes pin on my nose, and every fifth word I spoke was interrupted with 'and a-a-ah... and a-a-ah...'"

Then a flash of inspiration hit me. "We have fifteen minutes before we need to be at *David's*. Sit down in my recliner and let's see if we can get rid of some of your stage fright and microphone phobia by hypnotizing you...."

Rich and I arrived back at *David's* just in time to get everything set up, and as we moved among the crowd, hooking up the extension microphone and getting a supply of fresh lemons and napkins, we were frequently interrupted with congratulations on our earlier performance. They were as complimentary about Rich's contribution as mine.

As we were setting up the stage chairs Rich said, "I don't understand why they are complimenting me. All I did was catch a few people before they hit the floor, then just stood around and watched the audience."

I replied, "Well, I wondered the same thing while assisting Eric. I got numerous compliments for the fine performance, when in fact I did almost nothing. I guess just the fact that a person is on stage leads the audience to think they played a major part, regardless of what they actually did."

David must have caught bits of our conversation because when he approached us he said, "That was a fantastic show. Both of you guys did a wonderful job and put on a grand performance. I've heard nothing but compliments about it."

He looked at me and continued, "You didn't seem all that enthusiastic about doing the show when I said you had better get ready to stand in for Eric, but once you got started you didn't look nervous at all. If you'd been wearing Eric's tux, and if you hadn't told everyone that it was your first performance, they'd have thought you'd been doing stage shows for years. I don't know why you think you need Eric!"

And then he turned to Rich (I am sure to bolster his courage) and said, "And you, Rich, I didn't know you had it in you. I didn't think you had the courage to even go up on the stage, let alone do that catching thing with all of those people looking at you, especially since we've talked about your anxieties about being in front of an audience. You do an excellent job managing this place when I'm not here, but I never thought I'd see you on stage. You really looked comfortable and confident up there."

David gave me a curious look (as did Rich) when I said, "Just wait until you see him do the telepathic routine with me. That's what we have been doing between shows—establishing a psychic link between our minds. If you think he was good at catching people you will never believe how good he is at receiving telepathic messages! I'm sure that he'll turn into a real showman once he gets into it."

In fact, Rich's desire to be a performer, and to be comfortable on stage and to be rid of his microphone phobia, coupled with the fifteen minutes of hypnotherapy and the suggestions—"You are as outgoing and as comfortable on stage as you are around your friends. On stage you are uninhibited and you view the audience as being your closest friends. You use your natural wit and creative talent to find ways to entertain the audience and make them laugh. And you like hearing the sound of your voice when talking into a microphone"—had made an astonishing transformation in him.

So when the music stopped and we were on our way to the stage I asked Rich, "Do you want to introduce me?"

But he turned white and said, "No!"

It wasn't until after the performance that I realized that all of the suggestions I had given to Rich were contingent on "while you are on stage" and since we were not yet on stage he was still in his timid, inhibited mode.

So the DJ handed the stage mic to me. I took it and said, "Ladies and gentlemen, may I have your attention, please..... May I please have your attention?"

When things had quieted down a bit I said, "Dr. Eric is still among the missing so you'll have to put up with Rich and me for this final scheduled hypnosis stage-show performance here at *David's*—now the most popular nightclub in the Salt Lake Valley!"

I knew that I had been lucky to have selected the right subjects for the right routines at the earlier performance—the show went better than I could have ever dreamed—but I was shocked at the enthusiastic applause and shouts of approval when I announced that Rich and I would be doing this show, too.

I responded to the applause with a slight bow and a few thank you's and then I gestured toward Rich, who, to my surprise, made a deeply exaggerated bow that drew smiles and laughter from the crowd—it seemed so much out of character for him.

After the applause and tittering had quieted down I said, "On several occasions some of you have requested that Eric and I do the telepathic demonstration routine again—which we did. I think that some of you believe it involves some kind of trickery and you've been trying to figure it out. To demonstrate that such a link can be established between any two minds (if you know the secret), Rich and I have been practicing to create such a connection, and I think we've successfully accomplished it. So in a moment I will come down among you, ask one of you for a dollar bill and see if Rich can successfully distinguish my messages from all of the other thoughts that are going on and correctly reveal the serial number."

I made my way down to the crowd, asked a fellow for a dollar bill, gathered a few people around me and then asked them to shout "Yes" or "No" depending on the correctness of Rich's response.

"Are you ready?"

"Yes."

I put my fingers to my forehead while "sending" Rich the "message" and said, "For this first number take your time... Tell me when you have received it."

Rich put his fingertips to his head as though he was in deep concentration. Although he was doing exactly what I had just said—"take your time"—his hesitation was much longer than I thought it should be. Fearing that his stage fright had kicked in and his brain had frozen up (and that the fifteen-minute hypnosis session hadn't made any difference, after all) I asked, "Do I need to send it again?"

I was very relieved when Rich cleared his throat a couple of times and said into his mic, "No! I mean, yes I have received it; the number is 'four.'"

Not only did the group gathered around me shout, "YES," but there were other "yes's," coupled with a few "he did it's," coming primarily from the bartenders and cocktail waitresses. I think they were amazed that Rich was on stage to begin with and were flabbergasted that he possessed "psychic powers."

This enthusiastic response seemed to spark something inside Rich—it was almost like a switch had been thrown that sent shock waves into his psyche and had awakened a quiescent entertaining genius that had been sleeping inside his being.

"Are you ready?"

"Yes."

"This number should give you no problem, either."

His "receiving" act was a little more dramatized this time, he said, "You are right, you sent this number loud and clear. The number is 'two.'"

"Are you ready?"

"Yes."

"If our telepathic link is open you should have this one by now."

He responded, "Debbie (Debbie was a cocktail waitress who had joined in with the group of 'confirmers'), stop trying to send the wrong number like you did when Eric was here! Try being nice or I'll have you fired!" Still talking to Debbie, Rich said, "The number is not 'eight'; the right number is 'six.'"

Debbie was amazed that he knew she was thinking eight. I put my mic close to her mouth so the audience could hear her response: "How did you know I was thinking eight? You really *are* telepathic!" (Rich told me afterward that "eight" [her birthday] was her favorite number and that she had been trying to send me the number eight while *I* was doing the "receiving." He just took a chance that she was using it again.) As you can imagine, the audience whooped with delight. Many of the clientele knew Rich and seemed to be astounded at what they were witnessing.

"Are you ready?"

"Yes."

"Once in a while someone is successful in sending a different number, just as you did with Eric and me that one time, but I think you have already sorted out the right number this time. Am I right?"

"Yes I have it, but I am still wondering how this is possible. I never before believed in mental telepathy or thought that I had any telepathic powers. But the number is 'one.'"

After that response, it was evident that even some of the skeptics in the audience were becoming believers.

"Are you ready?"

"Yes."

"Everyone, I am sure, is amazed by your psychic powers by now. What is the number I am sending?"

Rich was even more animated now. He put both hands to his head, looked upward and then closed his eyes. "I think I have it now. The number is 'three.'"

"Are you ready?"

"Yes."

Because Rich was getting into making the routine more theatrical, I did too. Mimicking Rich's animation I said, "Think, as I send this number. I'm sending it now."

"You've got to be kidding! You sent me another 'two,' didn't you?"

"Are you ready?"

"Yes."

"In everyone's telepathic career a person is bound to make at least one mistake. I hope this one isn't yours!"

"If you send it right, I'll receive it right. Are you trying to justify that one time you messed up? The number is 'six.'"

"Are you ready?"

"Yes."

"Get this last number right and you'll be batting a thousand. Do you have it?"

"Yes, I do. If people only knew how easy it is to receive telepathic messages, they'd be doing it all the time. The number is 'eight!'"

The audience applauded and cheered as Rich took a deep "chivalrous" bow. And then I heard someone in the audience say, "What about the letters? What about the letters?"

I always thought that Eric had just feigned that someone had asked for the letters, just to give the routine a little more flair, but in this case I didn't have to.

I said into my mic, "So you want the letters, too? Rich, are you up to receiving the letters of the serial number, too? If not, we can stop now and the audience will still be amazed at your telepathic powers."

Rich replied into *his* mic, "Are you kidding? I'm on a roll.... Isn't this fun? Yes, I think I can easily do it if you will just send the letter instead of babbling on about it."

"In that case... Are you ready?"

"Yes."

"Now, having put all of that effort into establishing our telepathic communication, don't mess it up. Do you have the letter yet?"

Rich hesitated, rolled his eyes back, closed his eyelids, and began, "Did you send... ah... ah... I think that it just came through... it is... is 'h!'"

No one even shouted, "Yes!" They just howled and cheered.

"Are you ready?"

"Yes."

"If anything is going to make you famous it will be getting this last letter right. Did you receive it yet?"

By this time Rich was more than going with the flow of the routine and, in my opinion, went to the extreme on this last letter when he dropped to his knees, stretched out his arms towards heaven, as though looking for inspiration from some deity, and said, "Thank you, oh telepathic spirit who dwells in the ether. The letter is 'a!'

Needless to say, the crowd had been more entertained by Rich's antics than they were by the demonstration of "telepathy" itself.

It was at that moment that I understood that there are naturally gifted entertainers and then there are those of us who are not. *I* could have employed that same kind of creativity when performing with Eric, but it didn't even enter my mind and even if it had, it would probably have been forced and awkward—but for Rich it was free and natural.

For the remainder of the show I did a few of the routines that I had memorized. I used Eric's routine of the "lemon tastes like an orange," Reveen's routine of "you can no longer remember or say the number six" (the subject counted his fingers but kept coming up with eleven of them) and for the finale did the "cats, dogs, chickens and ducks" routine.

All of the routines went especially well, but it wasn't the volunteers or me who were responsible for the audience's delirium; it was Rich! He not only helped me with the show; he *was* the show!

When I asked him to gather up the lemons and napkins he not only gathered them but as he took the slice from one of the volunteers he squeezed a drop on his tongue, turned to the audience and mouthed *"lemon"* as he pointed to it and winced dramatically. And when he picked up and tasted Ann's (the subject who thought the lemon was an orange), he looked at the audience and spun his finger around his ear in a gesture of lunacy as he nodded in her direction, squeezed a drop of her "orange" on his tongue and said, *"lemon."*

And when Homer kept coming up with eleven fingers, Rich, to no avail, tried to coach him by counting Homer's fingers and coming up with ten. Homer shook his head with a gesture of confusion, tried again, but still came up with eleven. Rich's gestures, facial expressions and physical animations turned *David's* into a madhouse.

And when I suggested the barnyard scenario, Rich was in his element. He patted the St. Bernard on its head and mouthed "nice doggy." And then for a moment, squatted down, put his hands into his armpits, flapped his imaginary wings and waddled around trying to out-quack a duck that was waddling around the stage.

He took the mic out of my hand, went over to a crowing rooster, pointed to his watch and said, "It's almost eleven o'clock at night, you're not supposed to be crowing in the middle of the night," and handed the mic back to me just before he checked under the clucking hen to see if there was an egg and said, "Nope!"

As I observed Rich's antics, I realized that when I had hypnotized him earlier I hadn't bothered to go through any kind of waking up procedure. I had just said, "Open your eyes and let's get over to *David's* and make this last stage-show a blowout." *I wonder if Rich is acting this way because he is still hypnotized*, I thought. *He's acting exactly as I suggested he would act. I wonder if he will continue on with this same uninhibited stage presence for the rest of his life, even when I wake everyone up–I hope so.*

As I was thinking this, Rich was attempting to calm down a squabble between a Persian cat and a yapping terrier. He stroked the cat on the head and shook his finger at the terrier and said, "Bad doggy... bad doggy!"

And then I snapped my fingers and said, "Everyone, WIDE AWAKE!"

Everyone on the stage and in the audience went silent. When each volunteer left the stage they were greeted with a round of applause. But when Rich walked off, the jubilation hit the roof with a deafening standing ovation. Halfway down the stage steps Rich did a few of his deep bows and waved to the crowd. *I guess the hypnosis stuck*, I thought.

As Rich was trying to make it to David's office amid the congratulations I said into the microphone, "Wasn't he great?" I intentionally delayed leaving the stage by busying myself, replacing the mic on its stand and moving the chairs off stage, in an effort to not distract from Rich's triumphant performance.

While doing this I thought to myself, *Maybe I'm not made of the right stuff to be a great stage-show entertainer. I think I can be an okay performer, but I'm not sure I have the personality to be a great entertainer. Eric and Rich are naturals at entertaining but for these two performances, for the most part, I just went through the motions... Maybe I can learn to loosen up and become as creative and entertaining as Eric and Rich.*

Eventually I made it to David's office through the congratulations and backslaps and question after question. It was then that I understood why Eric, when he was at the top of his form, made straight for the door after the performance—to avoid the endless questions people have if you hang around.

When I entered David's office he was shaking his head in disbelief and vigorously shaking Rich's hand as he was saying, "Now that was a *real* performance. Really, I had no idea that you were such a ham. And where have you been hiding all of that wit? I think you ought to bring in your guitar and entertain the crowd sometime."

David turned to me and said (with no mention of the performance), "Stop by Monday morning and I'll have a check ready for you. By then I will have had a chance to go through this week's receipts and figure the bonus I owe you, but I'll have to deduct several hundred dollars to cover Eric's tab from the last two nights and this afternoon's bender. I don't know how we ever let him run up that size of a bill. He was buying drinks left and right for all his biker friends the last couple of nights as though there was going to be no tomorrow."

He then added, "If you are still doing stage-show hypnosis in six months, give me a call and I'll make the same deal with you, so long as Eric is not involved. But I think the hypnosis stage-show for the time being has run its course here at my club."

After shaking his hand and thanking him for his business, and especially for manipulating me into doing my first stage-show performance, I headed straight home with a sense of accomplishment for having achieved a feat (performing hypnosis on stage) that only a month and a half earlier was hardly a flicker in my imagination as a possibility.

Sunday was a day of peace and contentment, but then came Monday—a shocker.

CHAPTER 22

Parting
of the Ways

When on Monday morning I stopped by David's to pick up the check he asked, "To whom should I make this out to, Eric or you?"

It seemed strange that he had to ask and when I told him to make it out to Positive Suggestion Institute he acted a little confused but then said, "Oh you mean PSI." I told him yes and left with a check for around $800 in hand (Eric had engaged in much more drinking and intoxicating his friends than even David had guessed—over five hundred dollars!) and headed for my office.

I don't remember if I was hoping Eric would be at my office or hoping that he wouldn't be there, but when I opened the door what I saw shocked me to the core—my office had been trashed. It looked like one of those scenes from a spy movie after the bad guys had ransacked the heroine's apartment looking for the microfilm.

The incriminating evidence that Eric was the culprit came from his missing certificates that had been torn off the wall. He must have hung them with extra-heavy-duty sticky-on-both-sides tape because not only had the paint come off with their removal but chunks of the plaster had been pulled out in the process, leaving big pock-marks in the sheetrock.

Fortunately, or maybe unfortunately, two days before I had received in the mail PSI's first month's bank statement and, just on a whim, had taken it home unopened, along with the PSI checkbook, with the intention of reconciling them over the weekend (which I had neglected to do).

Probably the checkbook is what Eric was looking for when he emptied all of the drawers and the bookshelves of their content, I thought.

I surmised that Eric had heard from his cronies (some of whom I had noticed in the audience Saturday night) that the stage-show went on without him, and in a drunken (or hung-over) rage went to the office in search of the checkbook and when unable to find it took out his frustrations on my belongings.

After I had put my office back in order I began reconciling PSI's checkbook and the bank statement. When I opened the checkbook at first glance it appeared that no checks had been written and the only entries in the checkbook registry totaled $1150 ($100 initial deposit, $50 for two of my clinical sessions and $1,000 from *David's* for the first week's performance). Thinking that Eric had deposited David's other checks as he received them (and had just neglected to enter them in the checkbook register) I figured that there should be at least $3,150 in the account and maybe more with our override... and then I opened the statement. To my dismay, I not only discovered the statement but three canceled checks and an ending balance of only $147.50!

In that era the actual canceled checks were returned in the envelope with the bank statement, so to my consternation all three checks had been made out to Eric and endorsed by Eric for cash. But the first three checks in the checkbook were still in place. Upon closer examination, I discovered the returned checks were from back further in the checkbook. It appeared that Eric had used checks from the middle of the checkbook to camouflage the fact that he had written them.

The first two canceled checks were for $450.00 each with the notation: Tuxedo rental $150/night—three nights. I knew that Eric owned his tux but probably justified the rental (although greatly inflated) because he would have had to rent one if he had not owned one—so he rented it from himself. The third check was for $100—Travel expenses and props.

As I thought it through, David's confusion about to whom the check should be written now made sense: The first check for $1,000 had been made out to PSI so Eric had to deposit it in the account but then I surmised that he asked David to make the other checks out to him personally and then cashed them!

I was dumbfounded. I couldn't believe my gullibility and my naiveté for having not kept better track of what was going on with PSI's finances. I had just *assumed* that Eric was depositing the checks from David and that he had written no checks—*there you go assuming again*, I said to myself.

As I considered my ransacked office, it dawned on me that Eric was not only looking for the checkbook, because it was large enough to be easily found, but he had probably been searching for the statement that he knew would contain incriminating evidence. He probably justified his actions by rationalizing that he *was* PSI's treasurer and should have access to both the checkbook and the statement.

But, it was really strange that I wasn't angry. And then I realized why: Since, in my mind, I am dead at the bottom of a cliff, then the occurrence of this experience really doesn't matter much!

There was one factor in Eric's favor, however: He had taken no money that *he* had not personally propagated—the $100 of my personal money used to open the account and the $50 from my private sessions was untouched—less a $2.50 "service charge." He had not committed a crime (except possibly for destroying my office) because he had complete authority to write checks for whatever amount was available. His behavior certainly displayed questionable ethics but he had broken no laws that I could tell.

So I was at peace and grateful for the things I had learned from Eric in a very short time. Besides that, I *did* have in my hand the $800 check from David.

Everything seemed well until later that afternoon: While engaged in a pre-hypnotic talk with a client, the door to my office flew open and there stood Eric in his white painting jumpsuit, with a pale of spackle in one hand and a spatula in the other hand. He looked at me and then at my client and apologetically said, "I didn't mean to burst in on your session; I just stopped by to patch-up your wall and to see if *we* could patch-up our affiliation."

I had made a decision earlier that if, or when, Eric ever showed up in my life I'd treat him civilly but rebuff any attempt to reestablish a personal or business relationship. So I asserted my decision and said, "It would be nice if you would come back and patch my wall when I'm not in a session, but any association with you personally or in business was terminated last Friday as a result of your behavior and I want nothing more to do with you from now on... is that clear?"

He looked shocked at my bold frankness, recoiled and said, "Yes," as he slammed the door shut.

That was the last time I saw Eric. However about six months later, just by chance, I happened upon Linda (the one female that Eric had invited to be a surrogate stage-show subject).

"Aren't you Linda?" I asked. She may have had a vague recollection of having met me some place but I was sure she didn't remember my name or who I was, so I introduced myself. "I'm Lindsay Brady; you were in my office six months ago when Dr. Eric was teaching me how to do stage hypnosis."

A light flashed on in her memory bank and she said, "You looked familiar but I couldn't remember where I knew you from, but I do now."

When I asked if she had seen or heard anything of Eric she responded, "No, I haven't seen 'the Dr. Eric' since shortly after I was in your office that one time and I hope I never see him again."

I had no idea why she held such vehemence toward Eric. As I could best recall they seemed to have had an amenable relationship back then.

"By the way," she said, "did you know his real name is not Eric? That is just a stage name he uses when doing stage-shows—along with several other aliases I've heard he uses from time to time."

We parted, and with this new revelation, a few nagging questions fell into place. I pondered: *I think that Eric must have been trying to turn over a new leaf when he made his way here to Salt Lake City, after all he was looking for a job as a painter, not a job doing stage-show hypnosis and he hadn't had a drink for nine months. And I am sure he was very sincere, at least in the beginning, about passing on to me his vast store of knowledge and experience about stage-show hypnosis and hypnosis in general... but maybe his past caught up with him. I wonder if the "friends" he was buying drinks for at David's were really all that friendly. They looked and acted more like people wanting to get something from him more than wanting to be friends with him. And, I wonder if his past had anything to do with the way he reacted when I went over to David's to rescue him and I mentioned the police?*

Come on Lindsay, I said to myself, *don't go reading things into stuff that you know nothing about. Just let go of all the speculation and get on with your own life!* So I did.

For the next nine months or so after Eric and I had parted ways, I successfully booked a few more stage-shows at second-rate nightclubs (bars) for only a night or two at each establishment. I called Rich to assist me and even a few times, and as part of a "package" agreement with the nightclub owners, arranged for him to play his guitar and sing a couple of his "joke songs" as an added bonus. He had lost none of his entertaining zeal since that last show at David's—he only got better with each performance.

I guess that the 15 minute hypnosis session stuck because Rich seemed to be having the time of his life when performing...but I was not! And one night after one of the shows (when the audience had been particularly rowdy and seemed more interested in drinking than in what was happening on stage) I realized that it was the "bar scene" environment and the late nights and coming home smelling like cigarette smoke that had dampened my enthusiasm about doing stage-shows.

I had completely lost all interest in performing in nightclubs, but I secured several engagements for private parties and a couple of high school fundraising events that I loved doing. They were very rewarding and enjoyable to perform. Besides that, working with small groups (private parties with 15 to 25 people and using only two or three subjects who had volunteered) I found myself in a position where I could gain insight into what makes hypnosis work, and how to improve its effectiveness, by grilling the subjects after each show: "What was going on in your mind while hypnotized? Why did you do those unreasonable things just because I suggested that you do them? Would you have ever acted that way or done those things in your every-day life? Although you may not now remember everything you did while hypnotized were you unconscious at the time? How would *you* explain the experience of being hypnotized...?"[3]

My private sessions picked up considerably. Most of them came as spin-offs from the stage-shows at *David's* and my other performances. So I began to employ Eric's "right way" to do clinical hypnosis:

1. You *must* do a pre-hypnotic talk so the client knows what to expect during the session.

2. After your pre-hypnotic talk you *must* spend at least twenty minutes on the "induction" to make sure that they have reached a deep state of hypnosis.

3. The induction *must* include "progressive relaxation" starting with the muscles and joints of the client's toes; then to the arch of each foot; then their ankles; then their calves and continue moving on up to the client's head and then back down through their arms to their fingertips. And as you progress through each muscle tell the subject that you "want them to" relax that particular muscle.

4. After getting the client body relaxed you *must* get their mind relaxed by taking them to an imaginary place: A beach, a forest, a park, a retreat, an inner room.... A place where they are safe, secure and peaceful.

5. Once their body and their mind are relaxed, you *must* regress them back to the event that is causing their unwanted behavior; whether the event happened in this life or some other life. No matter the reason for the session they *must* be regressed back to the sensitizing event.

6. Once the sensitizing event is discovered they *must* re-experience the emotions of the event that is responsible for their self-destructive behavior and then "vent" it all out through any method you want to use. And then suggest that the event no longer troubles them.

7. To make a person stop smoking you *must* make cigarettes taste and smell terrible. But you must discover why they started smoking in the first place (regression).

---

3 I will be referring back to the insight gained from these small group performances and private sessions as my story unfolds.

8. To make a person lose weight you *must* make fattening foods that taste good, taste terrible and you *must* make food that is good for them taste delicious, and anytime they overeat you suggest to them that they feel nauseated. You *must* also regress the person back to the event that makes them think they need to eat fattening food and why they feel they need to eat so much.

9. You *must* see people several times to accomplish the desired results. Besides that you earn more money by having people come back many times.

10. *Always* give the suggestion at the end of the session that each time they are hypnotized they will go into deeper hypnosis and that they *cannot* be hypnotized by anyone but you or someone that is PSI certified.

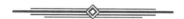

So I started to employ Eric's "Ten Commandments" of nine "musts" and one "always," and my success rate began moving backwards.

Doing hypnosis the "right way" (as Eric had defined it—i.e., a 15-minute pre-hypnotic talk, a 30-minute induction and then regressing a subject back to a "sensitizing event") necessitated seeing each client several times, and many of the sessions stretched out to several hours. In addition to the time requirement, it was also discouraging to find that my success rate (for achieving the behavior for which the clients initially made the appointment) dropped off.

From the beginning, my interest in hypnosis had been to discover how the process works and how to best use it to enhance a client's behavior (as well as my own), rather than to confirm some predetermined agenda or belief system. Many hypnotists start out with a belief or philosophy and then use their preconceived notions to explain hypnosis and even manipulate the hypnotic process in an attempt to confirm that their erstwhile premise is true.

While the personal philosophy and belief system that I now embrace are a spin-off of my investigation into the hypnotic process, it was never my intention to directly use hypnosis to establish them. Many times (and probably many more times in the future) I have had to scrap some of my most cherished ideas and convictions when they no longer held true after experiment, research and empirical observation, or when they got in the way of successfully helping a client achieve his or her objectives.

Even with Eric's "right way," I felt that my approach was helter-skelter and lacked organization. So in an attempt to establish a structured approach for conducting a hypnosis session, I wrote down a self-critique of each session when it was over. Then, when time permitted, I would take it into my "inner room" and thrash out my questions and observations with "Socrates." Early on in my attempt to organize my ideas I almost daily used this method of sorting things out, and occasionally still do.

I want to make it perfectly clear that *although* when in my inner room it is truly like being in a conversation with another person (Socrates), I never lose sight of the fact that I am conversing with myself. (An unexpected benefit of having Socrates to converse with is the ability—while writing the narrative of this book—to say "Socrates said" instead of "I said to myself"!)

The procedure I use for my investigations is based on the edict that if a principle (an idea or premise) is to be accepted as being true (valid and reliable), one must define the principle, describe a process for testing it and then replicate the process several times to confirm that the expected outcome is consistent.... And then accept the outcome even if it is different from personal bias and what *was* expected. If a principle cannot be consistently replicated, with the same outcome, it is not a valid principle and as such must be relegated to some theoretical or metaphysical niche.

I am completely willing to accept that my approach to hypnosis is based on only a few principles that truly meet the above criteria; the rest fall into the theory department. And if an idea or theory falls into the realm of metaphysics I leave it to the mystics to sort out.

So keep in mind that much of what follows is *not* etched in stone.

CHAPTER 23

Preface to Regressive Hypnotherapy

Eric's stage-show regression demonstration created in me a serious inquisitiveness as to its validity: With hypnosis, can a person, in truth, remember what happened on their second birthday and actually go back beyond that and recall what happened in a past life? Did we truly live past lives, and if we did, how much do they influence how we behave in this one? And for that matter, how much do earlier experiences in this life influence how we behave now?

For more than a year after Eric and I parted company, I blindly believed that it was necessary to regress a client back to the core events that shape present behavior. I suggested to every client that they return to the event that initiated their unwanted behavior, regardless of the issue they wanted to resolve at the outset. Whether it was an emotional issue, smoking, weight loss, school, sports, profession, public speaking, relationships—you name it— I'd regress you back to the episode that had been getting in the way of being how you wanted to be.

With these two questions in mind (Did we live past-lives? and can we remember what happened on our second birthday?) I began an exciting but challenging adventure into what I thought of at the time as the subconscious mind.

In the next two chapters (*Regressions-This Life* and *Regressions-Past Lives*) I will recount a few case histories of regressive hypnosis sessions that exemplify what a "hypnotized" person can come up with when asked to return to a memorable event out of their past. These (and hundreds more) have shaped my present view on regressive hypnotherapy.

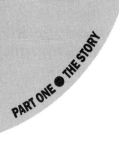

CHAPTER 24

Regressions
This Life

RUTH – FEAR OF MAKING SALES CALLS

Ruth made an appointment to get over her fear of making sales calls. She had fallen heir to a successful packaging company but could not make herself go out and call on existing customers, let alone make cold calls to acquire new customers.

After leading her through the hypnotic process I instructed her, *"Return back to the experience that has created your fear of making sales calls."*

She responded, "The only experience that comes to my mind is when I was 12 years old and my brother threw a snake into the swimming pool with us. I've always remembered this experience and for some reason that is the only thing that came to mind."

It seemed to me that my question and her answer were completely unrelated, so I asked, *"What in the world does a snake in a swimming pool have to do with your fear of making sales calls? Tell me about the experience and how it relates to your call reluctance."*

After contemplating my request she answered, "Well, my sister and I were swimming in the family swimming pool and as a prank my brother threw a water snake into the pool with us. I swam to the steps and climbed out but my sister (who had a phobia about snakes to begin with) just froze there in the deep end and started to sink under the water. I screamed at the top of my voice for someone to come and save her. My father heard the commotion, ran out of the house, jumped in the pool with all of his clothes on and saved my sister from drowning."

I waited for a few moments for an explanation of how this story related to having a fear of making sales calls but none was forthcoming so I asked her, *"What does this event have to do with your fear of making sales calls?"*

After some introspection Ruth said, "This is really bizarre, but I think it fits: After my father saved my sister he turned to me and harshly criticized me for not saving her myself. My sister is older than me so I felt that she should have been able to jump out of the pool and save herself, just as I did. I didn't like snakes either, so I wasn't about to jump back in the pool with a snake swimming around in it, so I did what I thought I should do—I screamed. My father's criticism was so harsh that I didn't talk to him for a month."

"Okay," I responded, "but what does that have to do with your fear of making sales calls?"

She said, "I hadn't thought of this before and it seems irrational, but I did what I thought my father would have wanted me to do—scream for help—and then he criticized me for it. Just before he died he sat me down and told me he wanted me to take over and manage the company. I already knew how to manage it; I'd been doing it for the last ten years. But then he gave me a lecture on how important it is to, 'go out there, make your sales calls and keep the customers happy—that's what I want you to do.'"

I responded, "I still haven't made a connection between a snake in a swimming pool and your fear of calling on customers. Can you help me?"

"That's the irrational part," she answered. "I have worked in the company office and out in the production line since I was a teenager. I am familiar with the business inside out and know exactly what to do, but my father's lecture about running the business like he wanted me to triggered in me the notion that I couldn't measure up to his expectations and that I would be criticized for doing what I thought he wanted me to do! Just like the snake incident, when I thought he wanted me to scream for help to save my sister, but instead he criticized me for it. I know he wants me to go out and make sales calls to our customers, and to make calls on prospective customers, but when I try to make a call I get this sick feeling that I will be criticized for doing it the way I think it should be done. So I just sit in my car in the customer's parking lot and, after a while, drive away. Does that make any sense to you?"

I told her that it didn't seem rational, but admitted that I could understand how the idea that she would be criticized for doing what she thought she should do could trigger those emotions.

I told Ruth that I used to be terrified of making sales calls, too, but that my selling experience changed from fear to enjoyment because I stopped thinking of selling as selling; rather, I started thinking of it as an opportunity to visit with friends (or to make new friends) by showing them how my products and services would benefit them by making their business or their personal situations easer and more profitable.

I asked her, "Is there anything else that comes to mind when you think about calling on customers or prospective customers?"

She opened her eyes and said, "Yes! I just thought of it when you talked about thinking of customers as friends.

"Our customers *were* all friends of my father's—many of them took off work to attend his funeral services—but they were never my friends and they are all much older than me. I have this notion that all of them think of me as being my daddy's little girl and that I know nothing about the packaging business, which is not true at all. I run the office, design the packages, order the boxes and fillers, manage the help and can operate the equipment—but they don't know that. How can a twenty-eight-year-old (me) convince an older person (the customer) that they are as capable as an older person (my father)? In my mind, in their eyes I'm just a shadow of my father. When I try to get out of my car to make a call, all I can see is a twelve-year-old screaming for help."

To make sure Ruth didn't have any lingering concerns, I asked her one final time, "*Is there anything else that comes to mind when you think about calling on customers or prospective customers?*"

I could see the wheels churning in her head and finally she said, "No, I think that's all. Just talking about it makes me feel better."

Earlier, after opening her eyes, our exchange had become conversational, so I asked her to close her eyes again and led her through the induction process for a second time. Then I suggested, "*The experience of being criticized by your father when twelve years old no longer troubles you, nor does it get in the way of doing what you think you should do. You are an attractive, intelligent and capable young woman and you no longer feel that there is an age barrier between you and older people; you are as comfortable around older people as you are around young people. You no longer walk in your father's shadow. You think of yourself as being an extension of your father's legacy and realize that your father's friends take pleasure in you treating them as your friends. Since you are highly knowledgeable of the packaging industry you confidently serve your customers by showing them how you and your company can provide them with greater benefits than any of your competitors. You feel good about yourself and radiate that feeling to your customers.*"

When Ruth opened her eyes she said, "Wow! That was wonderful. I feel like a great burden has been lifted from my whole being."

I received a note from Ruth a few months later thanking me for helping her to discover that her father's friends were her friends, too. She said that business was thriving.

CATHY - FEAR OF WATER

"I have a fear of water. Can you make it go away?" The voice on the telephone said.

"I'm not sure that I can, but I have been able to help a number of people overcome their fears and phobias," I answered.

Cathy was in her early thirties, seemed to have all the confidence in the world, looked athletic, sported a healthy suntan and didn't appear at all like a person who would be suffering from aqua-phobia.

I started out the session by asking, "Tell me about your fear of water. You don't look like a person who would be threatened by anything, let alone water."

"Well, my fear of water isn't what most people would think of as being aqua-phobic. I swim 20 laps a day. I'm not at all afraid of deep water but I get this panicky feeling when I am taking a shower and the water in the shower-stall begins to puddle up; even a fraction of an inch sends me into a tizzy. I still shower every day anyway, sometimes twice; I just worry that I might flip out."

I said, "I know that this issue must be a problem for you or you wouldn't be looking for a way to resolve it. You say that you *feel* like you are *going* to 'flip out,' but how often does it actually happen—you flipping out?"

"Oh, it only happened once. I haven't gone into hysterics while in the shower since junior high. It's just that whenever I shower I am *afraid* that I will," she said.

I must have looked puzzled so she went on to explain, "I wasn't even aware that it was an issue until I was in junior high school and PE was one of the required classes. Up until then I had never showered before and that's when I discovered I had a problem.

"I grew up out in the country and our family had only a bathtub for bathing. On the first day of school after gym class was over I went into the shower and turned on the faucet, and I liked the feel of the water spraying on my back. I guess the drain was plugged, though, so the water backed up in the shower stall and when I looked down and saw the water creeping up over my toes I flipped out.... I mean I *really* flipped out! When the other girls heard my screams they were sure a predator had been lurking in my stall and had grabbed me. It was so bad that I was sent to the school shrink who gave me a special permission slip that exempted me from having to shower after gym class from then on. I didn't shower once right through high school. This presented somewhat of a problem—sometimes I was aware of my body odor, but I still rationalized that I'd rather stink than shower! I did go through a lot of deodorant, however.

"After high school, I moved out of my parent's house and into an apartment that had only a shower. I finally got so I could use it, but I always felt anxious.

"Have you ever heard of anything as crazy as that? I mean, going bonkers over a puddle of water in a shower stall?"

I assured her that I had and said, "I've had many clients wanting help to get over some pretty irrational fears, and all of them admitted that their fear had no coherent basis, but I haven't had anyone tell me of being afraid of water on the floor of their shower—you're the first."

I went through all of the preliminaries of hypnotizing her and then asked, "*What comes to your mind when I ask you to return back to the event that is responsible for your fear of water puddles in your shower?*"

When Cathy finally began speaking she spoke in baby talk and used very short sentences as she described the event. "It's raining. I can feel the rain on my bare body. I like how it feels. I'm only a baby, maybe only a year and a half old. I wobble when I walk. I can hear Mommy calling my name. 'Cathy, Cathy where are you?' I can hear her calling. She sounds frantic. She sounds angry. I'm afraid she is going to slap my bare bottom. Sometimes, when she sounds like that, she swats me on my bottom. I'm running away from the sound of her voice. I'm running through puddles of water. I just stumbled. I can't see anything. It's dark and wet and black. I can't breathe. The water is in my nose and my mouth. I can't get up. My face is in the water. Ouch! I just got slapped on my bottom. Ouch! Mommy slapped me again. Mommy is holding me upside down and swatting my bottom. I'm coughing. I'm breathing again. I'm crying. Mommy is hugging me. Now *she* is crying." And then Cathy started crying as she sat in my recliner.

I encouraged her to "*just let out all of the emotions that have been pent up inside of you*" and suggested, "*As you cry you are venting all of the negative emotions of that experience—let it all out now. You are also venting all of the fear that you might go into hysterics when showering. You realize that your mother was not punishing you but rather trying to get you to start breathing again. And now there is a complete disassociation between falling in a puddle of water when you were little and puddles of water in a shower stall. When you feel that all of your emotions have been released, you will feel a sense of peace come over you; when you do, open your eyes and you will be wide awake feeling a sense of amusement about the whole episode.*" And then I slipped a couple of tissues into her hand.

She continued to sob for only a few minutes. When she stopped she opened her eyes, dabbed the tears from her cheeks, looked at me, smiled and said, "For someone who has been crying their eyes out, right now I feel very peaceful.... What's been happening?"

Cathy had no recollection of the tale she had just divulged, so I retold it to her scene by scene. As I recounted each piece of the narrative Cathy said, "Oh, I remember saying that now." By the time I had finished she was laughing about it.

She said, "I know now that my mom wasn't swatting my bottom because she was punishing me, but to get me to start breathing. I'm going to call her and see if she remembers that experience."

When Cathy returned for her second session she told me that her mother recalled the event almost to a tee as she had related it to me. The only difference was that her mom didn't find it funny. "Not only that, but she became upset with me because I was laughing as I told her what I had remembered!" Cathy told me.

I asked Cathy if she had taken a shower since her last session. She thought for a moment and said, "Yes, but I didn't feel panicky, nor did the thought of it even enter into my mind."

Since she felt that her problem had been completely resolved I could see no reason to go through another session.

After she was gone I deliberated: *I guess that we can recall experiences from when we were very young. Cathy's mom not only remembered the event but also confirmed that Cathy's recollection of it was correct—even though she didn't find it amusing!*

GREG - ALIEN ABDUCTION

Greg was a walk-in client. "Can you help me remember something that happened to me less than a week ago?" he asked.

When a male client asks that question it usually means that he was out partying one night and either got a telephone number from a beautiful blonde and can't remember it, or he woke up in his own bed with a headache, an awful taste in his mouth and no recollection of how he got there.

So when I asked Greg, "What is it that you want to remember?" I was surprised when he answered, "Well, I was abducted by aliens and I have no recollection whatsoever about what happened—it's a complete blank."

Not intentionally *trying* to be cynical I asked, "If it is a complete blank, then how do you know you were abducted by aliens?"

He responded, "There are eight hours of my life that are missing and I even have evidence to confirm that they downloaded stuff from my body and brain and then deleted my memory of those eight hours."

Greg unbuttoned his shirt and showed me two abrasions, one on each of his shoulders.

"See, this is where they hooked me up so they could download the stuff about my body. After the abduction I had a terrible headache and then noticed

I had lumps on each side of my head just in back of my hairline—that's where they attached their other probes and extracted information from my brain."

He took my hand and directed my fingertips so I could feel them. He winced as he brushed my fingers over each "memory-extraction" point.

He went on, "I remember nothing between the time that I walked out my door at mid-morning and when I was awakened by my friends shaking me and shouting, 'Wake up, Greg! Wake up, Greg!' late that evening. They had even thrown ice water on me, so when I woke up I was cold and soaking wet and had a headache."

Greg went on to explain, "I was supposed to have been the best man at Jerry's wedding—he's my best friend— but I never made it.

"It was Jerry who came up with the explanation that I must have been abducted by extraterrestrials—he's into all that kind of stuff. Over the years there have been reports of UFO sightings and abductions in Eastern Arizona— that's where I work, up on the Mogollon Rim near Clay Springs. It really makes sense because of the evidence on my body and besides that, I'd never under any other circumstances miss my best friend's wedding and the chance to kiss his wife right in front of him," he quipped. "But that day I just didn't show up."

When I asked why he thought that hypnosis could recover his memory he said, "I've heard that while hypnotized that you can recall everything that ever happened. I read that in a book someplace so I figured I'd give it a try. I really have no adverse physical effects from the experience, except for the bruises on my shoulders and these tender spots on my scalp; it's just the mental anguish that troubles me—it bugs me that I can't remember any of it."

I had no other sessions scheduled for that time slot so I agreed to hypnotize him on the spot.

He took a seat in my recliner and we went through the preliminaries. After he was hypnotized I asked Greg to go back to the day of his memory loss and to tell me what happened on that day. He began speaking in his normal voice, but it was as though our conversation just moments earlier had never occurred.

He said, "I had two hours before I needed to clean up, put on my rented tuxedo and ready myself for my best friend's wedding. I was *supposed* to have been his best man, but I never got there. Not showing up is completely unlike me, so when I didn't, everyone started worrying about me. It's about a two-hour drive to the church and they thought for sure I had been in a serious accident and was lying dead in a morgue somewhere. The last thing I remember was thinking that I have two hours to kill so I will.... And that is the last thing I remember. I cannot for the life of me recall what I was going to do, but I do remember going out the door to do something or go someplace. It's making me crazy not being able to remember.

"I'm a wrangler for a horse stable up in the high country on the Mogollon Rim near Clay Springs, and I have my own little bunkhouse—just enough room for me and a guest if they want to sleep in the upper bunk. My last memory is going out the bunkhouse door and heading towards the.... That's it."

When Greg had finished his narrative I suggested, "*Return to the day of your best friend's wedding. You are in your bunkhouse and have a couple of hours to kill. Returning now to the moment when you are thinking that you have plenty of time to do something or go someplace. You are walking out your bunkhouse door. It is as though you are actually there. You can see, smell, hear, taste, and feel the event. What is happening now?*"

This time when Greg responded he spoke in a more typical soft monotone hypnotic voice. "I'm standing at my bunkhouse door," he said, and as is typical for a hypnotized person, he said nothing more.

Each step along the way I had to drag out a response. "*What are you thinking about while standing at the door of your bunkhouse?*"

"I'm thinking it is a cool fall morning and since I have the day off of work I ought to take advantage of it."

"*What are you thinking of doing on this cool fall morning?*"

"I think I will get on my three-wheeler [this was before quad ATV's were on the market] and take a ride up into the aspens. The leaves are turning yellow and it is beautiful up there. I'd rather ride old Stumblefoot—she's my favorite mount; she doesn't really stumble but when she was a filly she tripped over a log once and that's how she got her name—but it would take too long to saddle her up, get up there and get back in time to get ready for the wedding, so I'll just jump on the three-wheeler."

"*What is happening now?*"

"I'm heading up the canyon. The road is good, for being just two tracks through the grass—the tracks are too wide so one of the rear wheels and the front wheel ride through the grass between the tracks. It's beautiful up here. I love being out of doors in the fall when it's cool. The leaves are turning and the wildlife watches as I approach, then they scurry away. I was made for this."

"*What is happening now?*"

"I think I'll lie down in the grass and just enjoy everything that there is to experience in this majestic scene—just for a few minutes. There is nothing as grand as stretching out on the grass, closing your eyes and enjoying the cool fresh mountain air and listening to the sounds of nature at its best."

"*What is happening now?*"

"Oh no, I must have fallen asleep! I've got to get back or I'll be late for the wedding."

"What is happening now?"

"I am racing down the road. The front wheel of the three-wheeler is bouncing through the grass between the tire tracks. I'm crouched down over the handlebars. I'm going lickety-split. I love speeding through the cool fall air like this, there is nothing more exhilarating. Whoops, I just hit something hard, like a big boulder, with my front wheel. My shoulders just hit the break handles on the handlebars and I'm flying through the air. I must have hit my head on something because everything's blank."

"What is happening now?"

"My friends have just thrown a pail of ice water on me and they are shaking me and demanding that I wake up."

"Return back to the event of your crash. How did you get down off of the mountain and back to your bunkhouse?"

Greg just sat there in my recliner and said nothing, so I tried a little different approach. *"You have already recalled much of the experience that you had previously forgotten, and so that means that you have the ability to recall things that have escaped your memory. So return to the event of getting off the mountain. How did you get back to your bunkhouse? What is happening now?"*

Greg said, "I can't remember a single thing. I guess when I banged my head.... I just remember flying through the air headlong at that tree that is coming at me; but I remember no more. I must have been knocked out and just unconsciously ridden my three-wheeler back, but I can't recall any of it. From the time I crashed into that tree and I woke up in my bed cold, wet, with a headache and being shaken by my friends, I have complete amnesia."

I suggested to Greg, *"I'll count up from one to five when I reach the number five open your eyes and you will be wide awake remembering everything you have told me, and sometime in the near future you will remember the rest of the story, how you got down off of the mountain, and why you didn't make it to the wedding–it appears that after the crash you still had time to make it there–how you got back to your bunkhouse will just come to you. Now that you know that you were not abducted, the events of that day no longer trouble you in any way."*

After he opened his eyes I asked, "How do you feel?"

He replied, "I feel great–just like I had a nice nap. It's like I don't have to worry about what happened anymore. But I don't think I was hypnotized because I remember everything that I told you. I thought that I was supposed to be unconscious and afterwards wake up and then you would have to tell me what I said."

Not wanting to get into a prolonged discussion about whether remembering or not remembering determined if a person had been hypnotized I said, "The reason you remember everything is because I gave you the suggestion that you would.... But at least now you know what happened."

He responded, "Yes, but I am disappointed that I wasn't abducted. That would have been awesome. It is going to be embarrassing when I have to tell my friends what really happened—I mean crashing my three-wheeler. Losing control of your three-wheeler and crashing into a tree doesn't make much of a plot for a book. When I get back up to the high country I'm going to take a good look at my three-wheeler and see if there is any evidence of damage and also see if the break handles match up with my bruises. I haven't ridden (or even looked at it) since the day of the wedding. I'll call you and let you know."

A few days later Greg called and left a message on my answering machine: "My three-wheeler was in good shape except for the dent in the front wheel rim and the break handles were knocked catawampus and matched up perfectly with my bruises. It wasn't until today that I remembered how I got back to my bunkhouse. I must have lain there unconscious for three or four hours, because the sun was in the west when I came to. The three-wheeler was on its side, so I rolled it over and road it back down off of the mountain. When I got back to my bunkhouse it was too late to go to the wedding and besides that my head hurt and all I wanted to do was lie down and go back to sleep."

And then he added, "Everyone is disappointed, as am I, that I wasn't snatched up by aliens. Before you helped me find out what really happened I was planning to have you help me remember everything about being abducted by aliens and then write a book about how the hypnotist helped me remember it all—then I'd be rich and you'd be famous. Oh well."

MARIA - REMEMBERING MOM

"I was adopted when I was three years old. That was twenty-one years ago and I have been searching for my birthmother for the past five years but I keep running into a dead end," Maria told me.

"My adoptive parents *say* that they know nothing about my natural parents except that my mother was a single parent working as a bartender at a club and one day she just disappeared, leaving me an orphan... so *they* adopted me. Beyond that, whenever the topic comes up they are mute and very standoffish.

"My dad has always been kind and loving when at home, but he has a mafia type personality at his job. I'm not saying that he has ever engaged in illegal activities but he is a union boss and has a reputation of using strong-arm tactics to get done whatever he wants done. You'd much rather have him as a friend than an enemy.

"I've heard that people have regressed back to the experience of being born and even while in the womb, so going back to three years old doesn't seem all that unlikely, does it? Do you think you can help me?"

I told Maria that I had occasionally had clients regress back and tell of experiences when they were very young and that their memory seemed to be accurate. I also explained that not everyone is able to regress back to those very early years, but if she still wanted to try I'd be happy to work with her.

It took a little while for Maria to get into a state of mind where she was able to let go of her analyzing and to just go with the flow of what came into her mind as I asked questions. Once she did, however, her recollection was vivid and her story was very interesting and enlightening to her.

"Maria, return back to a significant experience when you were very young. Go back to being with your birthmother. What came to your mind when I asked that?"

"I hear the tinkling of glasses. I'm wrapped up in a nice comfy blanket. I hear people talking and laughing. There is the smell of alcohol. I hear my mother's voice; she is laughing. I like to hear her laugh. I'm lying in a little basket. It's under a shelf. Now I can see my mother. She is wearing a short black skirt and a white blouse."

Maria broke away from being there and began talking to me in the present, "She was a bartender and I think that she had me tucked away under the bar counter, probably because she had no one to take care of me. It seems like it was a constant occurrence."

When I asked her to return back to the bar scene and to tell me what was happening she said, "My mother has taken me from the shelf and has set me in my basket *on top* of the counter. There are loads of people around, fussing over me. I like the attention. My mom has just shushed them all away and is carrying me out the door. She is beautiful. I think everybody likes her—and me. The air is cool and fresh now that we are outside."

"What is happening now?"

"I'm bigger, far too big to fit in a basket. I am standing up in a child's crib and leaning against the side rails that keep me from falling out. My mom is sleeping and I'm looking at her. I'm happy and trying to get her to wake up and play with me. She likes to play with me and to tease me. Now she is awake and smiling at me. She is really beautiful. She has long dark hair, sparkly dark eyes, clear olive skin and is wearing a lacy nightie."

"What is happening now?"

"I'm back in my crib again. I'm much bigger; I must be almost three years old. I hear voices. My mom is talking with a man who is in bed with her. They forgot to pull the curtain all the way closed. They are arguing. I think I recognize the man's voice; I've heard it before. Usually it is soft but now he is yelling at my mother. He is saying that he is not going to leave his wife for her because it would ruin his life, especially if anyone found out that his mistress is a barmaid and that he has an illegitimate daughter. He's saying, 'She's getting old enough that if she sees me here at your place she might recognize me at the club and tell people. If you don't start adoption proceedings today I'll take care of this matter myself. I'll do whatever it takes to not have my marriage and reputation tarnished by a bartending slut. Do you understand what I mean? Do you get the drift of what I am saying?'

"He just slapped her face and she is crying. He's getting out of bed and I can see him. Oh no! I recognize him. He's my adoptive father!"

Maria opened her eyes and said that she could probably fill in all of the details and implications with her own imagination.

"This answers a lot of questions. After all, my birth mom just dropped out of sight and my adoptive dad is a union boss who used strong-arm tactics to accomplish whatever he wants. I'm going to go back home to New Orleans and ruffle a few feathers," she said.

I never heard back from her.

Regressions
Past Lives

CINDY - "I DON'T WANT TO STARVE AGAIN"

I had been skeptical about past life regression, and so I had *not* seriously considered trying to get a client to return to one. Then Cindy came into my office one day and unexpectedly (for both of us) regressed back and told of having lived and died in a past life.

Cindy was a teacher who had arranged for me to perform an afternoon assembly stage-show at her junior high school. Even with the extra weight she carried, Cindy dressed well and was a striking young woman. When I returned to my office after the performance, I picked up my messages; one of them was from Cindy. "I want to be hypnotized to lose a lot of weight," the message said. "A lot" turned out to be 95 pounds, although she didn't appear to me to be that much overweight. I contacted her and we arranged an appointment.

After she had filled out my intake information sheet I asked her, "What do you think you are doing wrong? What are you doing that is causing you to weigh more than you want to? Do you think that it is because you overeat at mealtimes or because you eat the wrong kind of foods?"

"Both," she answered. "Not only do I eat too much of the wrong foods at mealtimes, but I graze all day long—it seems that I'm afraid I will get hungry. I can't remember being hungry since I was a kid. I'm always trying out new exotic foods and at the same time trying to follow a diet—and the food always wins. I've tried every diet under the sun but I just can't stick to one for more than a few days. I even wake up and make a trip to the refrigerator a couple of times a night. The more I try not to eat, the more I eat. I'm five foot seven and weigh 230 pounds and I want to get down to 135 pounds—that's where the doctor tells me I should be for my height and bone size. I'm desperate!"

I went through my induction procedures and when she was in a hypnotic state I instructed, *"Return back to the event that makes you feel that you need to eat so much and need to be snacking all the time."*

It took a while for her to answer. When I asked the question, the possibility of a past life experience wasn't even in my mind, so I was surprised when she said, "I don't want to starve to death again! I'm so cold and weak... "

"Where are you?" I asked.

"Denmark," she answered.

"Why are you cold and weak?"

I was even more surprised when she answered in the present tense—like it was happening at that very moment. "I have retreated to Father's hunting lodge."

"Why?" I asked.

"I want to join the Mormon Church and go to America but my whole family is furious about it and they have all ostracized me. My father—he's a duke, you know, and very rich—is very hostile toward the Mormon missionaries because he thinks they are not preaching to convert members to their faith, but rather to recruit women so they can take them off to America, marry them and add them to their harem."

"What happened? How did you end up at your father's hunting lodge?"

"I snuck out at night and hiked here for refuge from all of the persecution of my family. It took me two days to get here—it's high in the mountains. Thinking that I would stay for only a few days, I didn't bring many provisions. It is fall and an early snowstorm has set in—the snow is so deep now that I can't walk through it to get back home. Surely my father will know where I am and come and save me. I know he is angry with me but he won't knowingly just let me starve."

"What happened after you found yourself marooned and abandoned? What is happening now?"

"I have run out of firewood and it is so cold. I've been burning the furniture to keep warm. And I am hungry. What little food I brought with me is all gone. There was a little salted venison left over from this fall's hunt but it's all gone now, too. I managed to catch a couple of rats, and I cooked and ate them. I even tried boiling some tree bark and a leather hunting pouch but it just made me sick."

"What is happening now?"

"I'm starving to death. I'm so weak and so cold and abandoned. I don't want to die. I'm so scared!"

She stopped talking so I asked, *"What is happening now?"*

"Nothing.... Nothing at all... Nothing at all matters now."

"What do you mean when you say 'nothing matters'? Are you dead?"

"It's really strange. I know I am here with you now and that I have been telling you about living an experience of dying, but the story just stopped and there is nothing—no being in it. It just stopped."

"What does this experience have to do with your overeating in this life?"

She crossly responded, "Obviously, you don't understand; I don't want to starve to death again! I don't want to ever be hungry again! Don't you understand? I don't want to starve to death!" and then she burst into tears.

When I had recovered from her rebuke, and from my embarrassment over having not grasped the obvious, I blundered out (digging an even deeper hole) *"Do you really think that you are going to starve to death in this life? It's obvious that you have plenty to eat now; surely you are not going to starve, are you?"*

She didn't answer but just erupted into another round of sobbing.

I still get an uneasy feeling of embarrassment when I think back to my bungling insensitivity. For Cindy (at that moment) the experience was as real as any memory—as though it happened this afternoon. She was already sensitive about her weight and when I said, "It's *obvious* that you have plenty to eat now," I wasn't thinking that she might take it as criticism—inferring that she was fat.

After she had settled down I suggested (as I had been taught by Eric), *"Now that you know the experience that has been causing your uncontrollable eating behavior, and have experienced the emotions associated with it, you can now eat healthfully. As a matter of fact, fattening foods taste terrible so you don't even want to try eating them and healthy foods taste delicious and you enjoy eating healthy foods. At any time if you eat more than you know you should you will feel nauseated."*

I counted up and said, "Open your eyes now. You are wide awake!"

I asked Cindy how she felt and she responded, "I feel angry. I feel angry that my father in that other life abandoned me, and that my father in this life abandoned me and I don't care that I am fat. I don't want to ever again feel hungry. And besides that, if I am fat I don't have to worry about having someone get close to me and then abandoning me. I don't even care if *you* think I am fat and ugly!"

I thought again, she *is* overweight but for someone who wants to lose almost a hundred pounds she certainly is not ugly. She dresses well and her face is attractive... when she loses those extra pounds she'll be stunning.

I apologized for my earlier inference about her obesity and told her that it may take a few more sessions to successfully change her eating behavior, and so we set up another appointment for the next week.

When I called Cindy the following week to confirm her appointment time I asked, "How has your eating been since you were in?"

She responded, "Not very good. I may have even put on a pound or two, I think. One good thing though, I haven't eaten any junk food, but food that is healthy tastes so good I can't stop eating it. It's really odd. The only time I don't feel nauseated is when I wake up in the morning. I haven't thrown up or anything, but after I've eaten just a little bit of healthy food I start feeling sick to my stomach~but I just keep on eating, anyway. I'm really disappointed. I thought that hypnosis was going to make me not eat so much, but it seems to have made it worse."

I replied, "It may take several sessions to get to the bottom of your eating problem. There may be other experiences that need to be uncovered. So are we still on for tomorrow?"

She agreed.

When Cindy arrived the next day, it was apparent that she was not in the best of spirits. After sitting down in my recliner she said, "This has probably been the most miserable week of my life. I've not only been eating non-stop but I feel sick to my stomach most of the time. And worst of all, I keep thinking about what I told you about having lived a past life. I don't believe in past lives. I believe I lived as a spirit with Heavenly Father before I was born and we live only one life (to prove ourselves worthy) and then return to Heavenly Father when we die. I think I just made up that whole past life story because that's what I thought *you* were expecting. Besides that, I don't think I'd ever get hungry enough to cook a rat and eat it!"

"Well, you surprised me, too, when you told me that the reason you overeat is because you don't want to starve to death again. You really caught me off guard. That's the first time in my practice that a client has regressed back to a past-life experience. I witnessed a person telling of living a past life one time, but your experience last week was the first time one of *my* clients has done so. I'm very curious about past lives, but I don't know if we did or didn't live them. For me, the jury is still out. How would *you* explain what you experienced last week? I'm searching for answers about the topic and maybe you can shed some light on the subject and give me some insight."

She answered, "Well, now it seems more like a bad dream but at the time it seemed real—like I was really there. I usually don't remember my dreams when I wake up, but I can still see the snow outside piled up to the windowsills of the lodge, and I can feel the anguish of having nothing to eat and the pain of no one caring enough to come and save me. I don't know where it came from but the feelings are the same as when I think about my dad (in this life) abandoning me and I had nothing to eat. I survived only by begging for food from strangers and rummaging through garbage cans.

"When I was five, my mom died and my dad and I lived in a little rundown shack. He would leave me home alone when he went out to find work and one day he just didn't come back. A few weeks later when I was begging for food, a woman took me to the police station and they sent me to a foster home. My foster parents were kind and loving and eventually adopted me. When I was growing up they gave me any kind of food I wanted... and as much as I wanted. I remember them saying to me, 'You've got to get some fat on those little bones of yours. We love pudgy little children and you need to eat well so you don't die."

Cindy paused for a moment in contemplation and then continued, "I often think of them saying that to me, but right now it has taken on a different meaning. I feel that if I don't have fat on my "little bones" my adoptive parents won't love me. On the other hand, I know if I do have all of this fat on my little bones I'm going to die an early death. What a paradox."

I replied, "So you *know* that by being fit and trim you will live longer and that your parents would probably be pleased about that. Do you agree with that?"

She said, "Yes I do, and I feel much better now that I have talked about it. I think I can lose a lot of this fat if I will just keep reminding myself that fit and trim is healthy, and I will be all the more loved by my parents if I am. They've been telling me in recent years, 'You need to go on a diet and get some of that fat off of your bones.' I already know that but I have resented them telling me; it has just made me want to eat all the more—the resentment. That doesn't make much sense either, does it?"

I said, "It does seem a little paradoxical, as you put it earlier: You want to overeat because when you were young, overeating and being pudgy pleased your parents. Now, you could please your parents by eating less, but when they tell you to stop overeating you just eat more. That *doesn't* seem like sound, rational thinking, does it? It would appear that our behavior has little to do with logic or rational thinking. So what kind of suggestions do you think I should give you this session that would change your eating habits?"

After thinking for a few minutes Cindy said, "I think it would be helpful if you tell me that I'll be healthy by eating less and that eating healthy foods only three times a day will please my parents and that they will love me all the more if I do. And tell me to exercise three times a week because I will be healthier and will live a longer life if I do. And tell me that I like myself because I am losing weight and that I no longer have a feeling of abandonment. If you give me suggestions like that I think it might work. Oh yeah, and also tell me that my natural father didn't abandon me because he didn't love me. I found out a few years ago as I was researching my genealogy that the reason my father didn't come home that day was that he was killed in an industrial accident. No one but my dad knew that I was home alone and would be waiting for him to return."

So I hypnotized Cindy and, without doing any more regressions, the suggestions I gave her were precisely as she had asked.

"You now think about being healthy and loved because you eat less, and eating healthy foods only three times a day pleases your parents and they love you all the more because of it. You exercise three times a week because it will make you healthier and you will live a longer life by doing so. You like yourself because you are losing weight and you no longer have a feeling of abandonment. You love your natural father because you now know that he didn't abandon you, but rather he was out working and earning money because he loved you. The reason he didn't return was because he couldn't and you love him because he was out there working so you wouldn't be hungry. Now you feel, behave and act as a trim and healthy person."

Still locked into the "right way" to conduct clinical hypnosis, after she woke up I asked, "What day next week would be best for you to come in for your next session?"

She replied, "I think I'm going to do fine. Why don't we wait for a few weeks and I'll call you if I think I need any more help? I really feel good about it right now. Your suggestions were exactly what I wanted and if I just keep in my mind the thought that I behave as a fit, trim and healthy person and that my parents love me because I'm losing weight, I think I can stick to my diet."

Cindy called back two weeks later and told me she had lost fifteen pounds. She was elated. She said that she was sticking to her eating and exercise plan, didn't feel sick to her stomach, hadn't eaten between meals and was happier with her life than she could ever remember. She told me she would call me if she fell off the wagon and needed more help. I never heard back from Cindy so I assume that she was successful in achieving her weight-loss goal.

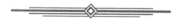

After Cindy left my office, I wanted to resolve some questions about what I had witnessed during her sessions. I sat down in my recliner, closed my eyes, took in three deep breaths and imagined myself at the top of a staircase leading down to my inner room.

In my imagination I was sitting across the table "interviewing" Socrates and asked, "Was Cindy's experience of dying truly a recollection of a past life or was it something that was just happening in her imagination?"

Socrates: Does it matter? Whether or not it was really a past life, it was still an experience that came from *her* mind, and at the time she was telling of experiencing it, it was a real experience to her. She even re-lived the emotions of the event, so it may as well have been a real experience as far as she was concerned. But we need to examine what you could have done better during that first session.

Me: I think I should have said what I meant to say instead of blurting out '*It's obvious that you have plenty to eat.*' I should have said, '*In your life now there is plenty of food available, so is there any reason for you to worry about running out of food?*' Or something like that.

Socrates: That would have been much better, but that is not what I was asking about... I was asking about your interest in finding out about past lives. If you are interested in finding out about past lives, then why were you surprised when Cindy regressed back to one?

Me: Because I don't know if we did or if we didn't live past lives; I am just curious to find out if we did. I wasn't expecting a past life to just pop up.

Socrates: If you weren't expecting her to recall a past life, then why, during the pre-hypnotic talk, did you suggest that she return to one? Why did you tell her, '*Stored in the subconscious mind is a perfect record of everything you have ever experienced whether in this life or some previous life*'? That's why she thought you were expecting her to regress to (or create for you) a past-life experience.

Me: Because that is what Eric told me to say. And it wasn't a suggestion; it was just a statement I made during the pre-hypnotic talk before hypnotizing her!

Socrates: How long is it going to take for you to realize that Eric's "right way" for conducting clinical hypnosis is not necessarily the best way? With experience, *you* will develop a best way for you and your clients. A good place to start is to recognize that the words you use during the pre-hypnotic talk are as much of a suggestion to the client as they are after you have gone through the induction process. Actually, the session starts the moment you talk to people on the phone when you are setting up an appointment. It appears that you are still floundering, trying to make hypnosis into something different than everyday conscious awareness. Someday you will grasp that concept. Also, you gave Cindy the suggestion that she would feel nauseated after she had eaten enough of the right food. Can you discern what was wrong with the suggestion?

Me: Well, I gave that suggestion because Eric said that that is what to suggest. I know, I know, 'stop thinking Eric's "right way" is the best way.' But it worked! She said that she felt sick to her stomach after having eaten just a bit of the healthy foods.

Socrates: Think! What was missing from the suggestion? Why did she keep on eating even after she was feeling nauseated? Think!

Me: I think I've got it! I *didn't* give the suggestion that she would stop eating when she had eaten enough of the right foods. Is that it?

Socrates: That's only part of it. Think again.

Me: Let me see... Apparently, feeling nauseated didn't keep her from eating. As I said to her, *reason and logic must not have much to do with your behavior....* Then what *am* I missing? ...Oh, I think I've got it: Instead of suggesting that she would feel nauseated after eating a little of the right foods, why not suggest that when she has eaten a little of the right foods she feels filled and satisfied and she stops eating? Is that it?

Socrates: You are getting very close. Think a little deeper.

Me: Hmmm.... Let me think.... If she feels filled and satisfied after having eaten a little of the right foods.... Then what.... I think I've got it! *You continue to feel filled and satisfied until your next mealtime.* Is that it?

Socrates: Good, but still not quite there. Think! The amount of food Cindy ate had nothing to do with whether she was hungry, stuffed, filled, satisfied or nauseated, nor did the *knowledge* she had about eating right and exercising. She already knew *what* she should be eating, *how much* she should be eating, *how often* she should be eating and that she needed some exercise to have a healthy, trim body. So think a little more creatively and think back to why she still grazed all day long.

Me: I think I have it. I neglected to suggest that she no longer fears feeling hungry. How is this? 'Now *you eat because your body needs nutrients, not because you don't want to feel hungry. When you have eaten as much as your body needs for maintaining good health—as much as a 135-pound person would eat at that time—you feel filled and satisfied and you stop eating. You don't mind feeling hungry between the times you eat because that means you are losing weight, and feeling hungry produces a sense of confidence and high self-esteem—you like the feeling of having an empty stomach. Now your eating behavior is consistent with your knowledge of how much you should eat, when you should eat and what you should eat. Eating healthfully and exercising make you feel confident and cause you to feel good about yourself.'* Is that better?

Socrates: That's much better, but now what about regression? Whether the experiences are from this life, or what appeared to be a past life, or something out of the client's imagination, how does that effect how they behave now? Think of a suggestion that you could have given to Cindy so those experiences, whether real or imagined, do not negatively affect her eating behavior now. Be creative!

Me: I think I did a pretty good job with my last suggestions, but let me think how I could have said it better.... How about if I add, '*Regardless of whether the experiences you have recalled came out of a past life, this life or your imagination, they no longer have a negative influence on your present eating behavior. You are now free to feel, behave, and act as a trim, healthy, confident, 135-pound person*'?

And all of a sudden Socrates and my inner room were gone and I found myself sitting in my recliner again.

DEBBIE - LOST LOVER

"Hello, Mr. Brady, this is Debbie; I work with Rich over at *David's*. Can you help me find out why I can't find a guy to fall in love with, marry, have a bunch of kids with and live happily ever after? I'm almost thirty and all I have ever wanted is to be a mom. It isn't that I haven't had my chances. I have dated a lot of really nice guys but I have this feeling that I am waiting for someone— Mr. Right. It's kind of like I know who he is but I can't remember his name or what he looks like. I keep waiting and looking, but I just can't discover who he is or where to find him. I have this empty feeling inside of me all the time, like something is missing, but I can't quite put my finger on it. Can you help me get over this feeling so I can get on with my life and find romance in it?"

I had noticed Debbie working the tables at *David's* but I didn't know her name until Rich accused her of trying to send the wrong number (eight) when we were doing our telepathy routine. Debbie was slender and attractive with jet-black hair (or bleached blonde hair, depending on which wig she was wearing that day) and seemed to be very personable. According to Rich, she was the most popular cocktail waitress at *David's* and she made more in tips than any two of the other servers. So when she called and said, "I want to find romance and find a fellow with whom to fall in love and ride off into the sunset," it seemed a little out of character.

Intrigued, I asked, "I don't know if I can help you since I've never dealt with this kind of a request, but if you think that a few hypnosis sessions would help resolve your issue I'd be happy to work with you. Why do you think that hypnosis can help you find a solution to your dilemma, anyway?"

"Well, I've tried everything else—counseling, psychotherapy, astrology, fortunetellers.... I even went to my minister! But nothing has helped get rid of this feeling that I can't fall in love until I find out who the person is that I'm waiting for. I know it sounds foolish, but does it make any sense to you? Do you understand what I need help with?"

I wasn't quite sure what she meant by what she had said so I responded, "It sounds to me like what you are seeking is to discover who the person is that you have been waiting for, then you would be free to fall in love and get married.... Even if the person you fall in love with isn't the person you have been waiting for. Is that what you meant?"

"Yes, that is exactly what I meant to say! You are the first person who seems to get the drift of what I'm trying to accomplish. When can I come and see you?" she asked.

"How about right now?" I answered.

"I'll be right over."

Debbie turned out to be an excellent hypnosis subject. *Maybe it is because she witnessed all of the stage-shows at David's*, I thought.

After going through the pre-hypnotic talk and the induction process I instructed, *"Return back now to the event that causes you to feel that you are waiting for someone and that you can't fall in love until you discover who that person is."*

I waited for her to respond. When she finally did, she began speaking in what sounded like French!

I let her jabber on for a few minutes and after the amazement of what I was witnessing had subsided, I stopped her in mid-sentence and said, *"You will have to speak in English since that is the only language that I understand. In English, tell me what you just said."*

She responded, "I said I am the *Countess Anna Maria De Leon* and I am waiting for Richard to return from the war. When he left with King Richard of England, I promised to wait for him and then we would marry upon his return. My father does not want me to even see Richard, let alone marry him, since he is English and I am French, but I will marry Richard anyway when he returns. He is so tall and handsome, with dark skin and steel gray eyes. I love him with all my heart."

With that, Debbie stopped talking and just sat there so I asked, *"Where are you and what are you doing now?"*

"I am in London and I'm just sitting here, looking out over the city and waiting... just sitting and waiting for Richard to return."

"How long has he been gone?" I asked.

"It's been more than a year that I've been waiting."

"Do you hear any news about the war or when King Richard and your Richard will be returning?"

She answered, "They say the war is going badly and that many knights have been killed or captured and are being held for ransom. No one knows when King Richard will return or if he will at all."

I said, "*Move forward in time and tell me of your fate as Anna Maria De Leon and of Richard's fate. Did he return and if so, did you and he marry?*"

Suddenly, her emotions changed to horror and anger. "They just threw a blanket over me and men are carrying me outside. I hear them talking in French and I recognize one of the voices as being one of my father's captains. They say they are abducting me and taking me back to France to keep me from marrying Richard. I'm kicking, screaming and protesting, but there are too many of them for me to resist. I can't get away."

She stopped talking again, so I asked, "*What was the outcome of your abduction and did you ever hear from Richard again? What is happening now?*"

"I'm sick!"

"*Are you emotionally sick or physically sick?*" I asked.

"Both."

"*Describe to me what you are experiencing emotionally and physically and what led to your present circumstances.*"

"I have been sequestered in my bedroom for months. It's like being in a prison. I have only one small opening to see out and all I can view is the forest. The servants are kind and give me everything I need but they have been forbidden to divulge any information about what is going on in the outside world; but I think they intentionally talk loud enough to each other so I can overhear their conversations. Yes, I know much of what is happening.

"Many of the soldiers have returned from the war and have brought back the plague. I think that I have caught it and that's why I'm so sick. I am heartbroken, not only because I don't know what has happened to Richard, but because of how my father has treated me. I used to be his little princess but since he had me kidnapped he hasn't been to see me, nor has he spoken to me. I'm miserable. All I do is sob and I am burning up with...."

She stopped talking again so I asked, "*What is happening now?*"

"I died! I see myself lying on my bed and I am dead!"

I said, "*Debbie, return back to here and now with me and answer a few questions.*"

Although the answer to my next question seems obvious, I decided to ask it anyway—and I was glad I did.

"*What does this experience as Anna Maria De Leon have to do with being unable to fall in love in this life?*"

"Ever since I began dating, my father (in this life) has been scrupulous about the types of boys and men I have dated and I was always afraid he would put a stop to any long-term relationship. So why even bother? One time, when I was young, he even locked me in my bedroom to keep me from dating a boy that he didn't approve of."

I asked, *"But didn't you already know this about your father in this life? And what do Richard, England and France have to do with this life?"*

"I don't know. The story of France, England, and Richard all just came to me, like in a dream, when you asked why I can't fall in love. It seemed like it was really happening while I was telling you about it, but now it just seems like it was a dream that I can still remember."

"For a while you were speaking in what sounded like French, but then you switched to English so I could understand what you were telling me. Do you remember that?" I asked.

"Now that you mention it I remember, but I'm not sure that I was speaking French—I don't know French and I've never studied it. That's really odd, now that I think about it."

"In a moment I am going to count up from one to five when I reach the number five just open your eyes and you will be wide awake remembering everything that you have experienced while hypnotized however the events that you have told me, whether in this life or a past life, will no longer keep you from falling in love. One, two, three, four, five, wide awake!"

Debbie opened her eyes and said, "Now that was really uncanny. I wonder where all of that stuff came from? And speaking in French was really interesting. What do *you* think about it?"

I was a little taken aback because that was what I was going to ask her, so I responded, "I don't know *what* to think about it. It seems to me that there must be some correlation between your story of a past life and your romance dilemma in this one. Or, it might be the other way around: Maybe the quandary in this life (your father's scrupulous screening of your boyfriends) is what triggered the tale you described to me as a past life. I don't know, what do you think about it?"

"Well, until now, I have never told anyone about my father's protectiveness and I didn't think it had anything to do with my feelings about falling in love and getting married. Nevertheless, as I was telling you about my father in that past life, I got those same empty feelings of not being able to fall in love. But for some reason, those feelings are gone now. Right now it is as though those feelings were never there. This is the first time I haven't had that empty feeling hovering in the background that had been there for as long as I can remember.

"I mean, I'm almost thirty years old and my father is rarely involved in my day-to-day life, and I'm sure that now he'd approve of anyone I chose. As a matter of fact, just talking about it gives me a feeling of freedom. It's like a great weight has been lifted from my being. But I am still curious about speaking in French."

"I am, too," I answered.

To satisfy *our* curiosity I asked, "Debbie, I have a friend who is from France; would you be willing to come back and see if it was really French you were speaking?"

"Sure, I'd like to do that just to find out if I can speak French—and don't *know* that I can," she answered.

When Debbie arrived a week later, I asked her how she was doing since our session and she said, "This has probably been the best romantic week of my life. A fellow my brother introduced me to back when I was a senior in high school (whom I have dated a few times over the years) called me last week—the very evening I was in to see you in fact—and we've gone out every night since. You are never going to believe this—his name is Richard!"

After a brief conversation about her change in attitude about falling in love, I introduced her to Max.

Max grew up in France and emigrated to the United States, where he opened a restaurant, *The La Persian* (only a block from the once forbidding dungeon—the Salt Lake City Library). He was, of course, fluent in French.

I went through all of the induction steps with Debbie and then asked her to return back to her life as the *Countess Anna Maria De Leon* and to tell her story to Max. She gave an abbreviated recounting but spoke only in English.

So I suggested that she now tell the same story to Max in French and she just sat there. So I used a little different tack.

"Anna Maria De Leon, do you speak French?"

"Yes, I do," she answered in English.

"Will you then use French to tell Max of your experience?" I requested.

"No, I will not!"

"Why not?" I asked.

"Because he is a secret agent—a spy—and will turn me in to the authorities if I speak French. When in England it is dangerous to speak French."

So I suggested, *"Then move forward or backward to a time in this lifetime when it is okay to speak French and tell your story. Will you do that?"*

"No, I will not."

"Why not?"

"Because he is a spy and can't be trusted."

No matter how hard I tried to pry even a single word of French out of her I was unable to do so. I even asked Max to try to communicate with her in either English or French and she refused to respond in either language—not a nod or a frown.

After I had brought her out of hypnosis I asked Debbie what kept her from cooperating and she said, "I don't know how to speak French!"

And that was the end of it. But it did motivate an even greater inquisitiveness, wondering and curiosity, *I wonder what is really going on up in our head?*

MARTY - INDIANS & JOHANN STRAUS

It was 100 degrees outside when the door opened and there stood an anomaly that I certainly wasn't expecting: He was wearing padded black ski gloves, his heavy dark woolen shirt was buttoned to the neck, and his black pant legs were tightly clasped around the top of combat boots with bicycle pant-leg clips. He had a stocking hat pulled down to meet his ebony-black sunglasses and I could see sweat-soaked circles on his shirt under his armpits, perspiration dripping off of the end of his nose and beads of sweat glistening from his upper lip.... Marty appeared to be dressed for Antarctica!

I struggled to not react adversely to the oddity standing before me when I asked, "How can I help you?"

"Are you the hypnotist guy?" he asked.

"Yes, I am. How can I help you?" I asked again.

His answer was obvious. "I need help."

"Can I get you a glass of water?" I inquired. "You must be thirsty."

"No, I always carry a thermos of ice water on my bicycle and I just had a drink. But thanks anyway."

I asked, "Would you like to take off some of your things? You might be a little more comfortable."

"Yes."

He slipped off his stocking cap, sunglasses and gloves, he unbuttoned his shirt collar, pulled off his pant-leg clips and sat down on the chair I had indicated.

Although his speech was coherent, his choice of dress for a hot summer day gave me reason to believe that he might need more help than hypnosis could provide.

When he had settled in I asked, "So why are you looking for a hypnotist? Why do you think hypnosis can help you?"

He explained, "I have a fear of the sun shining on me. For as long as I can remember, if the sun shines on my skin I start to shake and go into a convulsion. It's mostly when the sunshine hits the back of my hands, arms, neck and my forehead. For some reason I don't mind if it shines right on the rest of my face. I wear sunglasses but I really don't need them; I just think they are cool looking."

With his protective clothing removed I could see that he was a good-looking young fellow. He used good grammar and seemed comfortable when looking square into my eyes while he talked; yet there was a hint of something strange in his manner.

He went on, "I've also been in and out of psychotherapy for as long as I can remember. They say I am autistic and I need special help to keep me on track. They may be right about that but it doesn't have anything to do with my sun phobia."

At the time I had only a vague notion of what being autistic meant, so I assumed his autism explained why he seemed to be a little off kilter.

He articulated his words clearly, although his thoughts seemed a little disjointed as he continued. "I'm twenty-one years old and very intelligent—straight A's in high school—and I am really good at the piano—mostly waltzes. I've never played in public. My mom thinks I could but she'd probably never let me. I know that people think I am strange because of how I have to dress to keep the sun off of my hands, arms and forehead. When I was in high school the other students thought it odd that I always rode a bike and that my mom wouldn't let me learn to drive a car (she's afraid I'll go into a convulsion and kill someone). But I don't care. I'm used to it. My dad committed suicide when I was young so I help my mom publish an advertising circular and we make a good living. Life is pretty good for me except for my mom wanting to run my life and this sunshine problem—it dominates my life—and I'd kind of like to find a girlfriend but my mom laughs at me when I talk about it. 'What girl would want to hold hands with someone who is wearing padded ski gloves!' she tells me. Do you think you can help me?"

I responded, "I don't know if I can. But let me ask again, why do you think hypnosis can help you? What makes you think hypnosis can help when psychotherapy hasn't?"

"The medical doctors can't explain why the sun gives me convulsions, and all the psychiatrists do is give me medication, so I think it is in my subconscious mind. They say that my body chemistry is out of whack and the medicine they give me is supposed to make it normal. The medication doesn't do anything for my fear of getting sun on my skin, it just makes me dopey—maybe it's the medication that makes me autistic."

I scolded him, "You still haven't answered my question. Why do you think hypnosis can help you get over your fear of the sun shining on your skin? How did you come up with the notion that hypnosis can get into your subconscious mind and then make it so you don't go into a convulsion when the sun hits your skin?"

He seemed to take no offense and said, "Well, my mom took me to the state fair and I saw a hypnotist show. It made me think if he can make people on stage do crazy things then maybe hypnosis can make me not have convulsions when the sun hits my skin. After seeing the stage-show I bought a book on hypnosis. In it, the hypnotist said that hypnosis can change a person's subconscious thinking. Once your subconscious thinking is changed, then how you act changes. The book also said that past lives sometimes determine how we behave in this life—something about having to suffer if we did bad things in a past life. I must have been really bad in a past life because it seems all I do (except when playing the piano) is suffer."

I agreed to hypnotize him to see if we could find out what was causing his sun phobia and why he went into convulsions when the sun hit his skin.

Once he was in "hypnosis" I instructed him, "*Marty, return back to the experience that has caused you to fear the sun shining on your skin; whether the experience occurred in this life or some other life, return back to the event that is causing you to go into a convulsion when the sun hits your skin.*"

"Indians!" he exclaimed. "The Indians are after me!"

"*Why are the Indians after you? Tell me what is happening.*"

"The Indians are my friends. I've lived among them for only a few months but have gotten to know them. Gray Bear is my best Indian friend but a white man raped his wife and since the guy that did it got away, the chief wants to take revenge on me because I'm white—the deed must be avenged or she will be deemed unclean, they believe. I'm hiding in this wash. I know what they do to white men when they do that to one of their squaws. I've seen it and it is a horrible way to die."

Marty stopped talking so I asked, "*What is happening now?*"

"The chief has me by my hair and is dragging me to the pit they have dug. Gray Bear is pleading with him to let me go because it wasn't me who did it. The chief isn't listening to him. He has me by the hair and is dragging me to the pit. They are going to bury me alive! They've stripped off all of my clothes and have bound my feet. They are standing me up in the pit and are filling the pit up to my armpits with hot sand they have heated with fire—so it will cook my male organs. They are tying a leather mask over my eyes and mouth so I can't see or scream. They have staked my arms straight out from my body. I can't move. I'm so thirsty. The sun and the sand are so hot. I think they have gone away; I can't hear them anymore."

Marty stopped talking again so I asked, "*What is happening now?*"

"My forehead and neck feel like they are being fried. My arms and the back of my hands feel like they have been broiled by the sun. The hot sand is cooking my body. My insides are shaking—boiling. All I want to do is to die."

He stopped talking again but his body began jerking and shaking like he was having a convulsion, so I asked, *"What is happening now?"*

The moment I asked that question Marty's body stopped shaking and he said, "I am outside of my body now and I am looking down at the scene. The sight is horrible but I am finally peaceful and nothing matters now."

I said, *"Marty, return to here and now with me and tell me if this experience is the root cause of your fear of having the sun shine on your skin and the cause of your convulsions."*

"It must be!" he answered. "When the sun hits my forehead, neck, arms, and hands I get that same feeling—like my insides are boiling—and I go into a convulsion! Yes, when I was telling you about it I felt exactly the same as I do when I have a convulsion."

I said, *"Then accept these suggestions: The experience of being tortured and killed by Indians now no longer has an influence on your present life. There is no need to feel that you are being punished because you were not guilty—you had nothing to do with the rape of your Indian friend's wife. You are free now to enjoy the sunshine. You take care, like the rest of us, so you don't get sunburned, but with the passage of time your skin will become accustomed to the sun's rays and you will even enjoy getting a suntan. You take pleasure in wearing cool clothing when out of doors and in the sun light. You behave now as though the experience with the Indians never occurred."*

As Marty departed he left the top two buttons of his shirt undone, put his sunglasses in his shirt pocket, handed me his stocking hat and said, "Thanks, you can have this." But I noticed that he slipped his gloves back on as he went out the door.

Two days after that session, Marty called back and said, "I no longer go into convulsions when I'm in the sun, nor do I have the fear of getting sunburned, but I still feel like I need to protect my hands—not from the sun, but just from them getting hurt. Can I come back so you can make me stop worrying about getting my hands hurt?"

When Marty returned, he made quite a contrast to the picture he'd presented when he first appeared at my door. This time, he was wearing cycling shorts, socks that barely came above his cycling shoes, a tank top, a cycling crash helmet—and black padded ski gloves! He looked odd, wearing cycling togs with a body as white as Moby Dick, with black ski gloves on his "flippers."

He said, "My mom put lots of suntan lotion on me so I wouldn't get burned. She told me to still wear my padded gloves, not to protect my hands from the sun, but just to protect them. I'd rather not wear them at all but I just feel that I need to.

"My mom thinks that a miracle of some sort occurred because I changed so much in a single day. She even asked if I had stopped to see the priest and if I was thinking about going back to church or something. But she still wants to control my life. I didn't tell her that I had been to a hypnotist because she thinks hypnosis is the workings of the devil."

With that, we began the session. I went through the hypnosis process with Marty, and asked, *"Why do you have this feeling you need to protect your hands, not from the sun, but just need to protect them?"*

He answered, "I don't know, I just feel that if I hurt my hands something awful will happen to me. Of course, hurting one's hands in itself would be terrible, but it's something more than that. I can't explain it very well but it seems like I will lose something valuable if my hands get hurt."

I suggested, *"Return back to the event that has caused you to feel that you need to protect your hands."*

He thought for a moment, and said, "I'm playing the piano. I'm really good at it. My orchestra and I are playing for a small group of very important aristocrats. They are dressed in 19th century clothing—the women are bejeweled and have their hair stacked on top of their head. And the men are in high-collared lace shirts and all that kind of stuff."

I encouraged him to talk a little more about it. *"Tell me more about this experience of playing the piano. Where are you? Who are the important people? What does this event have to do with feeling that you need to protect your hands?"*

His response was interesting. "I am in Vienna. The emperor and his lady are here along with other dignitaries. Wagner and Brahms are here. Wagner and Brahms are kind of like fans of mine. I don't know why they like my music so much, but it is nice that they do."

Before Marty could go on, out of pure curiosity I asked, *"Who are you?"*

"Oh, my name is Johann Strauss. I'm a composer and pianist. I'm very good at playing the piano but I mostly use it for composing. People call me the 'King of Waltz.' My father is a musician, too. He tried to discourage me from getting into music, but I did it anyway. My father—he's a famous violinist—and I battle all the time over getting recognition from the nobles. I think it's a deadlock. We are even on opposite sides of the war. I told my brother Josef that I'd like to punch my father in the face but he warned me not to because my hands are all I have. 'If you break some bones you will never be able to play the piano again,' he told me.... Did you know that I invented the street sweeper? My brother Josef got the credit for the invention but it was my idea. I thought of it because something had to be done to quickly remove the horse dung from the streets before people left my performances."

I responded, *"No, I didn't know that. After your brother warned you not to punch your father in the face, did you start wearing gloves?"*

"No, there is no need to because I'm not going to punch him in the face. I just wish he would come and see me play my music. He's an old man and will soon die, anyway. When he does I'll inherit everything he has, including his music business, so I won't be punching him in the face."

"Then what does this experience have to do with wearing gloves now?" I asked.

He suddenly switched from the 19th century to the 20th century and said, "My dad and my mom... in this life!"

He said nothing more so I asked, *"What do your dad and mom in this life have to do with wearing gloves?"*

"One day, after I had started playing the piano, I told my mom that I'd like to punch my dad in the face for killing himself and not being around to hear me play. Ever since then she has harped about the necessity to protect my hands. She often tells me, 'You are different from most people out there and if people taunt you, you might get mad and punch someone in the face. It could break your hands and since you are wearing gloves anyway, I'll get you some of those padded ski gloves, just in case. Your piano playing is all you have and you would really miss not being able to play—you would have nothing left to live for. The only time you seem happy is when you are playing the piano.' The first time she said that it seemed that I had heard it before, and now I know why it seemed so familiar—I am the reincarnate of Johann Strauss."

He continued, "I do play the piano very well, especially for having had no lessons. But no one has ever heard me play, except my mom. One day I just sat down at the piano and started picking out melodies—in three-quarter time. My mom went out and bought some music books, showed me how to read music and I started practicing. Playing the piano just came to me."

I asked, *"Have you ever punched anyone in the face or had an experience that could have caused injury to your hands?"*

"No. I didn't really want to punch my father's face, nor anyone else's for that matter—it was just a figure of speech."

"Is it wearing gloves that keeps you from punching someone in the face?" I asked.

"No. In fact, that has probably increased the likelihood of *me* getting punched in the face."

"Since wearing gloves hasn't served a useful purpose, is there any need for you to feel that you need to wear them anymore?"

After thinking for a moment he answered, "No."

"Then accept these suggestions: You no longer feel like you need to wear gloves. You still wear cycling gloves when riding your bicycle, just because it is more comfortable, but

you no longer feel that you must wear gloves. You are free to have your hands ungloved when out in public and are free to even hold the hand of a girl when the opportunity arises. Feeling you need to wear gloves is no longer an issue and now you feel, behave and act as though it never was an issue."

I counted up and sent Marty out the door.

I was curious enough about the validity of Marty's story of living in Vienna in the nineteenth century that I went to the encyclopedia and looked up Johann Strauss. Most of what Marty had told me appeared to be accurate, except I could find no reference to either of the Strauss brothers having invented the street sweeper.

From time to time, Marty would come in for another session—always dealing with his mother wanting to control his life.

"It seems if she is not telling me what to do and how to live my life, she's not happy," he told me. "She threatens to sell the piano if I don't do what she demands, to take away my bike if I don't comply and bullies me all the time. I told her about being Johann Strauss in a past life and she just laughed at me. I didn't dare tell her that I'd been seeing a hypnotist!"

All of the regressive hypnosis and suggestions about not letting his mother bother him helped only temporarily; Marty would be back in my office a month later with the same issue.

At one session he told me, "I think that my mom can't stand for me to not need her. I no longer wear gloves or protective clothing, and I haven't had a convulsion in many months (since I started seeing you), but she still won't consider letting me learn to drive; she wants me to be dependent on her. I met a girl and we're friends. She plays the violin and that's what we mostly talk about—music. We haven't held hands yet, but I think she likes me and she likes classical music, too. I even played the piano for her once and she was delighted. But my mom found out about it and forbid me to even talk to her. 'She's too good for you and she'll just hurt you,' she told me. I wondered if it wasn't my mother's constant badgering that drove my dad to take his own life."

Marty stopped coming to see me, but a few years later I heard a news report of a murder-suicide investigation. Marty had shot his mom in the face and then turned the gun on himself.

RAYMOND - STABBED IN THE BACK

Residing in a couple of small rented houses near our home in Salt Lake City was a group of "hippie" type people. One of them lived in a house with his live-in girlfriend and three guys lived in the other house with an occasional female guest or two. They nurtured a small number of marijuana plants that (they said) naturally grew here and there on their half acre and, as one would suspect, tended a couple of goats and drove Volkswagen busses adorned with peace signs—kind of a mini two-house commune.

Remember, this was the early 70's and this living arrangement and lifestyle was just a part of *their* segment of society. They all had jobs (of sorts) and a few of them were going to school (of sorts). They were friendly, kind, and loved interacting with Darlene, me, and our children. Many of their standards and behaviors were quite different from ours but they were still good neighbors that we enjoyed having around.

They knew I was a hypnotist and on one occasion as we visited, the subject of past-life regression came up. They were all of the same mind (except for Raymond, who seemed impartial): Having lived past lives was an inexorable fact. They pressed me to regress one of them so they could witness the phenomenon first hand. Unlike most of my past-life regressions there was no particular behavioral issue involved; they just wanted to observe someone returning back and telling what happened in a previous life.

I explained to them that *I* didn't "know" whether we lived past lives or we didn't, but that I had had a few clients who had regressed back to what appeared to be such and if they wanted to see what might come of their request I'd be willing to oblige them.

With such a small number of subjects from which to draw (seven, as I recall) I first wanted to see if anyone in the group would be a good candidate for the purpose of regression.

I asked all of them to find a place to sit down, make themselves comfortable and then to *"Look into my eyes...."*

Actually, this was my first private-party, small-audience gig, but I treated them like I would have had they been volunteers who had *chosen* to participate in taking "an adventure into the realm of the subconscious mind."

After concluding the induction and deepening suggestions ("...you can't bend your arm and you can't open your eyes...") I chose Raymond to be the regression subject, since he had responded very well to my suggestions and seemed to be neutral on the topic of past lives.

I woke up the other six and turned my attention to Raymond, who was sitting on a straight-backed chair.

"Raymond, everything you have experienced, whether in this life or some other life, is stored in your subconscious mind. Return back now to some significant event from a past life. You can clearly see, smell, feel and hear every detail of the event. What is happening?"

After a few moments Raymond quietly said, "I'm sittin' at an ol' pine table 'n my pa is teachin' me ta play poker."

247

"What is significant about playing poker with your pa?"

"Ma died last winner so when Pa 'n me get done workin' out in the fields 'n done with supper we sit at the table 'n play poker because Ma ain't here 'n we're both lonely 'n there's nuth'n else ta do."

"How old are you? And what year is it?"

"I'm goin' on twelve 'n when we get through harvestin' the crops this fall Pa says he's gonna send me back east to Aunt Martha in Tennessee so I c'n get some schoolin.' Pa says it's the year of the forty-niners, 'n since Ma died 'n I'll be off ta Tennessee, he thinks he'll join 'em."

"Do you mean the 1849 gold rush to California?"

"Yeah."

"What is your name?"

"My name is Jebzriha, but Ma 'n Pa jus' calls me Jeb."

"Return to some other significant experience in your life as Jeb. What is happening?"

"I'm all spruced up. It's my wedding day and I'm going to marry Jennifer Spaulding. She is the daughter of Jackson Spaulding; he's one of the richest men in Lebanon. She has got to be the prettiest girl in the whole world." (After the session was over and everyone critiqued what they had witnessed, everyone without exception~even Raymond~ noticed how his manner of speech went from backwoodsy to being relatively sophisticated but still with a little hokeyness—"all spruced up.")

I asked him, *"Did you end up going to school? How did you meet Jennifer?"*

Jeb continued to tell his tale as though it was happening, "Yes," he said. "After I graduated from secondary school Aunt Martha arranged for me to enroll at Cumberland University here in Lebanon. That's where I met Jenny. CU is not far from where I did most of my growing up—that is, from twelve on. I was planning to practice law after I graduated but Jenny is going to have our baby and as any honorable man would do I'm going to marry her. I'd want to marry her anyway even if she *wasn't* going to have a baby."

The six spectators' focus had been fixed on Raymond and the story he was telling until he stopped talking and just sat there; then they turned their attention to me. Steve leaned over and whispered, "Why did he stop talking? We want to know what happened after that."

"Jeb, what happened after your marriage to Jenny? What is happening now?"

"Don't call me Jeb! My name is Jebariah P. Bolden. And don't call her Jenny, either."

Raymond's eyes began to well up with tears and he began to sob and said, "Whenever someone calls her Jenny it reminds me of happier days. Jennifer is dead and so is our little baby girl. They both died shortly after childbirth."

"I'm sorry to hear that Jennifer died and I apologize for reminding you of the event. But move forward now to some other significant event in your life as Jebariah. Where are you now and what are you doing?"

"I'm playing poker in a bar in Elko. I'm on my way to California to see if I can find my father. I haven't heard from him for months and I'm worried about his welfare."

"What is significant about playing poker in Elko? What is happening?"

"Well, I'm winnin' a lot of cash from these ol' hayseed farmhands 'n cowpunchers. Pa taught me well on playin' poker—keepin' a straight face, drawin' 'n bluffin.' Gamblin' 'n poker is how I paid for goin' ta school back in Lebanon. These ol' cowpokes are so dumb it's like liftin' money out of a dead man's pocket."

His speech had slipped back into his childhood dialect. He stopped talking again so I asked, *"What is happening now?"*

"I'm playin' with a new bunch o' suckers. Guess I took all o' the ready money frum them other guys last night. They was really angry that I won all their cash. Said they'd get even 'n left in a big huff."

All of a sudden Raymond gave a lurch and said, "Oh, there's a pain in my back. I think I've been stabbed in my back. I think I'm gonna be a dead man!"

With that Raymond tumbled off of his straight-backed chair and crumpled onto the floor and pulled up into a fetal position as he grasped at his back. Then his body went limp.

The scene stunned all of us who witnessed it—especially me. For a moment I wasn't sure that Raymond hadn't actually died right on the spot in front of our eyes—he really looked dead!

I dropped down to the floor and with a clap of my hands near his ear I shouted, *"Raymond, WAKE UP NOW!"*

To my great relief (and I suppose to the others,' too) Raymond gave a jerk, opened his eyes, shook his head, looked around and exclaimed, "What happened? Why am I lying here all curled up on the floor?"

Raymond's friends were amazed at what they had just observed and then hit Raymond with a barrage of questions for which he had no answers, since he had no recollection of what he had just told us.

So I hypnotized him again and suggested, *"While remaining upright in your chair, return back to your life as Jebariah P. Bolden. And return back to the experience of being stabbed in the back while playing poker. Tell us what happened after being stabbed."*

"I'm on the floor and the room is whirling around. I'm coiled up in a ball and I can feel the knife still stuck in my back. I'm grabbing but I can't reach it. I hear a man saying, 'That'll show you, you cheatin' sidewinder.'

"And now there is only a sense of peace—nothing matters now. I'm out of my body looking down on the scene from above. There's a guy taking my billfold out of my jacket pocket and another one stripping off my money belt and another one scraping all of my money into his hat off of the table and saying, 'I guess he's not gonna be needin' this.' Everyone else in the tavern is just standing around and letting them do it. Nobody seems to even care that I just got killed. But none of it matters to me. Now I think I'll go find Jenny!"

With that, I concluded the session. *"When I reach the number five just open your eyes and you will be wide awake remembering everything that you have just told us as well as what you talked about earlier.*

"One, two, three, four, and five.... WIDE AWAKE!"

Raymond opened his eyes and said, "That was really interesting! That whole story seemed to be real—just like I was living it. I've never been outside of Utah but it *seemed* like I was in Tennessee and Elko."

Then one of his friends said, "I wonder if Cumberland University is in Lebanon, Tennessee and if it was founded before the mid 1800's."

We looked in a dictionary—and both were true!

CHAPTER 26

A Menagerie of Strange Requests and Memorable Sessions

During the course of my 38 years as a hypnotherapist, working with over 27,000 clients one-on-one and having conducted numerous hypnosis stage-show performances, I have encountered countless strange requests for hypnosis and many memorable experiences related to my profession. This chapter is devoted to recounting a few of them.

Many people have the misconception that hypnosis, or the hypnotist, can *make* anyone do *anything*. Early in my career, when I was starving for clients to practice on (and sometimes just because I was curious about their request), I accepted everyone who wanted to be hypnotized for any reason.

Now when someone calls with an impracticable request I respond, "Hypnosis can't do that."

————◇————

"Will you hypnotize me so I will pick the right numbers to win the lottery?"

————◇————

"I hate studying. Can you hypnotize me so I will know the answers on the test without having to go to class or read the text?"

————◇————

A common unrealistic request: "Will you hypnotize my girlfriend (boyfriend) and *make* her (him) fall in love with me?"

My response to this request is: Find what kind of a person or personality your friend would fall in love with and then *you* come in and we'll work on you becoming that kind of a person.

To date I have had no takers!

————◇————

"Can you make my wife believe me? I don't want you to hypnotize my wife; I want you to hypnotize me while my wife is present and let her ask me any questions she wants to, to convince her that I am telling her the truth. Lupe, my wife, says that if she can do that then she will believe me. We both want to do this. Will you help us?"

I can understand why people would think that hypnosis acts like truth serum and that the answer to any question must be the truth because the person is "hypnotized."

I thought the same thing, before I learned a little bit about the hypnotic process. The reason I didn't want Art Baker to hypnotize me was because I was afraid that he would get me "hypnotized" and ask some sensitive questions about my private life, and I'd be unable to resist answering—"spilling my guts," in effect. I know now that that is not true at all.

However, I agreed to Jose's request and while hypnotized I allowed Lupe to ask him her questions. She pulled a crumpled piece of paper from her pocket and began.

Lupe: "Have you *ever* been unfaithful to me since we have been married?"
Jose: "No."
Lupe: "Do you sometimes visit with other women, including your ex-wife?"
Jose: "Yes."
Lupe: "That girl at work, did you ever make advances towards her?"
Jose: "No."
Lupe: "Do you love *me?*"
Jose: "Yes."
Lupe: "Do you love anyone else?"
Jose: "Yes."
Lupe: "Who is she?"
Jose: "My two daughters from my previous marriage."
With that, Lupe turned to me and said, "That's all the questions I have."
I counted up and said to Jose, "*Open your eyes... and wide awake!*"
Jose sat up and said, "I'm glad that is settled now."
Lupe said, "But those are the same answers he has been giving me all along. I still don't believe him!"

I don't know whether Jose was telling the truth or not, but I do suspect that if Lupe had proof that he was telling the truth she still wouldn't believe him anyway.

This experience starting me thinking: *Maybe I am hypnotizing the wrong person, Maybe I should have hypnotized Lupe and suggested to her that whether Jose is telling the truth or not, it no longer troubles her.*

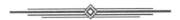

When Albert called to make a stop-smoking appointment for himself, I asked (as I always do), "Why do you want to stop smoking?"

Most people when asked that question say, "I want to stop smoking because it's bad for my health," or, "I don't want to get lung cancer," or, "I hate how it smells," or, "It's getting too expensive," or, "I'm just sick and tired of smoking...."

But, when I asked Albert why he wanted to stop smoking he said, "I *don't* want to stop smoking; I just want to make a stop-smoking appointment for myself!"

"Let me see, you have me a little confused," I said. "You are calling to make a hypnosis appointment to stop smoking but you *don't* want to quit. Do I have that right?"

"Yes, that is exactly right," he said.

"Would you explain that for me?"

"Sure, that's easy to explain. You helped my brother-in-law quit smoking and my wife told me that if I would come to you for a stop-smoking hypnosis session, even if it didn't work, she'd stop nagging me about me having to quit. I'm willing to pay your fee and come in for a session just to get her off of my back."

Maybe I needed the money, maybe I just wanted someone to practice on, or maybe I was just curious, but whatever the reason I agreed to work with him.

Albert had his wife with him when he came in and he instructed her to stay out in my outer waiting room.

When we got settled in my hypnosis room (and since we were going to be together for an hour and needed *something* to talk about) I asked Albert, "Well, why *don't* you want to stop smoking?"

"Because I enjoy smoking.... I think. But mostly it's because everyone is telling me that I have got to stop, and it really ticks me off. I'd like to quit, but as long as they are on my case about it I'm not going to do it—even if it kills me! Why can't they just leave me alone and let me enjoy my smokes? I'm a rebellious old cuss—and a very independent one, too—no one is going to tell *me* what to do!"

"Tell me, Albert," I asked, "what about smoking is it that you enjoy? Do you enjoy smoking because it is keeping you healthy?"

"You know better than that. Everyone knows that smoking is bad for your health."

"Is it that you enjoy having to go outside and stand around in the cold or the heat or the rain every half hour or so?"

"Well, I don't enjoy that part of it at all. It just wastes my time."

"Is it because you enjoy how it makes your clothing, hair and breath smell?"

"Well, no!"

"Is it because you like how much it costs to smoke?"

"Certainly not that," he said.

"Do you enjoy being ostracized and treated like you carry some sort of plague?"

"Don't like that either."

"Tell me then, what about smoking is it that you *do* enjoy?" I asked.

"Well it is like this. I know that smoking is not good for me and that I'd be much better off if I quit (for all of the reasons you just mentioned) but ever since I was a kid, smoking let everyone know that I was a tough guy—my own man—and that I was *not* going to do what they told me to do no matter the consequences. I guess that attitude has just stuck with me and that's what I enjoy about it—showing everyone that I'm my own man! But until right now I hadn't realized that is why I smoke."

"Let me see if I have this right: You *want* to stop smoking because you know it is not good for you and that you would be much better off if you did stop. Is that right?"

"Yes."

"But you are not going to stop because 'they' are telling you that you have got to stop, so even if you want to quit you are not going to. Is my understanding correct?"

"Yes, that's correct."

"Then reason with me for just a moment: If you want to quit smoking, but "them" telling you that you've got to stop makes you smoke, then they are 'making' you do something that you don't want to do. That's independence? Does that make any sense to you?"

"Well, it does but on the other hand it doesn't. Now you are confusing me!"

"Look at it this way: If 'them' telling you that you need to stop smoking makes you smoke, then they are making you do something that you don't want to do. But by being a *non-smoker* (just because *you* have chosen to be) demonstrates your true independence—you are a non-smoker even if *they* have been telling you to quit. It would appear to me that you being a nonsmoker for no other reason than you decided to be one would 'show them' that you are your own man. True?"

"Well, it would seem so."

"It's kind of like this: You are a non-smoker because you have chosen to be a non-smoker and you'll be damned if other people telling you that you have to quit is going to make you smoke; you are going to be a non-smoker anyway. Now that would demonstrate your true independence. Does *that* make better sense?"

"Well it does, but I hadn't thought of it that way before. So what you are saying is that by me being a non-smoker, even if they have been telling me to quit, and I continue to *not* smoke, then, in a sense, I'm showing them that they can't tell me what to do. Is that right?"

"Yes, at least that is how I see it. That is to say, you can maintain your 'tough guy' reputation by not smoking."

"I think I've got it!"

Believe it or not, the conversation was even more involved than the foregoing scenario depicts, but by the time we had finished, our hour had passed. But when asked if he wanted to come back for a "real" session he said, "Why would I want to do that? I'm going to go out there and show all of those miscreants that they can't make me smoke by telling me that I have to stop!"

I didn't hear back from Albert, but he and his wife referred probably a dozen new clients over the course of the next few months.

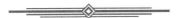

"My wife is shy and inhibited when we are out in public; she just sits there like a bump on a log, she hardly speaks and she spends a great deal of the time examining her fingernails. Can you *make* her more outgoing, and join in on the conversation and be a part of what is going on? She is highly intelligent and has a vocabulary like you'd never believe and in private, and around her family, she truly is clever, joins in the activities and at times even dominates the conversation. But when we get out in public and around strangers, she just clams up."

I answered, "Have your wife call me and if this is something that she would like to change I'd be happy to work with her.... Or I could hypnotize you and give you the suggestion that her inhibitions no longer bother *you*."

He declined, but his wife called back and made an appointment to overcome her shyness.

During the pre-hypnotic talk I asked her how she would rather be when socializing and around people with whom she was not acquainted. In response she said, "I'd like to be outgoing, join in on the conversation and speak my mind without being offended or upset if people don't agree with me; and I'd like to comfortably insert my natural wit on occasion just as I do in private.

In fact, I have a keen sense of humor and sometimes off the top of my head say some really funny thing, but when I am around strangers I just sit there as though I was a clam in a hermetic jar—sealed off from everything going on. I truly don't want to be a sequestered clam any more!"

After going through the induction, I gave her suggestions that repeated back word for word what she had just told me.

When I woke her up she began giggling and exclaimed, "Wow! That was just like going down a giant slippery slide right into a pool of whipping cream—scary at first but loving how it ends up. Thanks, that was great."

Two weeks later her husband called back and said, "Can you put my wife back to how she was before coming in to see you?!"

I responded, "Only if that's what *she* chooses."

Apparently she didn't, because she never called.

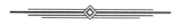

I grew up in an extremely protected environment. And even into my thirties I had had little exposure to people of varied ethnic groups or people who engaged in a liberal lifestyle. I was not only inhibited but I was naïve. For example, I had heard of people who liked people of their own sex (homosexuals) but I really thought I would never encounter one. I use the term "homosexual" because that is what they were called back then. *Gay* meant you were happy and joyful.

Gregory had been referred to me by Sonnie Shine, the client who worked at the employment agency. Sonnie had called a few days earlier to tell me that Gregory might be calling for an appointment. She said he was a client of hers and came in looking for employment as a salesman, but was apprehensive about going on job interviews, not to mention making sales calls if someone hired him. She told him how hypnosis had helped her get over her fear of being assertive and suggested that hypnosis might help him, also.

When Gregory came in he was immaculately dressed in a well-tailored suit with vest and necktie. It was apparent that he was particular about his appearance. However, he was carrying a purse over one shoulder and closer examination revealed that his cheeks were a little rosier than normal and his fingernails had been painted with clear polish.

My naïveté was still intact so I gave little thought to his anomalies.

Gregory was a very good hypnotic subject and seemed to be pleased with the result of the session.

The next day Gregory called and said, "I went for a job interview right after I left your office. I felt perfectly confident and they hired me on the spot. Then this morning I went out on two sales calls, with no reluctance at all, and closed on both sales. This hypnosis stuff is really wonderful. Can I come in for another session tomorrow just to make sure it sticks?"

I told him sure and we set up a time.

The next session went just as smoothly as the first one and Gregory told me that it was well worth his time and money.

The next day he called again and wanted to come in for another session just because he liked how it felt to be hypnotized. So we set up another appointment time.

This same routine went on for another couple of weeks—an appointment every three days and each time for a different reason, some of them trivial.

Then I got another call from Sonnie. "Lindsay, you really need to keep an eye on Gregory. You know that he is a homosexual, don't you? He has his eye on you!"

"What do you mean?" I responded. "Sure, he's a little feminine, wears make-up and carries a purse, but he isn't really a homosexual, is he?"

She laughed as she said, "You've got to be kidding me! I knew he was a homosexual the moment I laid eyes on him. You must have lived a very sheltered life. Don't you know that there are guys out there who are attracted to other guys?"

I admitted that I had heard of such people but never thought I'd meet one.

Sonnie went on, "Gregory came in this morning to pay his employment finder's fee. He told me that because of you he had overcome all of his inhibitions and in two weeks had out-sold even the old-timers. But he also told me that he really liked you and thought that he was falling in love; so I thought I had better call you and alert you as to his intentions."

Needless to say I was dumbfounded! I couldn't believe that I had been so naïve nor could I imagine that I would ever have to confront such a situation—this is crazy, I thought.

Gregory had already set up another appointment so when he came in I was loaded for bear and wanted to face the affliction head-on.

Before Gregory could say anything I asked, "Are you a homosexual?"

He answered, "Well yes, isn't it obvious?"

"Well I'm not and I have no inclination toward becoming one nor am I inclined to engage in any homosexual activities whatever. In fact, I can think of nothing more repulsive, even the thought of it turns my stomach. It's fine with me if that is how you choose to be but I have no interest in that kind of behavior no matter what!"

"You certainly have made your position clear on the subject and I'm not offended by what you have just said." Gregory countered. "I have no intention of trying to get a straight guy to become a homo, but I do like flaunting my homosexuality in front of people—especially red-necks."

That was the first time I heard the term "straight" to distinguish a person who is not homosexual from one who is... but I did know what a red-neck was.

Gregory went on, "I really like to go into a 'straight' bar and hear the red-necks call me a 'faggot,' a 'queer' and a 'homo.' It gives me recognition and often leads to finding a new lover."

Before Gregory left, he thanked me for helping him with his sales performance and apologized if he had offended me.

I never heard from him again... thank goodness!

Since then I have had the opportunity to work with many gays (male and female) and have come to regard them as people who have just chosen a different lifestyle than I have and I have no prejudices towards them at all.

Of the gay people I have worked with few wanted to become straight; most of them just want to get over their self-consciousness about being gay or to not feel guilty or get angry when people tell them that they are evil.

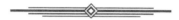

"I have back problems and the doctor has prescribed that I wear high-heeled shoes to correct it. When I wear them it helps my back, but these high-heeled shoes are killing my feet *and* I feel self-conscious when people look at me when I'm wearing them. Can you help me tolerate the discomfort and get over the self-consciousness?"

I explained to Rickie that I wasn't sure about his pain but I was confident that if he came in for a session we could resolve the self-consciousness issue.

When Rickie entered my office I was caught off guard: He was dressed in a fluffy silk blouse with a tight belt around his waist (an attempt to give the appearance of having a figure) that held up silk slacks with no zipper in front. His hair was pulled back into a ponytail, he wore earrings and he had a hint of makeup on his cheeks and lips.... And then I noticed his four-inch spike heels. I wouldn't say that he was totally dressed up in drag—but very near it!

Even before I could introduce myself Rickie handed me a prescription from his doctor ordering him to wear high-heeled shoes.

I ushered him in to my hypnosis room and had him fill out my intake form. In the section where it asks the reason for wanting to be hypnotized he had written: *Remove the discomfort of wearing high heels and not feel self-conscious when wearing them.* So I dealt with only those two issues.

After the session he stood up, slipped on his "four-inchers," smiled and said, "These feel much better." He paid me and swaggered out the door.

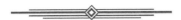

Early in my career I had established the habit of asking my client at the end of each session, "Is there anything else I can do for you?" The following incident quickly broke me of that habit.

From her manner of dress and the guitar slung over her shoulder she was obviously one of the flower children—a true hippie. She had made an appointment to quit smoking marijuana.

She explained that she had had an adventurous past five years and was thinking of changing her lifestyle.

She said, "I've hitchhiked across the country coast to coast more than once. I've lived in communes, slept in vans, smoked pot, sat in on protests, sung anti-war songs, experimented with drugs—you name it and I've done it. I just want to get back to a 'normal' way of life and thought that giving up smoking grass would be a good place to start... maybe!"

She was a good hypnotic subject and was pleased with the result of the session. After waking her up we visited for a few minutes and then I asked, "Is there anything else I can do for you?"

She answered, "Yeah, do you want to (bleep!)?"

After recovering from her blatant invitation to have sex with her I answered, "Yes I do, but not here, and not now, and not with you. I think I'll wait until I get home."

I don't ask that question at the end of the session anymore.

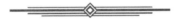

Another habitual response that I have fallen into (when a potential client asks what form of payment I accept—credit cards, debit card, checks, cash) is to say, "I'll take anything that spends."

One day when I used this clever response the fellow stopped for a moment, thought about it and then said, "Will you take my wife? She *really* spends!"

So I stopped and thought for moment and said, "No, I already *have* one of those."

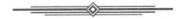

This unusual experience is not related to hypnosis, but since it happened at my hypnosis office and certainly was a memorable one, I'll recount it here.

My secretary was off for the day, so I was waiting at the receptionist's window for my next appointment when the door burst open and there stood a totally nude young woman—not a stitch of clothing on her body!

Not knowing what else to say I asked, "Can I help you?"

She just stood there glassy-eyed and said nothing.

So I asked, "Can I get something to cover you up?"

She nodded yes. So I slipped into my hypnosis room and secured the blanket that I keep just in case a client feels cold. When I returned to the waiting room she was curled up on the waiting room couch and just at that moment (before I could cover her up) in walked my next client who, understandably, seemed to be quite taken aback at the sight!

I quickly explained the situation to her and, although shocked at the spectacle, she seemed to quickly grasp my predicament. I asked if she would mind sitting with the girl while I called 911. She agreed, and sat on the couch and began talking to her with a kind, soft voice. Then I ran to the psychiatrist's office next door and asked one of the girls to come and watch her until the police arrived.

Luckily, just as I returned from next door with help the police arrived. After they had asked a few questions, taken down everyone's name, and left, I invited my client into my hypnosis room and asked, "When I left to get help I heard you visiting with her. Did she give any explanation of how she got into this pickle?"

My client answered, "She told me she just got into town last night and met a fellow at a bar who asked if she had a place to stay. She told him no, so he said she could stay with him in his camper. Before retiring he offered her some 'very special' mushrooms to eat. She said she took some and remembered nothing until she woke up in the camper this morning" (he had parked it in my parking lot overnight) "with no clothes on. So she jumped out of the camper and your door was the first one she came to. And that's how she got here."

I never heard back from the gal or the police so I don't know how it all turned out.

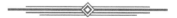

Another event also occurred that was not directly related to a hypnosis session but was certainly a memorable experience and confirmed to me that I had achieved a substantial degree of emotional independence—not letting other people's behavior have a *negative* influence on me emotionally.

"This is Len. I'm just calling to make sure that you are in your office so I can look at you face-to-face. I'll be there in a few minutes."

I could tell from the sound of Len's voice that he was not in the best of moods so I was curious as to what his issue was. As it turned out, it was me!

When he came in I could tell that he had been drinking. He was a good-looking guy, probably six foot two, and he was casually dressed but his clothes were a little disheveled and he had one hand in the pocket of his open jacket. "I've got a gun in here," he said with a bit of a slur. "My wife is divorcing me and there's a bullet here with your name on it!"

I had no idea who he was or who his wife was or how I might be involved in his wife's divorce proceedings. So I asked, "Who are you? Who is your wife? What do I have to do with her wanting to divorce you? And I don't believe that you have a gun in your pocket."

To prove me wrong he pulled out a revolver, cocked back the hammer and pointed it at me. I could see the cartridges in the cylinder!

Whoops! I thought.

He said, "I'm Len and you hypnotized my wife ten months ago. She lost a lot of weight, stopped doing what I tell her to do, got an office job, dresses up like she's a professional and is earning her own money now—and all because of you."

I responded, "You've told me your name but I still don't know who your wife is."

"Her name is Jeanie. She saw you and that Eric guy doing stage-shows at *David's* nightclub. She went there all the time."

I had to rack my brain and then I realized that Jeanie was the gal I had just hypnotized the day Rich called from *David's* and asked me to rescue Eric from the police.

I said, "Oh yes, I remember Jeanie now." I was sure that I had had only one session with her and hadn't seen or heard from her since. "So why do you want to shoot me just because she lost some weight and is now gainfully employed?"

"Because all I have been hearing about over the last ten months is how wonderful that Eric guy is and how you made her lose all that weight.... And when she got her figure back she got confident enough to go out and find a job. It used to be that she was always there when I came home. Even if I had been out working on business deals until two-thirty in the morning, she'd have dinner fixed or get out of bed and make something for me. She doesn't do that any more. She just tells me to go and fix it myself. That's why I want to shoot you—because of you, my life is miserable. So what do you say to that?"

After a moment of consideration I countered, "What I think is that I can't choose for your wife to divorce you or to not divorce you any more than I can choose for you to pull the trigger or to not pull the trigger. If you choose to shoot me I've got a real problem: I've never been shot before so I haven't had much practice knowing how to respond to that kind of an event."

My reply seemed to relax his tension. He un-cocked his gun and put it back into his pocket. I asked him to have a seat and we talked for another twenty minutes, mostly about how one person can't choose for another person their behavior and how no one else can choose ours for us. Finally he stood up and as he left he said, "I really mean it. If this divorce goes through I'm coming hunting for you—there's still a bullet in here for you," as he pointed to his coat pocket.

As I reflected on the event, Socrates and I came up with two significant points: First, we (all people) truly cannot choose for someone else how to behave (how to think, feel or act) and we can *choose* how to respond to the events in our day-to-day life—either in a positive way or a negative way. And second, it was curious how the experience had had no negative influence on me emotionally—Len may as well have been a magazine salesman who had stopped by making cold calls, as far as any adverse emotions were concerned. When Len left I felt peaceful and had no ill feelings about what had just happened—after all, I'm dead at the bottom of a cliff. Had the same experience happened before my imagined self-termination, I would for weeks have had a lump in my throat, felt sick to my stomach and been out there peeking around corners.

This event led to one of my very basic philosophies of life (which will be explored in depth in a later chapter) that I have termed *Emotional Independence*—being free from *negative emotions* when dealing with the behavior of other people, events that occur in our daily life or the uncertainties of the future; i.e., choosing to maintain a sense of peace regardless of events of the past, the present or what might happen in the future.

But the story isn't over yet: A few months later Len stopped by my office again, reached in his pocket, pulled out a slug that he had shot into a sand bag, tossed it to me and said, "This is the one that had your name on it and this is the one that had my name on it," as he held open his other hand.

"When I came in here a few months ago I had every intention of shooting you and then shooting myself because I was so miserable (and drunk), but what fun would it be to shoot someone who isn't pleading for their life? I wanted to make you feel as miserable as I was before shooting you."

He went on to explain, "Some of the things you said really struck home, particularly that you couldn't choose for me not to shoot you any more than you could choose for my ex-wife not to divorce me. And what really struck a chord in my rational mind was when you said that she was not divorcing me because of you; she was divorcing me because of me. Thanks for rationally talking it all out with me and bringing me to my senses. So rather than shooting you and myself I went out and shot a sandbag. If I would have followed through with my initial plan it would have messed up the lives of a whole bunch of people. And one last thing: Now that I'm divorced I don't have to falsify what I'm doing out there until two or three in the morning!"

As he was going out the door he turned and said, "Thanks again."

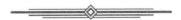

"I really love my new girlfriend, but if it just wasn't for the men that she has been with before I met her... It angers me when I think about her being with another guy. I don't want to feel this way; it's getting in my way of having a long-term relationship with her. I mean she is beautiful, confident, and well mannered; she has a great job, dresses neat as a new pin and is really great in bed. But I just can't stand to even think of her having been with someone else."

During the pre-hypnotic talk, among other things relative to being rid of his anxieties about his girlfriend's past relationships, I explained, "Did you stop to think that if it hadn't been for her prior experience with other men she wouldn't be all that great in bed now?"

I could see an immediate change in his countenance and he said, "I hadn't thought of it that way before. It's strange how when I think of it that way I already no longer have those yucky feelings. I think you've cured me!"

He stood up, handed me my fee and left without ever having to do any "hypnosis."

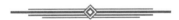

This last experience may deserve its own entire chapter!

"I'm ninety-three years old and I think it is time for me to stop smokin'," Zack told me over the telephone. "Can you get an old geezer like me to quit? You helped my son to stop and he's almost seventy."

I thought about it for a moment and then asked, "Why in the world do you want to stop smoking *now?*"

He scolded me, "Because it is bad for my health. You been livin' in a cave someplace, sonny, don't you know it's bad for you?"

I admitted that I did and we set up an appointment.

On the day of the appointment, after Zack was seated I asked, "What motivated you to think about giving up smoking at ninety-three and to use hypnosis to do it?"

"My wife passed a month ago and my son and I promised her on her death bed that we'd quit. My son did after he came and saw you and that's why I'm here—I've tried but I just can't do it on my own."

"I started rollin' my own back when I was eleven years old. Then when the tailor-mades came out I started smokin' them and I've been goin' through a pack and a half every day ever since... never stopped once, never wanted to, 'til now."

After the session he reported that he felt "really good" and was sure that he had successfully achieved the promise he had made to his wife.

Two years later (at ninety-five) Zack stopped by my office and told me he hadn't smoked a cigarette since his session. He said, "I'm on my way to the airport to get on an airplane to Hawaii. I just wanted to stop by and thank you for helpin' me to stop smokin'. This is something that I should have done fifty years ago. I haven't felt this good for as long as I can remember.

"When I was a young man working in the mines down in Douglas [Arizona] a fellow brought a brochure to work about Hawaii. I took it home and from time to time my wife and I would pull it out and dream of goin' there someday. But we had ten children so we never had the time or the money to do it. Since I came in to see you two years ago, every cent that I would have spent on cigarettes I put into a jar. I didn't have quite enough for the airfare and the accommodations, too, so my family and some of my friends chipped in a few dollars each (and I did, too) so I could fulfill my lifetime dream. I only wish that my companion of 71 years could have been here to enjoy it with me."

I never heard back from Zack but I like to think that when he arrived in Hawaii he found a new companion and "rowed" off into the sunset with her.

CHAPTER 27

Finding Stuff

Quite often someone will make an appointment wanting to remember where they hid something of value and can't recall where they secreted it away—most of the time they had hidden it for safekeeping. Almost always, if the client was consciously aware of what they were doing when they stowed the item, they are able to go back and remember its hiding place.

However, sometimes a client can't find their treasure because it was either lost or stolen. If an item unknowingly slipped out of their pocket during the course of a day they *can* return back to where they last had it, but they are rarely able to recall the exact place and what they were doing when it slipped out. And if the item was stolen, of course hypnosis can't cause them to recall where their property is now, but they may be able to come up with some good ideas about who might have done the pilfering.

Nevertheless, hypnosis is very good at ridding the client of the anxieties of having had their valuables misplaced, lost or stolen and can produce peace of mind in spite of the fact that they no longer have their belongings.

Many people (and even some hypnotists) hold to the belief that the subconscious mind stores every scrap of information a human being has ever been exposed to, whether consciously aware of the details or not, and that while "hypnotized" they can recall every bit of it.

I am convinced that this is not true at all. What is true is that while in a state of "hypnosis" a person's ability to recall the information that has been stored in their brain is significantly enhanced. It appears to me that in order to retrieve a memory from its storage place in our brain it is necessary to have been consciously aware of the information when it was stored.

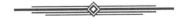

To illustrate: I had a client who had been involved in an automobile accident and wanted to recall the license plate number of a vehicle that was passing through the intersection an instant after the accident occurred.

I asked if he had looked at the license plate on the car before it disappeared down the street, and he answered, "No."

"Then how do you expect to remember the plate number if you didn't see it?"

He said, "I thought that the subconscious mind records *everything* around us at all times and once a person is in hypnosis they can recall it all—everything. I mean, not only the make of the car and the license plate number, but the lines painted on the street, the rocks in the pavement and each blade of grass between the cracks in the sidewalk."

"That is not true," I replied. "The only way we can recall such details is if we are consciously aware of observing them.... Were you aware of grass growing up through the cracks in the sidewalk at the accident scene?"

"No, I am sure that I wasn't."

"Your attention was probably focused in on the accident. Do you remember a car passing by just as the accident occurred?"

"Well no, but one of the witnesses said she thought she saw one."

"Now, if you had consciously looked at the car and the license plate number there would be a high likelihood of recalling it. But since you were not consciously aware of the car and the plate number, it was never recorded in your brain so there is nothing to recall."

I had just talked myself out of an appointment!

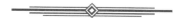

Our sensory system has a huge capacity to store a great deal of information in our brain. We can grasp the big picture of an event (like where an accident occurred, the time of day, or whether it was hot, cold or raining) but it appears to me that we don't recall the details unless we are conscious and aware of them at the moment.

Most of the requests to recall something involve the client wanting to remember where they placed an article for safekeeping but being unable to remember where they hid it. I have selected only a few out of the hundreds of case histories that are typical of this type of request.

The most common lost property is jewelry.

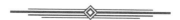

Brenda was sure that she had put her wedding and engagement rings some place where they would be safe just before going on a week's vacation to a beach house. She told me that her rings fit loosely and she didn't want them to slip off and end up in the Pacific Ocean. "I'm sure that I put them someplace so if a burglar broke into our home they would for sure not find them. I did such a good job that now I can't find them."

I was only halfway into the induction process when Brenda's eyes opened and she said, "I know exactly where I put them!"

She explained that she had placed them in her basement on one of the floor joist spreaders and went on to say, "I've been so frustrated about being unable to find them and the more I've tried to remember the more stressed-out I've become. But while you were hypnotizing me I could feel all of that stress and anxiety just evaporate, and when all the stress was gone, the hiding place just popped into my mind."

This scenario illustrates a couple of valid points: Stress inhibits clear thinking and clouds our memory, and often times *trying* to recall something (if we are stressed out) gets in the way of recalling it.

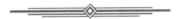

Most often people are able to remember where they put things by the end of the session, but if they are unable to remember before ending the session I suggest: *"In the near future, when your mind is engaged in some routine activity or you encounter some stimulus, where you put your things will just pop into your consciousness."*

Randy had hidden several guns ten years earlier. He told me, "I can't remember *where* I hid them but I do remember that I put them someplace where I would find them if I ever needed them."

Randy was not a gun collector or an avid hunter but he was an ultra right conservative; he had built a bomb shelter in his basement and had stored enough food and provisions to feed and clothe his family for a year, "just in case the Russians drop a bomb on us."

After going through the hypnotic induction I said, *"Randy, return back to the last time you had your guns in your hands. What are you doing now?"*

"I am in my shelter with the guns in my hands and I am thinking that I need to hide them because I don't want my children to find them. I don't like the thought of having guns in the house but if a disaster strikes I'll need them to protect my family and my food storage.

"I used solid concrete blocks to construct a 25 x 15 foot room behind a basement wall, so the room is pretty big. It's full of canned goods, dry-pack food and drums of grain and a bunch of other stuff. It's really well stocked but I've searched in every nook and cranny and I still can't find where I hid them. I've camouflaged the shelter door so it looks like it's just a cabinet and except for my wife, no one knows the room exists, so I know they have not been stolen."

He went on, "You know, if there is a major disaster and people start running out of food they'll stop at nothing to find people who have planned ahead; that's why I bought the guns—so I can protect my food and other necessities in the event of a calamity. And now for the life of me I can't remember where I hid them."

During the session I tried every trick I could think of to jar his memory as to the disposition of his guns and he always ended up in his shelter with the guns in his hands, but he could not recall exactly where he had concealed them.

Just before awakening Randy, I suggested, *"In the near future, when you are not even thinking about your guns, something will jog your memory and where you hid them will just come to mind."*

The very next morning Randy called. "I found them! When I got home after leaving your office I told my wife that the hypnosis didn't help so I guessed I'd just put it out of my mind and not worry about it. 'I'll just go and buy some more guns,' I told her.

"My wife said, 'That would be fine. It's been over ten years since we stored most of that stuff so it is probably time to rotate the wheat.' And that's what triggered my memory—I had hidden my guns in one of the wheat drums!

"I remember now thinking when I hid them, *'If I hide them in the wheat drum, and if there is ever a disaster and I need the wheat I'll find my guns so I can protect my family and our food.'"*

Randy may have remembered the hiding place without hypnosis if the conversation about rotating the wheat would have come up on its own, but he told me that if he had not been hypnotized the topic would have never come up so it must have been the hypnosis.... Who knows?

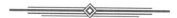

Howard was a student at Arizona State University. He had lost an heirloom ring that had been handed down from father to son for several generations. He said, "I'm sick inside. I can't sleep, I'm not eating, I can't concentrate on my studies and I don't listen to my professors' lectures. All I do is mope around and obsess on the wrath I'll suffer when I have to tell my dad that it is lost—a centuries-old legacy down the drain. Trying to remember when I last had it is ruining my life."

Howard turned out to be an excellent hypnotic subject but no matter the questions I asked or tactics I used to jog his memory, he always returned to standing at the counter in the bathroom of his dormitory as being the last time he had the ring in his possession.

In an effort to console him I asked, *"Could it have been washed down the drain?"*

"No, but I thought of that so I had the plumbers come in and take apart the p-trap and nothing was there. Thinking that it may have made it past the p-trap I put another ring of lesser weight down the drain and turned the water on full force, had them take the plumbing apart again and the 'test ring' was there in the p-trap, so that brought a little relief. How in the world could I have ever found it if it made its way into the sewer system?" he said.

I asked, *"Could it have been stolen?"*

"Don't think so. My roommate is as honest as the day is long and no one else was in our room between the time I had it and when it came up missing. I must have put it some place but for the life of me I can't remember where."

So I suggested, *"In the near future, when you are not even thinking about your ring, someone, some event or some object will trigger the recall of where you last had your ring. But in the meantime, you have a sense of peace of mind as the result of knowing you have made every effort to find it so now you are back in the flow of your daily routine. You are enthusiastic about school, your mind is clear, you are focused in on what your professors are saying while in class and you eat healthfully. When studying, all that matters is the material you're studying. The information that you acquire is stored in your brain for accurate and immediate recall when it is needed and since all avenues of recovering your ring have been pursued, you have a sense of well-being knowing that eventually you will discover its disposition."*

When Howard left my office he said that he felt "really good" even though we had not discovered the whereabouts of his ring.

But I had a gnawing feeling in the pit of my stomach for having suggested that, "eventually you will discover the disposition of your ring." From all of the evidence it was gone forever.

Six weeks later Howard called and said, "Well I didn't find my ring but all of those other suggestions about school really sank in—I just aced my physics test! Thanks for your help."

Six months later I got another call from Howard. "My ring showed up!" he said. "My roommate was arrested for fencing stolen property and my ring was found among his loot. I still can't believe that he was the culprit, but I guess that a really good thief needs to put on an air of honesty... Oh, by the way, I finished at the top in every one of my classes last semester!"

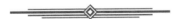

Dean, a day earlier, had lost his keys. One of them was to a secure room at his work and he told me he'd be in "deep doodoo" if he had to advise the company that he had lost it. "It wouldn't be all that much trouble if they had to change the lock but it may have a negative reflection on my security clearance."

He explained, "I drove my car home from shopping with my kids. I unlocked the tailgate of my station wagon and that's the last time I remember having them. I probably put them in my pocket and just set them down someplace, but I'll be darned if I can remember where. We've looked everywhere: Between the cushions of the sofa, under the beds, in all of the clothes hampers, in every pocket of every pair of pants and jacket, but they are nowhere to be found. They've got to be at my house—somewhere."

After the hypnosis induction I asked Dean to return back to the last time he was *aware* of the whereabouts of his keys.

I don't know why I used "aware" or "whereabouts" but they were the right word for the purpose because he responded, "Chink!"

I asked, *"What do you mean when you say 'chink?'"*

He gestured with his head as though the "chink" came from above and behind him and he said, *"chink*, up there," with another nod of his head, indicating behind and above himself.

I asked him to explain what the *"chink up there"* had to do with his keys.

He said, "I don't know, but as I thought about unloading stuff from my station wagon I remember hearing this 'chink' sound, kind of like keys on the roof of the carport."

"If the 'chink' was your keys on the roof of your carport how do you suppose they got up there?"

"I have no idea, but it's the best clue I have had so far!"

After I brought him up he said that he'd give me a call when he got home—either way.

An hour later Dean called and said, "When I got home I put the ladder up and there they were, lying on the carport roof. After I found them I interrogated my sons and finally the youngest one admitted that he had taken the keys out of the station wagon's door and was playing with them by tossing them up in the air. The last time, they didn't come down. He told me that he was afraid to tell me because I had often threatened them with the pain of death if any of them even touched my keys!"

It's interesting how we are able to remember subtle things like the "chink" of keys on the roof, but Dean had to be aware of the "chink" in order to recall having heard the "chink."

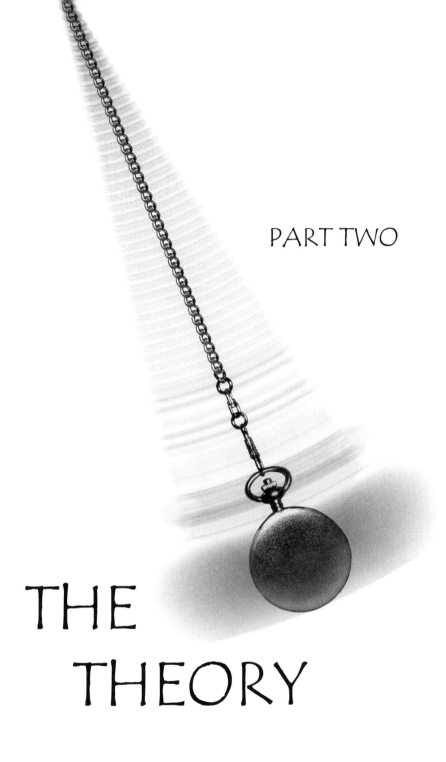

PART TWO

THE
THEORY

CHAPTER 28

Organization and a Move Back to Phoenix

It was really not until I had been practicing for six or seven years that my approach to hypnotherapy began to truly take shape. Up until this time in my career it was a hodgepodge of disjointed ideas.

I learned a great deal about hypnosis from my mentors (Art Baker and Eric) and the few books had I read, but the greatest impact on developing a coherent approach came from my clients, stage-show volunteers and even from people who had witnessed other people being hypnotized. When a client, volunteer or spectator asked a question or made an observation I would, to the best of my ability, answer the question and comment on their observation but more often than not they were the same questions and observations that I had been wrestling with myself. But sometimes they were questions and observations that had never entered my mind. So I would make a mental note of each query and at my next opportunity take it into my inner room to see if Socrates could come up with a rational answer.

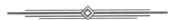

Thinking that I needed to bring myriad disjointed ideas to a semblance of order, I sat down in my recliner, made myself comfortable, went through my self-hypnosis routine, descended my spiral staircase, entered into my inner room, sat across the desk at which Socrates sat and asked:

Me: Many people with whom I talk about the hypnotic process have insightful questions about hypnosis itself; the subconscious mind, human behavior, past-life experiences and what happens after we die, and more often than not I have no clear-cut answers to their inquiry. Even more puzzling is finding a way to explain the driving force behind what they observe during the course of a stage-show or a clinical session. How can I resolve this quandary?

Socrates: Organize your (and their) questions and observations, write them down and consider them one at a time. Remember that the answers may come from sources other than your own rational thinking and introspection. And also remember that not all of the questions have been asked. So never stop wondering, listening and asking.

Me: Okay. A few of the questions I think I have pretty well resolved, but I will give you a list, resolved or not. I know that some of them are controversial and may have no absolute answers.

I got out of my recliner and went to my desk drawer where I had stuffed the scraps of paper, napkins, backs of calling cards and a few pieces of cardboard on which I had jotted down the questions and observations that had arisen over the past several years. I then wrote them down in a spiral notebook in the random order that I picked them up:

- What is hypnosis and can everyone be hypnotized?
- Can a hypnotist make a person engage in a behavior that would violate their moral or ethical standards?
- Do we have a predetermined purpose to accomplish in life? If so, can hypnosis help me to discover what it is?
- Does a person have to *believe* in hypnosis in order to be hypnotized?
- Do events earlier in our life determine our present behavior? If so, can hypnosis change it?
- Can the hypnotist make a hypnotized subject do something that they normally wouldn't do?
- Do we need to go back and discover unconscious events in order to change our present behavior?
- Did we live past lives?
- If we lived past lives how much do they influence our behavior in this one?
- Why do some people think hypnosis is Satanic?
- What does the human soul or spirit have to do with hypnosis?
- How does God fit into the hypnotic process?
- How did we become human beings and the only creatures on earth that can be hypnotized?
- Did God create us in the twinkling of an eye? Was the hypnotic process included in God's breath of air when He breathed into a lump of clay and made man a living soul?
- Did we evolve through a process of natural selection and the survival of the fittest and is the hypnotic process a part of that evolution?

- Is the state of hypnosis something different than other everyday states of mind?
- Is a subject truly asleep while hypnotized?
- What is an unconscious mind?
- If the hypnotist is talking to the unconscious or subconscious mind ("sub" meaning below the level of conscious awareness) how can the unconscious mind "know" what the hypnotist is saying?
- Is there a way to easily demonstrate that visualization can change human behavior without having to be hypnotized first? (This was my question.)
- What is the subject thinking about while hypnotized—if anything?
- When a hypnotized person is hallucinating (like seeing little people having a party in a cigar box), do they really believe that the hallucination is reality?
- Is hypnosis a state of mind or is it a process of the brain? (Another one of my questions)
- Do we have two minds: a *conscious mind* that we intentionally use to make decisions about our daily behavior and a *subconscious mind* that is operating on its own and we have little to say about the behavior that it produces?
- What does the brain have to do with hypnosis?
- Is hypnosis a relatively recent phenomenon or has it been a part of the human experience from the moment human beings became rational, logical, thinking beings?
- Can a hypnotist hypnotize a person without them knowing that they have been hypnotized?
- How long does it take to hypnotize a person?
- Does hypnosis wear off with the passage of time?
- What kind of schooling do you need to be a hypnotist? Do you need a degree or governmental certification to be a hypnotherapist?

After making my list I sat back down in my recliner, went back into my inner room and said:

Me: Okay, how is that for a list of questions?

Socrates: Now you need to break them down into categories and work on the categories one at a time. Many of your questions are the same questions but just asked differently. For you to successfully answer most of your questions it

might not hurt to consider going to college and getting a formal education so you can draw on the experiences and thoughts of countless other people who have had many of the same questions and spent a lifetime pondering them.

I had already considered going to college but this conversation with Socrates motivated me to take action.

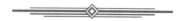

In the summer of 1975 (I was still living in Salt Lake City at the time) I received a call from a friend and former business associate (Clark Allen) whom I had met when living in the Phoenix area five years earlier. Clark asked me to come to Tempe (a suburb of Phoenix) and work with him as an associate in his thriving insurance business. Clark was the general sales manager for American Savings Life (a small but well established and well managed family-owned insurance company) and made me a financial offer I couldn't refuse. By accepting his proposal I estimated that I could wipe out all of my debts in six months, rather than the three years that I had anticipated. There were two stipulations that Clark agreed to: First, that I could still pursue my interest in hypnosis, and second, that I could return to SLC once a month to service a few of my most lucrative industrial supply accounts.

So Darlene and I loaded up our five children (we had added Patrick and Laurel—and the next January, Amber—to the clan) and established residence in Gilbert, Arizona.

It took a little longer than I had predicted, but nine months after returning to the Phoenix area my only financial encumbrance was the mortgage on my home—no credit card debt, no delinquent utility bills, no car payments and (a new experience for me) a growing savings account!

Once I had learned the ropes of the insurance business and was settled in to my new job, I opened a hypnosis office in Tempe where I still have my practice.

I placed an ad in the *Penneysaver,* an advertising circular similar to the *Little Nickel* in Salt Lake City. The *Pennysaver* produced only a few clients—not nearly as many as I had hoped. So I made a phone call to the *Arizona Republic and Gazette* classified advertising department to place an ad in their personals section for hypnosis—the *Arizona Republic and Gazette* was the only major newspaper in the Phoenix area at the time.

When I called to inquire about advertising hypnosis, to my astonishment, I discovered that the narrow-mindedness and bigotry against hypnosis was no less in Phoenix than it was in SLC at that time—the 1970's: they refused to accept my ad because it was in violation of the *Board of Ethical Advertising* guidelines. I don't know that I have the name exactly right but I believe it

was the same organization that I had encountered six years earlier when I sent away for my "LEARN HOW TO HYPNOTIZE–PUT PEOPLE UNDER YOUR SPELL–Get whatever you want" mail order pamphlet.

The lady on the phone with whom I talked about placing an ad must have quit her volunteer job at the SLC Library and secured a position with the newspaper's classified department. She explained to me that the newspaper had a standard policy to not advertise séances, voodoo, fortune telling, witchcraft, and other Satanic practices like hypnosis.

"Why in the world would you want to be advertising hypnosis in the first place?" she rebuked. "Don't you know that hypnosis is the same as devil worship? Don't you know that once a person is hypnotized the devil can get in and possess their body, mind and soul? Haven't you ever seen one of those hypnosis sideshows where the hypnotist makes people do things that they don't want to do–that's evil. And no, you cannot advertise the devil's work with this newspaper!" [CLUNK]

So I looked in the Yellow Pages under hypnotists. Although there was only one hypnotist advertised (Don Weldon) I was relieved to discover that here was at least one major advertising source the Board of Ethical Advertising hadn't gotten to.

When I had looked in the Yellow Pages six years earlier there was only one hypnotist listed; in all likelihood this was the same Don Weldon whom I didn't have the courage to call back then. I never did meet Don in person (his office was on the west side of Phoenix and mine was on the east, about 30 miles apart) but for several years he and I were the only hypnotists listed in the Yellow Pages–now there are sixty-five! However, I gained a great respect for Don because of the good reputation he had established over his many years of practice and the positive influence he had on the public's attitude toward hypnosis.

I placed ads in the Yellow Pages under several listings: Hypnotists, Smoker Treatment, Weight Control and Stress Management. It took three months before the new phonebook was distributed but when it was I began getting new clients and it was not long until I had enough business to cover my office and advertising expenses with a little to spare. And, I was getting more valuable experience.

It was fortunate that I still had my business in SLC as well as my hypnosis practice, because a year after arriving in Tempe, American Savings Life was served a cease and desist order by the Arizona State Attorney General's office ordering us to stop selling insurance policies. It turned out that one of the policies that we were selling (the policy that accounted for 95% of our business) was deemed to be in violation of the laws governing the sale of insurance. So once again my financial bubble burst, and my income was reduced by one-half. But I still had my SLC accounts and my hypnosis practice—and I was out of debt and there *was* a little money in my savings account. So this time I had a safety net to catch my pecuniary fall.

For some reason that I could not explain, my hypnosis clientele was of a higher social and economic class than it had been in SLC. Maybe it was because I was no longer doing stage-shows in nightclubs or maybe it was because of the proximity of my office to Arizona State University (ASU). Whatever the reason, a substantial number of my clients were college educated and of a higher economic class. Often times during the course of a session I would become self-conscious about my meager educational background when a client would introduce into the conversation topics of which I had little or no knowledge—such as principles of psychology, philosophical views, science and history.

So I decided to go to college and get an education!

I trust that by now the reader has a sense of my minimal education and my reading deficiency. Even though my reading ability had been significantly enhanced from what it had been five years earlier (as a result of self-hypnosis and practicing reading skills) my reading speed was probably still at a junior high level. I had little trouble retaining what I read; it was just that there seemed to be a great weight holding me back as I attempted to increase my reading speed. And reading out loud was even slower. But I decided to enroll at Mesa Community College (MCC) anyway.

I thought I was over all of my inhibitions about institutions and learned people but when I entered MCC's admissions office I experienced some of the same anxieties that I had met with when entering into the "house of doom"—the Salt Lake City library. But when I reminded myself that "I am dead at the bottom of a cliff, so nothing can threaten me," those feelings of dread vanished.

After taking the entrance examination, to my surprise, I qualified for enrollment at MCC but I would need to include in my schedule remedial math and English.

That semester, in addition to English and Math 001 I enrolled in Psychology 101 and Philosophy 101. To my complete wonderment, at the end of the semester I boasted a GPA of 4.0! It was the first time in my educational history that I had received a grade in English or math higher than a D+ or C-. But the best part of going to college was that I was learning things that I had missed out on back in the forties and fifties when struggling through K to

12. But better still, I began satisfying many of my curiosities about topics that most people my age just took for granted.

I was still a little self-conscious about my limited exposure to topics with which many of my classmates were current. Most of them were just out of high school and what they had learned was still fresh in their minds... and most of them were 19 years younger than me. So here I was, 40 years old and 22 years since I had been in a classroom. Not only that, I was 12 years older than some of the professors.

I was especially self-conscious in my psychology classes not knowing how my professors, who were academically oriented and university schooled, viewed hypnosis. From my limited exposure to highly educated people it seemed that most (if not all) of them thought of hypnosis as a bunch of mystical poppycock.

So when Professor Kurt Mahoney (with whom I had established a good rapport since we were about the same age) asked me what I did for a living I sheepishly said, "I'm a hypnotist."

His response was quite unexpected. "Wow, that's neat! I've always had a curiosity about hypnosis. As a matter of fact I wrote a short paper on the use of hypnosis for breaking bad habits. What kind of stuff do you use hypnosis for in your practice?"

With a little more confidence I said, "Oh, I help people to stop smoking, to lose weight and to overcome stress, phobias and anxieties—those kinds of things."

Dr. Mahoney went on to say, "In addition to teaching here at MCC I have a private psychology practice and I deal with many of the same kind of issues. I don't use hypnosis but I'm curious to know how long your sessions are and how much you charge."

By this time in my career my confidence as a hypnotist, and my confidence in the hypnotic process, had significantly increased and my fees had risen proportionally. I answered, "I am working on keeping a session to under an hour and I charge $85 a session."

Professor Mahoney seemed to be a little taken aback and said, "Let me tell you what I think you should do, Lindsay. Finish up here at MCC, enroll over at Arizona State University for another two years and get your bachelor's degree (like I did). Spend another two years and get your master's degree in counseling (like I did), then spend another two years and get a Ph.D. in psychology (like I did) and then after eight years of schooling and thousands of dollars in tuition fees you can charge $45 a session (like I do)!"

Until then I had no idea what psychologists charged for their services, or what other hypnotists charged for that matter, but what Dr. Mahoney said had a profound influence on my thinking about the true value of *me* getting a formal higher education. I'm not saying that a higher education does not hold great value in itself or that having some letters behind one's name does not present an air of credibility. But for me, having a Ph.D. tagged on to the end of my name would have little to do with successfully helping people to favorably make a change in their behavior. (Of course, a book written by a Ph.D. may entice more people to buy it!)

I graduated from MCC with an AA degree and a 3.86 GPA, and then completed another year at ASU with a 4.0 GPA. My major was psychology and after three years of studying the topic I discovered that there was only one consistency in psychology: Nobody agrees!

Because of the termination of my income from American Savings Life and the inordinate amount of time required to study and maintain a high GPA, service my industrial accounts from a distance, and raise six children who were in or approaching the expensive teenage years, I dropped out of school to satisfy my growing monetary demands, with the intention of finishing up at some later date. And it may still happen.

The classes during my tenure at MCC and ASU that held my greatest interest were psychology (discovering why people behave as they do), philosophy (what and why people think as they do), science (how and why nature works as it does) history (events and experiences in the lives of other people) and the other humanities (art, literature, music, theater, etc.). However, probably the two most useful discoveries from psychology were *classical conditioning* (Pavlov's experiment with salivating dogs) and *dyslexia* (a probable explanation of my reading deficiency).

CHAPTER 29

University Enlightenment

Not until I enrolled in college level education did I realize how miniature the cocoon was in which I had lived my life. I had been taught from youth that "to know the truth" one becomes free; however, this was always expressed within a Scriptural context and implied that freedom came only from knowing the truths of God's plan and the faith to blindly accept it.

Once I was exposed to secular opinions I soon discovered that there are never-ending truths outside of those found in the Scriptures and being unrestrained to investigate them is *true* freedom. I don't mean to imply that there is anything wrong with studying the Scriptures and the teachings of religious leaders but by studying them exclusively the investigator is confined to a very narrow spectrum of knowledge and is excluded from discovering other truths.

But my limited and delayed education had some advantages: I had not been indoctrinated in traditional academic thinking and I was mature enough in age (40 years old) and had gained sufficient confidence to not only question what my professors taught but to *ask* the questions—to challenge their point of view if *I* had a different one.

Another interesting discovery: Many of the questions and opinions that I had secretly harbored within the confines of my brain regarding human behavior, religion, science and philosophy (questions and opinions that I had considered to be uniquely my own) had been more than once pondered by great thinkers throughout the ages.

College level classes spawned as many questions as they resolved. Several dialogs with Socrates in later chapters will systematically address many of these questions as they relate to "hypnosis," my personal philosophy about life and psychology in general.

Here are a few of the significant things I gleaned from attending college:

History

I had only a fuzzy understanding of world and American history before starting college. Except for the very narrow historical information one can scrape together from the Bible, I had no idea of what was going on in the rest of the world before, during and after Old and New Testament times—any other historical events and the people who lived them were for the most part a blank slate. History has become a guiding light in my quest to understand the thinking and motivations of humanity.

I believe that my greatest personal benefit from history is having learned from those who have enlightened and elevated human understanding. And that we individually, by drawing from the thoughts and experiences of the "giants" of the arts, psychology, philosophy, religion and science, can not only elevate ourselves but are able to uplift, encourage and give hope to others.

And yes, from the giants involved in the development of this thing that is called "hypnosis" I have caught a glimpse of what makes it work and a practical way to use it. I have also learned from history that sometimes the giants don't always have it right—Mesmer and *animal magnetism*[4] for example!

Humanities

From my humanities classes I learned that the sole purpose of literature, art and music is to engender an emotional response in the reader, viewer or listener. Leonardo da Vinci wrote, "Painting is felt rather than seen." Literature, music, theater and art, good or bad, are created with the intent of stirring up "feelings." The ones that produce the emotions intended by their creator most often become classics and are performed or viewed over and over, but the ones that produce no emotions disappear. Most writers intend to evoke feelings of happiness, sadness, fear, anger, peace of mind or pleasure. Even some technical papers evoke pleasure or outrage depending upon whether the reader agrees or disagrees with the writer.

I learned to love the humanities once I began looking for the emotion that the creator of the work intended.

Science

I learned from science that it is quite okay to have differences of opinion and to be proven wrong. It is okay to say I made a mistake—I now see there was a flaw in the design of my study or my thinking. There is a great deal of disagreement and even animosity among scientists, and some even withhold their findings for fear that someone else will take them and develop a new

---

4. Mesmer and animal magnetism will be discussed in a later chapter.

theory that they themselves are seeking. Nevertheless, for the most part scientists freely share their discoveries and theories.

Frequently a scientist comes up with sound data that show an established and accepted theory is wrong and, although reluctant to do so, the scientist who created the theory most often is willing to admit that they made a mistake. Probably the most famous example of this is when Einstein inserted an arbitrary equation (the cosmological constant) into his general theory of relativity so his calculations would produce a stable universe (one that does not expand). Then, when Edwin Hubble's observations of galaxies proved that the universe is indeed expanding, Einstein quickly relented, removed the constant from his equation, and exclaimed that inserting it in the first place was one of his greatest blunders—which would imply that he must have made other blunders.

I remember reading somewhere that science is the study of things that *can* be *dis*-proven—unlike opinion, philosophy, politics, religion and the like.

I would define science as being the systematic study (through the application of the scientific method) of any phenomenon of the physical world that separates knowledge, general truths and natural laws from ignorance, supposition, false concepts, assumption, superstition, bigotry and hearsay.

Before *Psychology 101* I had never heard of the *scientific method*, which basically is a procedure of stating a hypothesis and then setting up an experimental procedure that uses empirical data to prove or disprove that a theory is (or is not) valid (one that produces the prediction of the hypothesis) and reliable (one that consistently produces the predicted result). Nevertheless, and more important, I learned that the experimenter must be willing to accept the results of the experiment—even if it is different from his or her prediction. If the results are different from the prediction then the experimenter is free to devise a new experimental method to confirm the theory or to accept the fact that what was originally thought to be true is not true.

Behavioral Science

Behavioral science is a branch of science that deals primarily with human behavior and includes psychology, sociology and anthropology. In addition, the fact that it is a science implies the need for controlled methods of study and a need to establish theories that can predict an outcome (or consequences) of a given event.

In the physical sciences, there are many well-established laws. For example, Newtonian physics reliably predicts that a massive object will fall towards the center of the earth when released (an event). However, it does not explain *why* it does—the mechanism or the process that causes it to fall.

In the case of *behavioral science*, however, things are not so black and white. Because human behavior is so complex and holds infinite possibilities for the ways in which an individual can behave, psychology has produced very few theories that reliably predict the response of each individual person to an event. The best behavioral science can do is to rely on statistical analysis, which will tell an experimenter the *likelihood* that a person will respond to a stimulus or an event in a predictable way. While many statistical models have a high degree of reliability, none is absolute, nor do they explain the mechanisms that drive a given behavior.

I approach "hypnosis" as being one aspect of behavioral science and, as such, I have searched for a method to reliably test my theories of how it works and how to use it.

Philosophy

In Philosophy 101, I met the *real* Socrates. I don't know why I chose him as my inner guide—I only knew that he was a wise person who lived a long time ago—but as it turns out I couldn't have made a better choice, especially since he, too, had an inner guide—his "daimon" (or spiritual guide). In addition, as I met other great thinkers I realized that, for the most part, they pondered the same questions that I had been pondering.

My philosophy classes taught me that a good place to start is to question everything (which is an aspect of my basic nature, anyway), or better still, to accept nothing that anyone has ever said, written or taught to be true *or* false— rather, start out with a blank slate! Then closely examine all of the available empirical evidence and through logic and sound reasoning create a philosophy of life that fits into the perspective of *my* world. Then find comfort in that perspective even if it goes against traditional thinking. However, always be ready to abandon any conviction when compelling evidence proves that it no longer holds true.

Psychology

The greatest discovery made as the result of studying psychology is that nobody agrees!

Everyone who has written a book or taught a class has their own ideas about why people behave as they do and how to manipulate their behavior. Therefore, I decided that since no one would agree with me anyway, I would construct my own model that describes what determines human behavior and how to change it when change is desirable and for the good of the person desiring the change.

Most approaches in psychology are eclectic—taking the ideas of many theories and then bringing them together into a form that produces a different unique model. Most certainly, my approach to explaining "hypnosis" is eclectic with just a few ideas being abstractions of my own mind.

From psychology I also learned about T. X. Barber, from whom (in addition to many other views) I learned to put quotation marks around "hypnosis"—a designation that I will quite often use during the rest of my narrative.

In the beginning, I took exception to T. X. Barber's views on "hypnosis," but with experience and experiment I have come full circle and embrace almost all of his conclusions.

T. X. Barber himself came full circle with his own conclusions. Starting out skeptical that "hypnosis" is a unique phenomenon of human behavior, he systematically conducted countless studies and traveled the world seeking answers as to just what "hypnosis" is, expecting to prove his theory that it was *not* unique. At one point he believed that "hypnosis" was a unique human behavior, but then, based on further studies, concluded that that there is little difference in the suggestibility of a "hypnotized" person and a person who has not been "hypnotized." Many experimenters who have since carried out numerous well-conducted independent studies have confirmed this conclusion.

Another contribution psychology had to my early ideas of "hypnosis" was that it is an *altered state of consciousness*. The chapter in my psychology 101 text on *altered states of consciousness* included dreaming, hallucinations, figments of imagination, out of body experiences, alcohol intoxication, drug abuse, and "hypnosis." This concept (that "hypnosis" is an altered state of consciousness) for several years was the nucleus of my pre-hypnotic talk when explaining "hypnosis" to my clients. However, after an intense debate with a colleague and a conversation with Socrates, it was a concept I had to discard (discussed in detail in a later chapter).

From psychology, I also learned about Pavlov and dyslexia!

I am not a pure "behaviorist" by any means but my eclectic approach certainly includes the fact that we humans sometimes get conditioned into behaving in a given way as the result of exterior stimuli like Pavlov's dogs—ring the bell and they salivate. Not only do we human beings respond to exterior stimuli with our five senses, but mental stimuli that we create with our imagination also trigger overt behavior and emotions.

Classical Conditioning

In almost every hypnosis session I talk about classical conditioning. Once I learned about Pavlov and then began mentioning his name to clients I was amazed to find that almost everyone had heard of him and his experiments with salivating dogs. This is just one example of the informational cocoon in which I had lived for forty years—Pavlov and classical conditioning were nonexistent.

Most people think that Pavlov, the Russian 1907 Pulitzer Prize winner, was a psychologist—not true. Pavlov was a *philologist* whose studies dealt with gastrointestinal processes in dogs and who serendipitously stumbled upon what is now called *classical conditioning*.

Pavlov knew that when his dogs smelled food, their instinctual reflex was to salivate (drool)—the first step of the digestive process. As part of his study he measured how much each dog would salivate when presented with food. Then one day he noticed that when the door to the food storage room opened, his dogs began to salivate—although there was no food his dogs could taste, smell or see. He then set up a controlled study to confirm his suspicions.

Over a period, Pavlov systematically presented food to his dogs (in his experiment he used meat powder). When their instincts kicked in and they started to salivate, he rang a bell. Once that association of the sound of the bell and salivation had been established, whenever he would ring the bell his dogs would salivate, even when there was no food present.

With this study, I learned the true measure of science: Pavlov established a hypothesis (dogs become conditioned to salivate with the rapacious sound of a bell) and both the stimulus and response were measurable and empirically observed.

Many psychologists (John Watson and B. F. Skinner among them) contributed to the branch of psychology termed "behaviorism." Behaviorism asserts that all behavior is learned behavior and gives little credibility to the idea of cognitive behavior—the theory that human beings possess the ability to *choose* their behavior.

We as human beings do become conditioned to respond to different stimuli and for the most part it is good that we do—the light turns red and we step on the brake without consciously thinking about it. But often we get conditioned to engage in destructive behavior—drink a cup of coffee, light a cigarette, get stressed-out and march to the refrigerator, or get angry when someone disagrees with us. However, I am convinced that we (us human beings) can change and alter how we respond to the stimuli that trigger unwanted behavior by application of this process that is *called* "hypnosis."

Dyslexia

It was probably in Developmental Psychology that I first heard of the condition called dyslexia. When the topic came up it was like an eye-opening revelation—could dyslexia explain my own reading and spelling deficiency? As it turns out, I believe that it does.

Dyslexia is a <u>neurological</u> or brain-based condition that has nothing to do with intelligence, creativity, or the ability to grasp ideas or to reason. Some studies estimate that up to 17% of the population is dyslexic. Many famous and highly successful people have been diagnosed as being dyslexic or have displayed related reading and writing problems found in the dyslectic: Robin Williams, Leonardo daVinci, Nolan Ryan, Henry Ford, Walt Disney and even Albert Einstein—just to mention a few. (For more go to Google search—*dyslexic famous people*.)

In the late 1800s physicians called the condition "congenital word blindness." Then in 1928, a neurologist named Samuel Orton called it "strephosymbolia" (meaning "twisted symbols"), which has been replaced by its current term, "dyslexia": from Latin *dys-* meaning difficult and Greek *lexis* meaning speech, or word.

In the 1940s, neurologists thought dyslexia was a visual (of the eye) dysfunction that stood in the way of a student attaining even mediocre scholastic accomplishments.

Probably from the first day of kindergarten I was aware of the fact that it was more difficult for me to read well than it was for *most* of the other students—in retrospect, maybe 83% of them. If I had enough time I could make it through a *Dick and Jane* book—actually, to avoid embarrassment, at times I took the books home and memorized them so when I got into class it would appear that I was actually reading the text. However, eventually the ruse caught up with me when it came to taking tests and sight-reading.

I have a vivid recollection of, when in the fifth grade, being kept after school for a special session with two teachers—fortunately, Miss Howard, who had kicked me out of the Sandy City Library, was not one of them.

I knew that this after-school meeting had something to do with reading and I thought that they were going to teach me *how* to read. One of the teachers was Miss Killian, who was the sixth grade teacher, and the other was a teacher I had never before seen—I deduce now that she was a specialist trained for testing students who displayed dyslexic symptoms.

I clearly remember my disappointment when the session lasted only fifteen minutes and there was no attempt at teaching or even a mention of how to read.

They had me sit in the second row of desks and Miss Killian drew a three-foot diameter circle on the chalkboard. She had in her hand a pointer and asked me to keep my eyes fixed on its tip regardless of the direction she pointed it. She moved it around the chalkboard circle clockwise for a few minutes and then counter-clockwise for another few minutes. She then moved the pointer up and down and then back and forth for another period. While this exercise was going on, I noticed that the "mystery" teacher did nothing but look at my eyes.

My suspicion is this: I "passed" the dyslexic test—I have it!

No mention was ever made about the results of the session—not by the teachers or my parents. However, I believe that my parents (both of whom were educators) were apprised of my condition and advised that nothing could be done about my state and were told the best they could hope for was that I would somehow squeak through the remaining grades and *maybe* even graduate from high school—which is exactly what happened. I suspect that this information was passed along from teacher to teacher because a few of my fellow students who had better grades than me were held back for a year. Nowadays schools make special provisions for dyslexic students, but not then; they just moved me along.

Understanding dyslexia has come a long way since then. Although not definitive, *some* evidence indicates that the condition has a slightly greater likelihood of occurring in children whose parents are dyslexic (neither of my parents displayed the slightest hint of the condition), who are left-handed (which I am not) or who have hearing problems—which could be a contributor to my condition (during my early formative years I did have frequent earaches and eventually a tonsillectomy to resolve the problem).

Regardless of the indicators, all evidence points to dyslexia as being a dysfunction of the brain and not necessarily caused by genetics. Researchers have discovered that the problem lies in the area designated as V5 within the mango cellular area of the brain, but they have yet to discover the actual *cause* of dyslexia.

Obviously, there are disadvantages for the dyslexic: Of course, slow and difficult reading is one of them, especially when attempting to read aloud. Spelling is another one—even as I am writing this text some words (although I have used them many times during the preceding chapters) necessitate using my spell-checker to get the letters in the right order—"obviously," for example. And some words sound different than they are spoken—pavement has always sounded like pathement and funeral sounds like funerl.

But there are compensations for the dyslexic. Studies have shown that a person with dyslexia tends to be more creative, physically coordinated, intuitive and empathetic than their non-dyslexic counterparts.

For me, being dyslexic provided an additional advantage: I have developed an excellent ability to memorize, conceptualize and store information about the large picture and to recall it when needed—in short, I have a good memory.

As mentioned earlier, I would memorize my grade school primers so when I got into class it *looked* like I was reading the text rather than reciting it. Not only that, I discovered if I was always in class (which I was) I could glean from the teacher a great deal of information just by paying attention. This ability spilled over into college level learning. As I refined this attribute it significantly enhanced my grade point average... it is, in a way, like cheating: I discovered that by always being in class and focusing only on what the instructor was explaining, in effect, the teacher was telling me most of the answers on the upcoming test. All I need to do was recall it when the time came. Once it was stored in my brain, recall was easy.

When growing up another fortunate advantage was that both of my parents were educators and university graduates—and my older siblings were exceptional students—so good grammar and a rich and varied vocabulary was used in our home and I intuitively picked up on it and it spilled over into grasping ideas and recognizing the meaning of explanatory words.

In my 9th grade English class Mr. Bitters conducted an exercise of presenting five descriptive words that he had taken from that morning's newspaper. He recited them one at a time and if any student knew what the word meant they were to raise their hand and give a definition. Of the five, I was able to comprehend and correctly define four of them. None of my fellow students did as well. The memorable part of this experience happened after class: Reece Jensen (who was one of the brightest students in the school) came up to me after the class and said, "Lindsay, how did you know what all of those words meant when you are so dumb?" I didn't understand it, either, but part of it may have been that I *heard* the words rather than having to *read* them.

Being dyslexic may have also contributed to my need for a point of view to be logical, which not only led to my obsessive skepticism and questioning but also led to my discovering new ideas and innovative ways of thinking and of doing things—particularly in the field of hypnotherapy.

CHAPTER 30

Arizona Society for Professional Hypnosis

A tall, distinguished-looking gentleman entered my office one day and introduced himself. "Hi, my name is Jon Pace. I am a member of an organization called the *Arizona Society for Professional Hypnosis* (ASPH) and we'd like you to join our group. ASPH is a nonprofit society that was incorporated in 1978. For the first few years we were a relatively active group, but a couple of years ago two of the members moved away, one retired from doing hypnosis, three lost interest and another died, so that left me (now the recruiting person), Bill Nelson (secretary/treasurer), Roy Martin (in charge of creating a certification test) and Leo Gagnon (ASPH's president). Under Leo's leadership our numbers are beginning to grow. We now have 12 members and usually 8 or 10 show up to our monthly meetings. Would you come and join us?"

I was surprised to discover that there were 12 hypnotists in the Phoenix area, let alone an assemblage of them.

Thinking that ASPH was a group of professionals with academic degrees, if not in psychology probably in medicine (doctors and dentists) and that they had had many years of experience doing hypnosis, I was a little reluctant to expose my limited education and training to the academics. (I had just started my first year at MCC.) So I said, "Jon, I am relatively new to the profession of hypnosis and have no university degree, so I'm not sure I would qualify to be a part of your group."

With a chuckle Jon responded, "You don't even need to be a hypnotist to be a member of ASPH. There are three classifications of membership: We have an *Associate* member. These are people who have an interest in hypnosis but don't do any hypnotizing. There is a *Professional Hypnotist* membership—people who, like you, actively hypnotize people for a fee. And finally, we have a *Certified Professional Hypnotist* classification for professionals who have successfully passed the ASPH certification test. To be certified, a candidate must pass a written and oral examination and then demonstrate his hypnosis procedure before a certification board.

"As a matter of fact, one of the orders of business at our next meeting is to iron out some wrinkles in the written examination. It should be a very spirited meeting since there seems to be little consensus as to the questions that should be asked and how to ask them.

"Will you at least come to our next meeting and meet some of the hypnotists in the area? You don't have to join if you don't want to, but at least come to this one meeting and then decide."

More out of curiosity than for any other reason I agreed to attend. *It would be interesting to witness a dozen hypnotists debating issues about "hypnosis,"* I thought.

At this point in my career I was not only questioning but sharply disagreeing with many of the opinions that my teachers and the authors of books on the topic of hypnosis had, so I could hardly imagine what it would be like to be in a room full of them.

So I agreed to attend just this one meeting. But as it turned out, I attended almost every meeting for the next 17 years and was elected ASPH president for 5 of them.

At this first ASPH meeting my curiosity was not to be disappointed as to the diversity of people and the opinions of each member of the *Arizona Society for Professional Hypnosis.*

The group ranged from the proper, prim Jon Pace to an un-kempt fellow, whose name I cannot recall, with rumpled clothes and disheveled hair who looked like he just rolled out of bed. A diversity of professions was represented, too: As I recall there was a dentist, an attorney, a construction worker, a couple of people who were working in the aerospace industry, a high school teacher/psychologist/counselor and a fellow who was unemployed and considering hypnosis as a possible profession. And to my surprise it turned out that, except for me, none worked out of an office nor did any make a living by doing hypnosis exclusively.

Among the cast of characters was Leo Gagnon, ASPH president, who conducted the proceedings in precise parliamentary form—recognition of members and visitors, minutes of the previous meeting read and approved by vote, new and old business to be considered at this meeting. Leo was the apparent leader of the group, not only by title but by demeanor.

There was a noticeable agitation once preliminary matters had been finalized and Leo turned the "floor" over to Roy Martin for the purpose of reconciling some differences of opinion that members had regarding questions on the ASPH certification test.

Question 1:

A subject can lie when under hypnosis. __True __ False

One group said true, another said false, and I thought, *Why is the question on the test at all?* So reluctantly, I asked, "Can you explain to me how knowing whether a person can lie or is unable to lie while hypnotized is an issue? Will knowing the answer, either way, make me a better hypnotist?"

Both camps—true and false—believed it would. The first group contended, "If a person *can* lie when under hypnosis then you will know not to place complete stock in the subject's answers, because they may just be making things up to mislead you. And if they *are* lying, then any post-hypnotic suggestions given in an attempt to help them with their issues will be of little value, since they are based on untruths. Being aware of this and adjusting your session accordingly will make you a better hypnotist."

The opposing camp agreed that the question was relevant, but used different reasoning. "Since you are talking directly to the subconscious mind when the subject is in hypnosis," they argued, "and since the subconscious mind does not reason, you know that the answers given by the subject are true; the subconscious mind is impersonal, therefore the answers have to be true. And because you know that what the subject is telling you is true, you are better equipped to deal with the client's issues and, thus, are a better hypnotist."

They are surely in disagreement as to whether a person can or cannot lie while in hypnosis but it appears that at least they agree that it is an important question to consider, I thought.

Their discussion on this issue continued for quite some time. A member named Ken, who believed that subjects have the ability to lie, said, "A few weeks ago I had a subject..." (The way he phrased it led me to believe having a subject to hypnotize was a rarity for him!) "And when she woke up she said, 'Where did all of that stuff come from? I don't remember of any of those things ever happening to me. It just seems like a dream. I'm not sure that I wasn't just making it up.'"

"That is exactly the point," responded a member named Bert, who believed subjects were incapable of lying. "Stored in her unconscious mind were suppressed memories and when her critical conscious mind was out of the way she was able to recall what happened. How could someone consciously make something up and afterwards declare that she didn't know where it came from?"

Leonard looked to me for help. "Lindsay, Jon told me that you have performed stage-show hypnosis. Don't people make things up during stage-shows?"

"Yes they do, but most, if not all, of what they make up is the result of the hypnotist's suggestions. It appears to me that regardless of whether a suggestion is intentionally given or is just inferred, people on stage say and do things just because it was suggested or implied. Lying or not lying has little to do with following and carrying out a suggestion."

"I've never performed a stage-show but I have witnessed several," noted Bert, "and some of the people afterwards remember nothing of what they said or did. Doesn't that tell you that if a person is in deep hypnosis, whatever they do or say could not have been a lie *to them* because they remembered none of it? Isn't a lie something that someone consciously distorts?"

"That certainly makes sense by your definition," I replied, "but reason with me further: The reason that the stage-show subjects, as you observed, didn't recall what they said or did was because the stage hypnotist suggested that they wouldn't—they must have been conscious of the suggestion when it was given or they wouldn't have known what the suggestion was. But on the other hand, even when a subject *claims* to not remember what they did on stage, once the suggestion "*with the snap of my fingers you recall everything*" is given, then they remember.

"So apparently, by your argument, at first the subject could not have been lying because he didn't remember what had happened but then he *could have been lying* since he then remembered what happened. That doesn't make a whole lot of sense, does it?

"I believe the question isn't whether a person can or cannot lie while hypnotized but, rather, why would a subject feel a need to lie."

The discussion went on for another twenty minutes until finally Leo slammed down his gavel (or maybe he just gave a loud clap of his hand) and said, "This discussion is going nowhere. Let's either drop the question or ask it differently."

After another lengthy discussion, the question to which the majority agreed was:

In hypnosis a subject *may* lie.   ___ True   ___ False

The time was up and Leo asked for a motion to adjourn the meeting; it was seconded and the meeting was over with just one of twenty proposed questions agreed on by the majority.

Note: When I took the ASPH certification test, on Question No. 1 I checked neither alternative but made a notation: *If my client feels a need to lie* during a hypnosis session then I have not done my job as a hypnotherapist. I have not created a rapport with the subject nor have I projected to them the perception that I am totally nonjudgmental and am accepting of them. Neither have I placed them into a peaceful, non-threatened state of mind where they have no need to lie.

My answer to Question No. 1, along with the rest of the written questions, the oral exam and my hypnosis demonstration must have been acceptable to the examining board, because they issued me a certificate as being qualified to be a *Certified Professional Hypnotist*, and to use the designation of *C.Ht.* after my name.

Over the course of the next two decades I acquired a broad insight into possible definitions and usages of "hypnosis" from my ASPH colleagues. ASPH is now the most active hypnosis organization in the United States (that is, has the greatest number of hypnotists attending meetings on a monthly basis).

For me, this first meeting was an exciting introduction to a long and rewarding relationship with hundreds of hypnotists over the next twenty-five years and an important source of many differing points of view about what "hypnosis" is and how a session should be conducted.

But the most important thing I learned was that in spite of an immense diversity of approaches and opinions about "hypnosis" and how a hypnosis session should be conducted, hypnotherapy has proven in most cases to have a faster and more effective rate in helping people make positive changes in their lives than any other therapeutic approach.

So my query became: Since it appears that every ASPH member uses a different approach, and since they all believe that their method is the right way to conduct a session, and since they report having reasonably good success, then what is the common thread that is woven into these countless dissimilar approaches used by hypnotherapists that gives hypnotherapy an advantage over other forms of therapy?

The answer to my query and my interaction with ASPH members will be addressed throughout the following chapters, but let me say that ASPH has had a major influence on my present views on the topic of "hypnosis."

CHAPTER 31

Simplifying the Induction

About the time of my first juncture with ASPH, I was having serious doubts about the "right way" to do the *clinical hypnosis induction*. Having been taught that it was necessary to lead a client through a lengthy procedure to get them hypnotized—a procedure that in itself consumed up to half an hour, not to mention a 15 minute pre-hypnotic talk, in addition to the time-consuming process of regressing a client back to some sensitizing event, then giving suggestions to desensitize them—a session could easily gobble up more than two hours. Not only that, but my newly happened-upon ASPH colleagues seemed to agree that the induction had to be a lengthy process. It was apparent that each ASPH member had differing views about "hypnosis" and how to use it, yet the consensus was that inducing a hypnotic state needed to be a protracted process, only reinforcing the premise that the "right way" is the right way. However, I was not convinced. Albeit nowadays, the idea of "rapid induction" for clinical hypnotherapy is a common topic for discussion, back then the idea had either not been conceived or had not caught on as being a viable approach.

So in one of my "inner room" discussions with Socrates I asked:

Me: Why is it that it takes 5 minutes to get 10 people hypnotized when doing stage-shows but it takes 20 to 30 minutes to get just one person hypnotized when doing clinical hypnosis?

Socrates: Why does it?

Me: I don't know. It's just that the hypnotists who have tutored me, the authors of the books, and now the ASPH hypnotists all seem to agree: when doing clinical hypnosis, the *induction* procedure needs to be a time-consuming process. The more I think about it the more it seems to me that it doesn't *have* to be. It appears that *they* assume that clinical hypnosis has to be performed that way because that's how *they* were taught and that's how *they* have always done it and because it seems to be relatively successful. They believe that it is not only the "right way" but the "only way." But I'm not convinced.

Socrates: Do you think just because a procedure has been successfully used by those who developed the procedure, and fashioned an explanation of why it works, that the procedure and explanation are the *only* valid ones?

Me: No. I am not inclined to think that way anymore.

Socrates: If everyone since the 1700s would have blindly accepted Franz Anton Mesmer's method and explanation, hypnotists today would be mesmerists and you would be talking about animal magnetism to describe the process. True?

Me: That's right.

Socrates: Mesmer ran in social circles with the likes of Darwin and Mozart, and because of his social and academic standing the procedure he used to "cure" people of their maladies and the explanation of what made it work, made him famous. This was the era of the naturalists and scientific enlightenment. Mesmer knew about recent theories of magnetism and used it to explain that his process involved a *magnetic force* that came from within him that was radiated into his subjects—it was magnetism that made the phenomenon work. So he called it *animal magnetism,* but his followers called it "Mesmerism."

If you think the "right way" is a long and drawn-out procedure you should consider Mesmer's approach.

Mesmer, when working with individual patients, would sit for most of an hour with *his* knees pressed against the *subject's* knees while holding their thumbs in his hands and gazing fixedly into their eyes. He would then pass his hand up and down the patient's arms for another 20 minutes and then press his fingers just below the subject's diaphragm for a time and while performing these procedures would suggest that the malady is in the process of being cured. He would go through this process several times until his patients felt a strange sensation or went into a convulsion; when they did, it was a sign that the procedure had worked and, if not immediately, would eventually bring about a cure. He would also frequently conclude his treatment by playing music. If you were going to have a session with Mesmer you'd better plan on all afternoon and well into the evening.

Mesmer's career began to decline when in Vienna he had assembled several influential people to demonstrate the healing powers of *animal magnetism* but was unable to cure a young blind musician. In 1784 King Louis XVI requested a commission of prominent academics, one of whom was Benjamin Franklin, to investigate *animal magnetism.* They concluded that any benefit that came from the procedure could simply be attributed to "imagination." Little is known about Mesmer's activities during the last 20 years of his life.

Me: That's interesting. Isn't "imagination" pretty much the same as "visualization?" It appears to me that the only difference between the two is that imagination is like daydreaming—just the wanderings of the mind—and visualization is the intentional use of the mind to create mental images for a chosen purpose.

Socrates: Yes, that is a good way to look at the differences.

Me: I guess the reason mesmerism fell out of favor is that the explanation of what made it work (animal magnetism) was wrong.

Socrates: That is correct.

Me: Then why is "hypnosis" still around? I have yet to find a reliable explanation of what makes it work.

Socrates: Probably because the word itself seems to fit what it looks like—sleep.

In the early 1800s, Viennese physician James Braid experimented with "mesmerism" and because his subjects *appeared* to be in a state of sleep coined the name "hypnosis"—a derivative of the Greek god Hypnos, the god of sleep and master of dreams—and referred to his subject as having been "hypnotized."

In the beginning, Braid's procedure to hypnotize a subject involved holding a bright object a foot in front of their eyes and then asking them to stare at it while he repeated over and over, *"Your eyes are becoming tired and sleepy."* He told them to keep their eyes open until they became heavy and tired and when they felt that they could no longer keep them open, to let them close. This seemed to produce a trance-like state that looked like sleep.

However, Braid soon discovered that he could achieve the same state by suggestion alone—without the need of an object to stare at. Then he concluded after more experimenting that the same conditions that he used to "test" to see if a subject was hypnotized (catalepsy, anesthesia, amnesia) could be achieved without "sleep," that is, while still conscious.

Since the phenomenon did not require the subject to be in a trance or sleep state he attempted to rename his procedure and called it "monoideism"— "the quality of a repetitive suggestion or command that creates an altered state of consciousness and transcends the limits of volitional control." But by this time "hypnosis" and "hypnotism" had become widely accepted terms, and besides that, people could *not* easily relate to what "monoideism" meant. So that's why you are a hypnotist and not a mesmerist or a monoideismist.

Me: So it seems that it is just a question of semantics that defines the process—the process is the same regardless of the words one uses to describe it–like Shakespeare's rose. But what I'm looking for is a way to speed up the procedure regardless of what it is called.

Socrates: Then discard what others have said and purposely try other approaches. Draw upon your experiences and your own creativity, and then experiment with anything that comes to mind–you will never know that some other procedure works better until you try it.

Me: Let me see if I correctly understand what you just said: I don't need to go through an imaginary peaceful scene and I don't have to go through a progressive physical relaxation routine to get a client into a proper state of mind before I can probe their subconscious mind and give suggestions about making a change in their behavior. Is that correct?

Socrates: That's not *exactly* what I said. What I said is that you don't *know* that you *don't* need to go through an established procedure to achieve the same or better result. Is that clear?

Me: I thought that that is what I just said.

Socrates: Maybe you *do* need to go through those steps to get a person hypnotized but *maybe* you don't. You won't know until you come up with different approaches and then put them to the test. Maybe after trying alternatives you will discover that the "right way" works best. But you won't know that until you have tested numerous unconventional options. Glean from your clinical and stage hypnosis experiences, come up with some untried approaches, and then try them. Is that clear now?

Me: Yes.

Socrates: Some of your ideas will work and some won't. But answer this: If you just keep doing hypnosis the same way you are doing it will you ever discover a quicker and more effective way to get a subject into a hypnotic state? If you never change your approach then your approach will never change. That seems elementary, doesn't it?

Me: True. It seems, Socrates, that I've been stuck in a rut by thinking that the experts are right; but I can see now that if I don't try something new (even if it is unconventional) I'll never discover new ways to get better.

Socrates: That is correct. But remember to also reap insight from your clients by asking questions that will force them to examine their thinking and cause them to come up with otherwise unthought-of solutions. By challenging the opinions of another person you force them to invent creative explanations as to why they think as they do and that will most likely lead to ideas that have not previously been conceived. Grasp those new ideas and see if they have a valid application to reaching your objectives.

Me: That's a good idea, but how do I think of the right questions to ask that will initiate creative responses?

Socrates: Ask! Ask your subjects at the conclusion of each session to critique your procedure and ask *what they think* could have improved the effectiveness of the session. After they have made their appraisal ask them why they think their ideas would work better. It may be uncomfortable for both you and your client when you challenge their observations but it *will* stimulate new ideas. And then examine their evaluations to see if they hold legitimate merit.

Creative ideas often come at unexpected times and from unexpected sources so be in tune and keep an open mind. And for sure, let go of needing to protect your ego. It's okay if someone has an opinion that differs from yours and to discover that your thinking has been defective. Keep in mind, however, that just because someone has a strong opinion about an issue, it doesn't mean that their conviction is based on fact. Sometimes hunting dogs bark up one tree when the raccoon is really in the one next to it!

Me: So it is okay to just try any idea that pops up even if someone who knows little or nothing about hypnosis comes up with it—I go ahead and try it anyway. And the way to apply and explain the hypnotic process may be in some tree other than the one everyone else is barking up—an idea that no one has yet thought of.

Socrates: Exactly! It's like when Einstein came up with his theories of relativity (*General Relativity* and *Special Relativity*) while everyone else was still stuck in Newtonian physics. True?

Me: True... but I'm no Einstein.

Socrates: That may well be true, but don't think that you cannot be creative in devising new ideas just because you are not a genius.

Answer this: What is the purpose of going through the physical progressive relaxation and the mental peace of mind procedures—why go through the procedures at all?

Me: Okay. The purpose of the *progressive physical relaxation* is to get the client's physical body relaxed and comfortable. And the *imaginary peaceful place* is intended to get the client into a peaceful state of mind in which their conscious critical mind no longer gets in their way of accepting a suggestion, thus the subject carries out the suggestion without questioning it. Is that right?

Socrates: Let your mind run wild and think.

Einstein let his mind run wild by wondering what the world would be like if he was riding alongside a beam of light—how would things appear from that vantage point? This mental experiment led to his theory of special relativity—in part, that no matter the direction or speed that an experimenter travels in a spaceship, and no matter the direction the experimenter chooses to shine a beam of light (in the direction of travel or behind the direction of travel) the light from the beam always travels at the same speed (186,000 miles a second). This theory flew in the face of traditional Newtonian physics and even present-day logic—it would seem that the speed of the light from a beam should be added to or subtracted from the speed of the spaceship. Not true. Experiments have proven that traditional thinking and logic relative to the speed of light are false!

When a quicker, easier and more effective way to produce a hypnotic state is discovered, continue to refine it. By continually fine-tuning your method of doing hypnosis it will never become routine and you'll never get bored doing it. But remember, be prepared to squelch any ideas or procedures, whether newly discovered or old established ones, when they no longer hold true. And accept new ideas when they hold up under close scrutiny and testing, even if they go against traditional thinking.

Me: Okay. But isn't that going to create a lot of friction between me and my colleagues—and the public in general for that matter—who have preconceived notions about what hypnosis is and how it should be induced?

Socrates: Yes, it will. The advancement of any new idea will always breed resistance and resentment if it goes against established beliefs and tradition, but it is well worth the consequences when eventually an idea or new way of thinking is advanced, even if it takes centuries, as is evidenced from *my* personal experience. The Athenians sentenced me to death for exposing flaws and inconsistencies in their thinking by closely examining their lives. Then they accused me of corrupting the youth of Athens by encouraging them to think independent of long-held traditions and beliefs. But now, over two thousand years later, I am revered for having established a powerful method of inquiry.

Again, answer this: Why do you go through the physical progressive relaxation procedure?

Me: To get every muscle relaxed so the client is comfortable and not distracted by physical issues.

Socrates: What I am asking is: Why does a client's body need to be relaxed in order to accept hypnotic suggestions?

Me: I don't know. I just thought that, in part, physical relaxation was hypnosis, but now as I think about it, being physically relaxed is not necessary for a client to accept suggestions. As with the "stretched out like a board between two chairs" routine during stage-shows: the subject's muscles are rigid and stiff as a board yet they still follow and carry out any suggestion that is given. So it would appear that physical relaxation has little to do with a person being hypnotized or accepting suggestions. I suppose that I could just as well suggest: *With each word I speak the muscles of your body become more rigid and tight and the more your muscles become rigid and tight you will go into a deeper and deeper hypnotic state.* Nonetheless, I suppose if a client had a choice between being relaxed or being stiff as a board they'd probably choose relaxed. Besides that, being relaxed is more like being asleep.

Socrates: Good. But why do you think that you need to spend so much time relaxing each little body part—each terminal member of the vertebrate's foot or hand, for example?

Me: Huh?

Socrates: You know, a single finger or each toe.

Me: Oh.

Socrates: The human mind has the ability to grasp the concept of a whole hand just as easily as it can conceive one finger. And consider this: Not everyone feels their stress in the same place. Stress causes muscles to tighten up but not everyone senses that physical tightness in the same part of their body. You didn't suggest to a guy stretched between two chairs to start out by making a finger stiff as a board—you simply suggested that his whole body was stiff as a board. Let me ask you this: When *you* feel stressed-out or anxious, where in your body do *you* "feel" it?

Me: I have never before thought of my stress or anxieties as being "felt" physically—in my body. But now that you ask, I guess I do; I suppose that if *somehow* I didn't have a body I wouldn't feel any stress.

It's been a while since I truly felt anxieties or stress, so I'll have to give this some thought.... A time when was I really uptight, stressed-out and anxious?

I reflected back to sitting in my car, with the engine revved and ready to drive off that "solve-every-problem-in-my-life" cliff in an effort to identify where I felt the emotions associated with the stress of the experience... as I reflected back it was as though I was there.

I feel tightness in my throat and my chest... and my hands. My hands are clenched so tight I think I'm embedding my fingerprints in the steering wheel. And my jaw, my jaw is clenched and tight and I'm grinding my teeth. I suppose my whole body is tight but I feel the anxieties primarily in my chest, hands and jaw.

Socrates: So, just as I asked you to identify where you feel stress and anxieties, ask your clients where in their body *they* "feel" their stress. Then use that information to simplify the physical relaxation part of the induction. Once several of your clients describe where they sense *their* stress, then, when working with future clients you can suggest that *those* parts of their body are relaxed, without having to ask.

So let your mind run wild and get on with your quest to find quicker, easier and more effective ways to induce the hypnotic state and discover a reliable explanation that describes what makes the process work.

So I did.

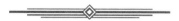

With each of the next 25 clients (it could have been 50, I didn't keep track), as part of the pre-hypnotic talk, I explained to them that the hypnotic process works best when in a relaxed physical state and that stress is felt physically, usually by the tightness of muscles. I asked, "Where in your body do *you* 'feel' *your* stress? When you feel anxious, in which muscles do you feel tightness?"

Sometimes I'd draw a blank stare, so I would ask, "Do you feel any stress or anxiety right now?" I would give them a moment to "look" and then ask, "Where in your body did you 'look' to see if you felt stress or anxiety?" That would usually get a response.

Although *most* of their answers were what I had expected, many came up with unexpected surprises:

- "My hands. When I feel stressed-out my hands are tense and sometimes even curl up and begin to sweat." (No one ever said, "I feel stress in my left finger or thumb.")
- "My arms. My arms feel heavy and tired, like it is hard to get them to move." (No one said, "My upper arms/lower arms/ biceps/triceps.")
- "My shoulders. They bunch up."
- "My neck. My neck muscles tighten up and sometimes if I move my head around I can get those muscles to relax for a while but then they just tighten up again."
- "In my head. It seems like there is pressure inside my head and sometimes I get headaches because of my stress."
- "My throat. When I am stressed-out and anxious my throat tightens up and I find it is difficult to speak—my voice gets all shaky."
- "My chest. When stressed my chest gets tight, I have trouble breathing and my heart races." This was the most common area of the body that people reported feeling their stress.
- "My upper back. The muscles in my upper back hunch up and get tight. I have to stretch my arms up and arch my back to get them to relax." (This is one of the areas of a person's body that

I had never associated with stress.)

- "My lower back." (I had never thought of stress as being felt in one's lower back, either.)
- "My stomach. When I get anxious, angry or stressed I feel it in my stomach. It feels like I need to eat something to get rid of it." (This was the next most common answer as to where people felt their stress.)
- "My hips." (I was surprised when several time hips came up as a place where people felt stress.)
- "My legs. My legs get heavy and tired. The muscles get tight and it seems that it takes a great effort to get them to move."
- "My feet. My feet hurt, the muscles in my feet get tight, my toes curl up and they get cold." (This was, for me, the most unexpected answer. I was surprised how frequently people said that they felt their stress in their feet.)

So to simplify the physical relaxation part of the induction I began suggesting that the client visualize each of those "chunks" of their body as being relaxed: hands, arms, shoulders, neck, head, jaw, throat, chest, upper back, stomach, lower back, hips, legs and feet.

By reducing the number of muscles to be relaxed to larger body parts, the relaxation part of the induction was cut from 20 minutes to 4 minutes. Not only that, but my clients appeared to become just as relaxed and were just as receptive to suggestions—if not more so.

But I still had the mental, peaceful ritual—going to an imaginary peaceful place—to shorten.

So I went back to Socrates.

Me: Okay, I have resolved a way to shorten the physical relaxation part of the induction process, but how do I shorten the mental relaxation part? How do I shorten the "peaceful place" part with the same result?

Socrates: Ask!

Me: What do you mean, "Ask"?

Socrates: Ask your clients what *they* think you could have done differently that would have caused them to enter into a peaceful state of mind.

So once again, I did as he had suggested.

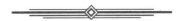

I remember having had little time between my conversation with Socrates and my next appointment so I reverted to my old established "right way." Nevertheless, as chance would have it, or maybe by divine intervention, I didn't need to come up with something new—the seeds of discovery were planted during my next session.

After having gone through my pre-hypnotic talk I seated Katie in my recliner. I pulled my chair close to her, held a pendulum a foot in front of her eyes then quietly said, "*Just make yourself comfortable. Look at this pendulum as it swings, and when your eyes become heavy and tired just close your eyes and listen to my voice. While watching the pendulum swing, take in a deep breath and hold it in while I count down, 5, 4, 3, 2, 1, then exhale. Now take in another deep breath and hold it in, 5, 4 , 3, 2, 1, and exhale. And now take in another deep breath and hold it in 5, 4, 3, 2, 1, and exhale.*"

Katie's eyes had closed on the second breath so I continued.

"*And now in your hands every muscle is relaxed. And now in your arms every muscle is relaxed....*"

I continued, "*And now every muscle is relaxed in your feet.*"

Once I had completed the physical relaxation I went on to the mental relaxation: "*The sound of my voice is relaxing to your mind and the sound of my voice produces within you a state of tranquility, calmness, a sense of security and peace of mind. It's really quite okay to let yourself relax and to experience a sense of well-being.*

"*Now imagine yourself on a sandy beach in a hammock that is stretched between two palm trees. You are swaying in the breeze on a beautiful quiet sunny spring afternoon.*

"*As you swing back and forth you relax deeper and deeper. The cool breeze feels good on your face and engenders a feeling of peace and tranquility. Nothing matters now except the serenity of this scene and the sound of my voice.*

"*The waves rolling in and the smell of the ocean breeze produce a sense of calm and comfortable composure. And as you experience this you continue drifting into a deeper and deeper sleep.*

"*Each word I speak and the scene I describe take you into a deeper and deeper hypnotic state.*

"*You are aware of the sound of seabirds in the distance and the breaking of the waves relaxes you even more....*"

To my surprise Katie opened her eyes, sat up in the recliner, looked me squarely in the eye and said, "I hate the ocean and the beach. My brother drowned in the ocean when I was a little girl. And besides that, every beach I have ever been on has trash and seaweed strewn all over the sand, and swinging in a hammock always makes me feel queasy and so does the smell of the ocean—it smells to me like dead fish. And besides that, I sunburn easily and I couldn't help wondering if there are birds up in those palm trees and, who knows, one of them may need to poop!"

Pow! What she said bolted me into a state of realization—a new insight flashed my mind: Just because Eric thinks, and me too for that matter, that the beach is a peaceful place, it doesn't mean that *everyone* thinks it is.

Once I collected my wits, I explained to Katie, "My purpose for having you imagine yourself in a hammock on a beach was because I mistakenly thought that it would be a place of peace and tranquility for you. Apparently I was dead wrong. What do you think would have been a better approach to create for you a state of peacefulness?"

She answered, "Why didn't you just continue on with how you started out?"

"Explain to me what you mean," I said.

"Well, by the end of your pre-hypnotic talk I already felt much more peaceful than when I walked into your office. For some reason the sound of your voice in itself seemed to relieve much of my stress and when you had me sit in your recliner and asked me to take in those deep breaths—I always do that when I want to relax, anyway—I just felt myself letting go even more. And as you gave me suggestions about my body being relaxed I could feel each part of my body relax just as you suggested. And then you said something like, '*My voice is relaxing and produces within you a state of tranquility, peace and peace of mind,*' and the sound of your voice did precisely that—caused me to feel peaceful and tranquil.

"I think that when you were talking *to me*—directly about *me*—I felt myself relaxing and truly experienced a sense of peace coming over me, but when you shifted to talking about things outside of me—seashore, hammocks, waves and birds—I felt myself becoming anxious. If you would have just continued for a little longer speaking in your soothing voice—assuring me that I was safe, and that it is okay for me to relax and be peaceful—I think I'd have easily reached a state of being completely at peace—a state in which I think nothing would have mattered except your voice."

Another thought occurred to me: In an attempt to shorten the induction process, I had for several months omitted from the induction procedure the exercise of having my clients take in three deep breaths. For reasons that I can't explain, I had led Katie through the breathing exercise and when she said that the breaths in themselves had caused her to relax it sparked my curiosity. So I asked, "Katie, did taking those few deep breaths at the beginning of my suggestion truly have a significant effect on getting rid of some of your stress?"

"Yes it did."

"Explain to me what taking in a deep breath has to do with relaxing?"

Katie responded, "Well, as I mentioned, that is something I always do when I want to get rid of stress. Taking in a deep breath or two relaxes me—it always works."

I questioned her further. "I understand that, but what I am asking is *why* does it relax you? Take a moment and really consider why you think that taking in a deep breath makes you relax."

Katie was very cooperative and seemed as interested in discovering the answer to my question as I was.

I deliberately allowed her to contemplate the question for a few minutes. Then she answered, "As I think about it, it's because my mother always did that when she was stressed-out. I can see her taking in a deep breath, and even holding it in for a moment and then exhaling. I think that I have been conditioned to do the same."

She went on to further explain, "I am an RN and as I think about it, many patients do the same thing when they are faced with an unpleasant procedure or are anticipating an unpleasant event—like a shot, giving blood or about to get the result of a medical test. It might just be an inherited human trait—like adrenalin shooting into our blood stream when we are threatened—a need to have more oxygen in our bloodstream and sending it to our brain so we are able to think more clearly. I'm not sure, but those would be my best explanations of why taking in a few deep breaths seems to be relaxing."

So I asked Katie to lean back in the recliner again and to close her eyes (without looking at a swinging pendulum) and said, *"Take in a deep breath. Hold it in while I count down, 5, 4, 3, 2, 1, then exhale..."*

When I had finished the breathing exercise I suggested, *"Just listen to my voice. The sound of my voice is relaxing to your mind and produces within you a state of tranquility and calmness, and a sense of security and peace of mind. It's really quite okay to let yourself relax and to experience a sense of well-being. You are safe and tranquil and experience a peace of mind that allows you to be receptive to my suggestions and a state of mind in which you freely answer the few questions I'll be asking in just a few moments. My voice continues to take you into a deeper and deeper mental state of peace. Your mind is relaxed and the only thing that matters now is my voice and what I am saying."*

This short, simplified approach for attaining the peace and tranquility part of the induction worked very well. A process that would have taken 15 minutes (by describing a peaceful scene) now took less than two... and coupled with the shortened physical relaxation procedure seemed to have even better results.

So, by reducing the time to get a client physically relaxed and disregarding the peace of mind *scene* process and replacing it with a peaceful statement related to the client's peaceful state of being rather than talking about things outside of their being, I had condensed a process that would have taken 20 or 30 minutes to 6 minutes!

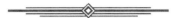

With the reduction of time required for inducing a hypnotic state settled, I turned my attention to resolving the question of what causes the process of hypnosis to work and finding a way to demonstrate that process.... I wanted to be able to quickly demonstrate that visualization has a direct influence on physical and emotional behavior.

The idea that visualization is involved in changing one's behavior was the foundation of Success Motivation Institute's concept and almost all of the self-help, positive-thinking books and recordings I had read or listened to.

In addition, I suspected not only that visualization held the secret for changing human behavior (because of my own experience) but that visualization was the root force behind the process of "hypnosis"—but I had no way to quickly or consistently demonstrate that my supposition was true.

I knew the benefits that "hypnosis" had produced on my clients and that those benefits could be empirically witnessed by overt observation—a client no longer smokes, has lost weight, comfortably speaks in public or has long, attractive fingernails. Nevertheless, I was looking for a way to *demonstrate* that visualization directly influences behavior, and I wanted to find a way to do it easily, quickly and consistently during the pre-hypnotic talk.

Once again, finding a way to accomplish my objective did not take long, once I engaged my mental energies, and Socrates, in the quest.

CHAPTER 32

The Pendulum Swings

During one of my training sessions, Eric had used one of his "practice subjects" (Linda) to demonstrate a technique for uncovering subconscious thoughts by using a pendulum to determine the answer to questions. The idea was to have a subject hold a pendulum (he used a marble attached to a 10-inch jewelry chain) with thumb and forefinger over the palm of the other hand, and whichever way the pendulum swings determines the answer to a question. The subject is then told that if the pendulum swings in the direction that the subject's fingers are pointing the answer to a question is "yes." If the pendulum swings crossways the answer is "no." If the pendulum swings in a circular direction it means, "I don't know" or "maybe" or "it's none of your business." And if the pendulum doesn't swing at all, either the question was asked wrong or the subject is not cooperating.

So Linda held the pendulum over the palm of her left hand and Eric asked, "Is your name Sam?" Immediately the pendulum began swinging crossways to the direction her fingers were pointing—"no."

"Are you in love with someone?" The pendulum swung in a circle.

"Does that mean that you don't know?" The pendulum swung crossways—"no."

Does that mean *maybe* you are in love?" the pendulum began swinging crossways again—"no."

"Does that mean that it is none of my business?" And the pendulum swung in the direction her fingers were pointing—"yes, it's none of your business."

It was obvious that Linda consciously knew the answers and it appeared to me that she was intentionally moving her arm to make the pendulum swing in the appropriate direction to confirm that the answer corresponded with her conscious knowledge. However, Linda said that she did not try to move her arm and that the pendulum just seemed to swing all on its own.

I had dismissed any thought that this "parlor trick" might have a useful purpose relative to hypnosis or demonstrating the powers of the human mind and brain, until I once again engaged Socrates in a dialogue.

Me: From my use of self-hypnosis—and my observations of stage-show subjects and clinical clients—it appears to me that visualization has something to do with the process that causes "hypnosis" to work.

Socrates: Reflect back to your SMI recordings. The foundation of the SMI concept was visualization. In *Psycho-Cybernetics*, for example, Maxwell Maltz based his theory of self-improvement on the premise that once he changed a person's physical appearance with his plastic surgery, the patient "saw" himself or herself as physically attractive and because this changed their self-image, their personality significantly changed. They were exactly the same person, with the same talents and abilities before the cosmetic surgery as they had after the surgery, but a life-long behavior of timidity and self-consciousness was transformed into an outgoing and confident person, simply by having changed the patient's self-image.

Me: So what you are implying is that how a person "sees" himself determines how he feels about himself and how he acts.

Socrates: Precisely, but you already know this and have personally experienced it. The issue of getting over *your* inhibitions about making sales calls was resolved when you changed your self-image *about* making sales calls. You changed your vision from "it's frightening to make sales calls" to visualizing that you are just out there making new friends (prospective customers) and serving old friends (existing customers). Isn't that the process you used to cause the change?

Me: Yes, this is exactly the process I used after I learned to "hypnotize" myself.

Socrates: So it was the change in how you visualized yourself that removed your inhibitions—you changed your self-image and once the new self-image hit your subconscious mind your subconscious mind changed how you felt about yourself and how you felt about making sales calls, true?

Me: Yes, you are right. I experienced a change in my own behavior once I changed how I visualized myself behaving. And I have observed significant changes in other people once they change their self-image (like Rich going from being afraid to talk into a microphone to loving it, for example). But what I am looking for is a way to *demonstrate* to my clients how their subconscious mind transforms their visualizations into overt observable behavior. That is, a way to demonstrate that the process works without having to wait for a day, or a week or a month to observe the results. Is that possible?

Socrates: Yes. And you have already witnessed the way to do that. However, you ignored its validity and didn't recognize it because until now you haven't needed it, and you haven't engaged your creative thinking to uncover it. Think back and see if you can discover the lesson that demonstrated how visualization produced an immediate, overt, observable behavior.

Me: I'm not sure that I have ever witnessed such an event.... but let me think. *What have I witnessed that I rejected as being useful to demonstrate that visualization causes a change in behavior? Let me think back....* I think I have it! It was Eric's parlor trick with Linda using a pendulum to answer questions.

Socrates: That's it. Now consider the implications of that, as you put it, "parlor trick."

Me: Well, by establishing a direction for the pendulum to swing beforehand, Linda chose to visualize it swinging in the appropriate direction and then her subconscious mind made her arm move to indicate the answer... and she wasn't even aware that it was her arm doing it. Could that be the answer?

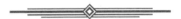

I didn't bother to ask Socrates any more questions because I was anxious to see if *I* could make a pendulum swing just by visualizing it swinging.

So I got up from my recliner and found the pendulum Eric had given me for the purpose of discovering subconscious answers to conscious questions. I held out my left hand with palm up, held the pendulum over the center of my hand and visualized the pendulum swinging crossways to the direction my fingers pointed. To my surprise the pendulum began swinging in the direction that I had visualized! Then I created a mental picture of the pendulum swinging in the direction that my fingers pointed and the pendulum changed and began to swing in that direction. And then I tried visualizing a circle and it swung in a circle.

Wow, I thought to myself. *That is really a strange occurrence. I don't think it was my arm, hand or fingers moving that made it swing because I was trying to hold them still and trying to* not *let the pendulum swing, but it swung in the direction that I visualized, anyway. I wonder if there is some kind of mystical energy or force that goes on between my subconscious mind and the pendulum that makes it swing?*

Being convinced that it was *not* my arm moving, and that it was an energy force being emitted from my subconscious mind that acted directly on the pendulum, I constructed a ten-inch high tripod out of some wooden dowels and hung the pendulum from its apex, then set it on my desk. I drew a cross on a sheet of paper (like the crosshairs in a rifle scope) and labeled the perpendicular axis A – B and the horizontal axis C – D and slid it under the pendulum so the pendulum hung over the center of the cross.

I sat down at my desk, took in a few deep breaths of air, conjured up mental images of my subconscious mind emitting its psychic energy and, without touching the pendulum, the tripod or my desk, visualized the pendulum swinging back and forth in the C to D direction.... To my dismay, my "visualization" did not have the slightest effect on the pendulum—it just hung there, perfectly still. I tried visualizing the direction A to B and then a circle, and still it did not show even a hint of a swing. I spent probably half an hour trying different techniques—visualization, imagination, picturing, calling upon divine providence, trying to conjure up a belief that I could make it swing just by willing it to swing—and nothing worked.

What a disappointment! Before the experiment, I thought I was on the verge of demonstrating that the human mind can cause inanimate objects to move. *If this experiment works*, I thought, *I will become famous by demonstrating that with enough psychic energy ancient Egyptians could have "thought" giant boulders up on to the pyramids...* so much for that idea.

So I detached the pendulum from the tripod and with my elbow braced firmly on my desk, and trying to hold my arm still, I held the pendulum over the center of the cross and thought about it swinging in the direction C to D and, immediately, it began to swing back and forth in that direction.

At the time, little did I understand the powerful implications this simple demonstration would have on revealing the powers of the human mind and brain, nor did I realize that it would be the foundation of a unique approach to explain the hypnotic process.

Wanting to get a clearer insight into this phenomenon, I slipped back into my inner room.

Me: What is the force or power that causes a pendulum to swing just by me imagining it swinging? I did not feel my arm, hand or fingers move; in fact, I was trying to keep them *from* moving, but the pendulum automatically swung, seemingly of its own accord, in the direction I chose to visualize it swinging. What a curious happening! What does this demonstration imply and how can I use it to enhance my effectiveness as a hypnotist?

Socrates: Your arm *was* moving and that is what made the pendulum swing. Just as you observed Linda's arm moving during that demonstration with Eric, even though she had no conscious awareness that her arm moved.

Just think about the powerful inference: You were trying to hold your arm still, you were not aware that your arm was moving, but your arm moved anyway and made the pendulum swing. Think! What does that imply?

Me: I guess it implies that my subconscious mind doesn't care what I am *trying* to do! It implies that my *visualization* (mental image) determines my behavior and that I'm not even aware that it is my visualization that makes me behave as I do! And also, it implies that my behavior is independent from what I am *trying* to do—if what I am trying to do is different than my visualization. My self-image determines my behavior, not what I want; consciously, I really *wanted* to make it swing when it was hanging from the tripod, and I really *didn't* want it to swing when holding it with my fingers.... If I had really wanted it to swing while holding it, why was I trying so hard to keep it *from* swinging? It would appear that *wanting* something to happen or *not wanting* it to happen has little to do with what happens.

Socrates: Now think of how this pendulum experience could fit into your hypnosis sessions.

Me: That's exactly what I've been searching for. I'll incorporate it into my pre-hypnotic talk and demonstrate to my clients that their subconscious mind responds to mental images... and not to what they want or what they are trying to do.

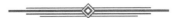

So I did just that. With every client from that moment on, during my pre-hypnotic talk I explain, "*I want to demonstrate the powers of your subconscious mind and how your subconscious mind will cause a behavior to occur, without you doing anything about it except to visualize it happening.*"

Although I was still skeptical that it was going to work with the first client I tried it on, I clearly remember the excitement that welled up in me when the demonstration was successful. And I was even more excited when I observed that it was his arm moving that made it swing. After the demonstration, I asked my client if he was aware that his arm was moving. His answer was "no" and he even argued that it couldn't have been his arm moving because he was trying to hold it still. Nevertheless, *I* knew it was, because I could see it moving.

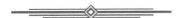

In the beginning, I used the above verbiage to explain the demonstration to my client, but over the years, my way of articulating it has evolved into a more accurate explanation of the demonstration and the process that makes it work.

With each session, I now take out of my desk drawer a sheet of paper on which I have drawn a crosshairss with its axes labeled A-B and C-D (a sample below). I place it on my desk in front of the subject, hand them my pendulum, have them hold the pendulum over the center of the cross, and then ask them to visualize the pendulum swinging back and forth in the direction C to D.

Try it yourself: Hook a paperclip to the end of a ten-inch long thread so it makes a simple pendulum. Hold the string end with your thumb and forefinger and position the paperclip end about a half-inch above the center of the cross so it can swing freely. Then imagine the pendulum swinging in the direction C to D or A to B, or a circle, or diagonally if you choose, and observe what happens. It really doesn't matter how much it swings, whether it swings an $1/8^{th}$ of an inch or if it swings four inches... that it swings at all is a phenomenal occurrence.

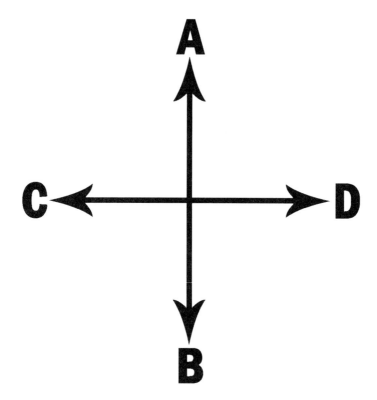

From that session until now (and that's over 25,000 of them) I have used this demonstration during my pre-hypnotic talk. In the beginning, the demonstration worked successfully about 95% of the time, but by refining and adjusting the wording used to describe the procedure, now it always works. Once the client creates a mental image of the pendulum swinging, it always swings in the direction the client chooses to picture. It never swings in some other direction!

This demonstration is central to my approach to the hypnotic process. But the power upon which this demonstration is based holds far more reaching implications relative to human behavior than I realized at the time. In the chapters that follow I will describe how this simple demonstration has evolved into a powerful principle that explains how the hypnotic process works and how any rational human being can use their conscious mind to intentionally change and alter their physical, mental and emotional behavior.

No Altered States of Consciousness

For more than a decade I thought of hypnosis as being an "altered state of consciousness." To the contrary, most people who have never been "hypnotized" believe that while hypnotized they will not be conscious at all—they will be "out" (unconscious) and under the complete control of the hypnotist. To put my clients at ease about this false opinion, I would explain that they would always be aware during the session. I would say, "In psychology, 'hypnosis' is defined as an *altered state of consciousness*, and that's why a hypnotist can't make the subject do anything that would harm them or go against their moral or ethical standards. Although you will be in an *altered* state of mind, you will always be conscious."

At one of our monthly meetings, I presented to my ASPH colleagues my thoughts on the hypnotic process. My approach to hypnosis was still in its early stages of development and I used conventional terms, phrases and methods as I demonstrated my approach; for example terms like trance, bypass the conscious analytical mind, subconscious mind, unconscious mind, regressive hypnosis, the subject goes into hypnosis or under hypnosis, and altered state of consciousness.

After my presentation Dr. Michael Preston, one of the most knowledgeable and respected members of the society and author of *Hypnosis: Medicine of the Mind*, took me aside and asked if I had a few minutes so that he could share an idea with me. The dialogue that follows is condensed into a few paragraphs, but we were engaged in a very spirited discussion about hypnosis *being*, or *not being* an *altered state of consciousness* for most of an hour.[5]

Dr. Preston: Lindsay, that was a fine presentation but I question your thinking about hypnosis being an *altered state of consciousness*.

---

5. Note: This dialogue took place 30 years ago. Dr. Preston's position on the topic may have shifted a little since then, but I remember the conversation well since it had such a profound impact on my way of thinking about hypnosis. Dr. Preston passed away in Ocotber of 2008.

Me: Thank you for your compliment about my presentation, I regard it as being particularly valuable coming from you, since I highly respect your opinion and I hold you in high esteem. I am in a continual process of refining my approach and understanding what makes hypnosis work, so I would appreciate any criticism you might have about my presentation. Please explain your views about hypnosis *being* or *not being* an altered state of consciousness.

Dr. Preston: It is not that hypnosis *is* or *is not* an altered state of consciousness; it's a question of there being such a state of mind at all. Even if there were such a state, it would be wrong to say that *hypnosis* is an altered state. The more correct way to state it would be to say that the hypnotized *person* is *in* an altered state of consciousness. Even so, a hypnotized person is *not* in an altered state of consciousness by any means.

Me: That is a very interesting thought. The reason I use the term is that hypnosis is defined in psychology, at least in my Psych 101 text, as being an altered state of consciousness along with dreaming, hallucinations, figments of imagination, out of body experiences, alcohol intoxication, drug abuse and all of those states that humans experience when *not* in their everyday, "normal" state of consciousness.

Dr. Preston: You are right about psychology's standard definition, and for many years I thought of those states of human experience as being such, but after close scrutiny I have arrived at a different conclusion.

Me: Go on and explain. If those conditions are not altered states of consciousness, then what are they?

Dr. Preston: You are missing the point. I am not questioning those conditions—what they are or what they are not—I am questioning *altered states of consciousness* particularly as it relates to hypnosis.

Me: Okay, but I think I am a little confused. What is it about *altered states of consciousness* that you question?

Dr. Preston: As I said at the beginning of our discussion, there is no such thing as an *altered* state of consciousness! Either consciousness is "on" or it is "off."

Me: I am not sure that I comprehend what you just said. I think you will agree there is an observable difference in the mental state of a person who is drunk and one who is not.

Dr. Preston: I agree, but you still don't quite get it. Sure, there is an observable and measurable difference in the physical and mental behavior of an intoxicated person, but the drunk who is staggering around and slurring his speech and whose thinking is fuzzy is still conscious; his view of himself and of those around him may be altered, but his consciousness isn't altered. Now, if he totally blacks out, then we could assume that he is no longer conscious.

Me: Okay, let me see if I grasp your assertion. A person's consciousness is either "on" or "off." Whether a person is drunk, hallucinating, dreaming or hypnotized they are still conscious. Their behavior and cognitive process may be altered but their consciousness is not. Did I get that right?

Dr. Preston: Yes, that is precisely right.

Me: So a person who is aware is conscious and if not aware is unconscious. Like a light bulb, it is either on or it is off, depending on which way the switch is flipped.

Dr. Preston: Yes, I think you have it but I am not sure you fully accept it. Sometimes it takes a while for a new idea to sink in. Those other conditions you mentioned are not the point. The point I want to make is this: for sure, a person who is in hypnosis is perfectly conscious and if a subject is *unconscious* they are in some state other than hypnotized. At any point during a session if a client no longer hears, understands or responds to your suggestions or questions, he or she has fallen asleep and therefore is not in hypnosis. If a subject is asleep and unconscious what is the use of giving them suggestions? Your suggestions are worthless if the subject is not conscious of them.

Me: I'm going to have to spend some time thinking about what you have told me. But I think the bottom line of your argument is this: When a person is in hypnosis they are not *unconscious*, regardless of the behavior hypnosis produces. Their behavior—how they act, feel and think—may be altered, but their consciousness is not altered; it is always "on" while hypnotized. This means if their consciousness is "off" (unconscious) they are not hypnotized.

Dr. Preston: That is correct.

I returned to my office, sat in my recliner and ventured again into my inner room for a visit with Socrates.

Me: Dr. Preston has asserted that there is not such a thing as an *altered* state of consciousness because consciousness is either "off" or it is "on." I'm having a little problem accepting that concept since I have been using the term to describe the state of mind in which a client should expect to be when in hypnosis.

Socrates: This is only one of the many treasured ideas you may have to abandon as you refine your approach and gain new knowledge. You must give up old ideas and cherished concepts when they no longer hold true, and when new ways of comprehending them become apparent.

Me: I think that I am getting better at accepting that change is necessary to advance my quest for better ways to conduct hypnosis and to understand the process that makes it work. However, if I embrace the idea that hypnosis is *not* an altered state of consciousness it means reworking most of my of thinking and the way I explain to my clients what to expect while in a hypnotic state. This idea shatters my approach and my whole way of thinking about hypnosis.

Socrates: You are right. With every new concept that you discover you will have to revamp established ways of performing hypnosis and explaining it. Review your conversation with Dr. Preston and find a creative way (and even a radical way) to explain to your clients that while hypnotized they are *not* going to be *unconscious* or in an *altered* state of consciousness.

Me: I think my brain is stymied but here goes. Dr. Preston said that *behavior* can be altered but *consciousness* cannot—we are either conscious or we are unconscious. He also said that while intoxicated, hallucinating, under the influence of drugs or dreaming, we are always conscious.

Socrates: No, that is not what he said. He said that in any of those conditions a person is conscious until they reach a state in which they are unconscious—they black out. That, however, is not what you are looking for. You are looking for a way to explain to your clients that they are not in an altered state of consciousness nor are they unconscious while in a hypnotic state. Think! While doing stage-show hypnosis what phrase do you use that seems to produce an instant hypnotic state?

Me: Let me think.... Well, when doing stage shows I say "sleep now," but I don't emphasize "sleep," or even talk about sleep for that matter, during clinical hypnosis. Is that what you are driving at—sleep? However, sleep is not a state of consciousness, is it?

Socrates: Are you sure that it isn't? You are on the right track but now hook it up with what Dr. Preston said about *behavior* being altered, but not consciousness.

Me: Let me think again.... I use "sleep now" when doing stage hypnosis and Dr. Preston said that hypnosis is not an altered state of consciousness and that behavior is altered while intoxicated, hallucinating, under the influence of drugs or dreaming, but consciousness isn't. I don't think I have ever really been drunk, nor have I ever had hallucinations or been under the influence of drugs, but I do dream. Is that it? Dreaming? While dreaming I am always conscious of my dreams so my consciousness is not altered—I am perfectly conscious of what is going on in my dreams while dreaming them—but I am asleep.

Socrates: So what does that imply?

Me: Are you saying that hypnosis is truly a state of sleep? But Dr. Preston said that a hypnotized person is *not* in a state of sleep... "If they fall asleep they are not hypnotized," he said.

Socrates: Maybe Dr. Preston has not wholly thought through the question of whether sleep is *necessarily* a state of unconsciousness or whether a "hypnotized" person is or is *not* in a sleep state. He may have neglected to consider that when a person is dreaming they are conscious of their dreams but at the same time, they are asleep.

Me: Well as I think about it, Dr. Preston cites cases in which people who are under general anesthesia during operations sometimes recall, after waking up, what the surgeon said during the procedure, even though they were supposedly "out"—asleep. So they must be conscious, but for all intents and purposes they are asleep. Most people (including me, until now) think that while asleep we are unconscious, but have never considered that dreaming isn't a state of unconsciousness.

Socrates: That may well be true, but once again what does all of this imply?

Me: It implies that sleep is not necessarily a state of unconsciousness! Apparently, there are stages of sleep when I *am* unconscious and not aware but while dreaming I must be conscious of my dream or I wouldn't be dreaming. If I were not aware and conscious of my dreams how would I remember them when I wake up? I don't remember all of my dreams but a lot of them I do. They may fade quickly, but even if I don't remember them I still remember, after awakening, that I dreamed *something.* I have never thought of dreaming as being a state of consciousness—a conscious state of sleep. That really sounds paradoxical: *a conscious state of sleep!* While I am dreaming I am not necessarily aware or conscious of what is going on in my surroundings, except that sometimes what goes on outside of me gets caught up in my dreams, like the sound of rain or wind coming through an open window or the temperature being hot or cold. However, I am still perfectly conscious and aware of what is going on in my dream at every moment.

Socrates: That is good thinking, but you are not answering the question about how to explain to your clients that hypnosis is not a state of being unconscious.

Me: When I am in this inner room with you I am not unconscious but I *am* oblivious to my surroundings, but if the phone rings or the door opens I immediately become aware of my environment.

Something that I have been wondering about for quite a while now makes sense. Sometimes I ask a hypnotized subject questions and they don't respond. Up until now, I thought that they were just in a very deep hypnotic state and were either not inclined, or maybe just unable, to respond. I didn't consider that maybe their subconscious mind wasn't even aware of or didn't understand my words. But when a subject's subconscious mind *is* comprehending my words then their subconscious mind must be conscious. How can that be—a conscious unconscious mind!

Some time I'm going to have to do some serious thinking about *that* idea. But maybe that would explain why sometimes clients don't get the full benefit they were expecting; they fell into an *unconscious* sleep and their subconscious mind didn't comprehend a single word of it.

Socrates: That's interesting speculation but not applicable to the question at hand: How can you use this insight to explain to your clients that they are always conscious during the session, although you are giving them suggestions to *SLEEP.*

Me: That *is* the question and I think I can resolve it right now. During the pre-hypnotic talk, I will explain that although they will always be conscious and aware, their physical body will be in a state of sleep. I'll say, "It's like dreaming—while you are dreaming a dream you are asleep but you are not unconscious because you know what is going on in your dream at every moment. So that must mean that you can be both at the same time—in a state of sleep but still conscious and aware."

Socrates: That sounds good but you may have to refine it so your clients fully comprehend its meaning.

Me: I am still puzzling about a couple of issues. First, does emphasizing the word "sleep" during the pre-hypnotic talk and during the induction make a difference in the effectiveness of the session? Second, how can the subconscious mind be subconscious (unconscious or below the level of conscious awareness) if it is "conscious" of hypnotic suggestions? I think that this last one may require some intense scrutinizing.

Socrates: To resolve your first question set up a controlled study.... Like you learned to do in experimental psychology. Randomly separate clients into two groups, and with one group emphasize "sleep" during the pre-hypnotic talk and during the induction process, and with the other group avoid using the word "sleep." Then establish a few tests that will determine how well they follow and carry out your suggestions. Keep a record of your findings and then apply the formulas you learned in your statistics class to see if there is a significant difference in the two groups.

Me: That is a good idea, Socrates.

CHAPTER 34

"Sleep" and Receptiveness

I began the next day using my newly conceived approach of introducing my clients to the idea that hypnosis is not an altered state of consciousness nor is it a state of unconsciousness but rather it is a state of sleep in which they are conscious. I explained to my clients, *"It is kind of like dreaming. While you are dreaming a dream you are not unconscious—you are completely conscious of what is going on in your dream—but you are asleep, so that must mean that we can be asleep and conscious at the same time."* I was surprised to discover that most of my clients not only understood the concept but also without reservation agreed with the idea, after thinking about it for a moment.

In fact, I learned from recent psychology courses that while in rapid eye movement (REM) state of sleep (actually, it turns out that REM is the deepest the state of sleep and the sleep state in which most of your dreaming is done) and while we are awake, our brainwave activity is very similar. Since EEG patterns are nearly the same when in REM sleep and while we are awake, it is referred to as "paradoxical" sleep. Interestingly, REM is easily observed during a hypnotic session, not only after the "induction," but also while leading a client through demonstrations that require the client's eyes to be closed during the pre-hypnotic talk.

It occurred to me that if indeed the hypnotic process works when the subject is in a conscious state of sleep then why not use the word "sleep" when doing clinical hypnosis. To satisfy my curiosity I designed a research study to determine if emphasizing the word "sleep" during the pre-hypnotic talk and using the phrase "sleep now" during the induction process *has* or *does not have* a positive effect on a client's receptiveness to hypnotic suggestions. From my stage-show experience, it *seemed* that it should, but I really didn't "know."

Actually, I received college credit for conducting this study since it met the requirements of an *Independent Study Program* offered by MCC. The faculty advisor for the study was Dr. Kurt Mahoney—the same professor who advised me to get a Ph.D. and then I could charge $45 a session like he did, instead of charging $85 like I did *without* a degree.

So under Dr. Mahoney's direction I created a hypothesis in the "null:" *The word "sleep" has no effect on a subject's receptiveness to hypnotic suggestions.* I had learned in experimental psychology that hypotheses are stated in the "null," meaning that the experimental condition to be tested (in my study, the word "sleep") has no significant effect. It is then up to the experimenter to accept or reject the hypothesis depending on the outcome of the study, regardless of the experimenter's bias.

The null hypothesis was fine with me, since in fact I didn't "know" if using the word "sleep" would affect the receptiveness of a hypnotic subject or if it would not.

The study procedure was straightforward: With half of my clients, I emphasized the word "sleep" during the pre-hypnotic talk and used the phrase "sleep now" during the induction. With the other half, I avoided using the word "sleep" altogether. I identified the groups as the "Sleep" group and the "No Sleep" group.

It took two months to accumulate 25 subjects for each group. I realized that the number of samples ("N," in statistical equations) was small, but in order to receive academic credits the project required completion by semester's end.

To test the hypothesis I used three tests.

Test One:

During the pre-hypnotic talk, I led each client through the pendulum demonstration—i.e., make a pendulum swing by visualizing it swinging—whether they were in the "Sleep" group or the "No Sleep" group. My plan was to discern the reliability of the demonstration, and record the amount of swing the subject was able to create by his or her visualization. I assigned a number determined by the distance the pendulum swung from center: (1) no swing, (2) slight swing (less than ½") and (3) large swing (more than ½").

After going through the induction procedure, I made the following two additional tests to determine how well each subject responded to my suggestions while in a hypnotic state.

Test Two:

I observed, measured and recorded the amount of arm movement and the heaviness/lightness that the clients reported in their arms after giving the following suggestions:

Place your arms straight out from your body at shoulder height with your palms downward. While trying to hold your arms level, visualize that there is balanced on the back of your right hand and wrist a big dictionary—you know how heavy a dictionary would be out there on your extended arm like that. Now visualize that the dictionary is pushing your right arm down lower and lower. Your right arm is getting heavier and heavier and the muscles in your right arm are getting more and more tired. The weight of the dictionary is pushing your right arm down lower and lower, and your right arm is getting even more heavy and tired. Now visualize that on your left wrist has been tied a giant bunch of helium balloons—like you would see at a carnival. In your imagination, visualize that those balloons are pulling your left arm up and that left arm and hand are floating up higher and higher. Visualize that all of the muscles in your left arm and shoulder are relaxed, and those balloons are now pulling up on your left arm. Your left arm is light, buoyant and floating up higher and higher.

I recorded the amount of movement of the subject's arms from their original level position and assigned a number determined by the amount of movement: (1) no deflection, (2) slight (less than 3"), (3) moderate to extreme (more than 3"). Some subjects' balloon arms ended up pointing straight up at the ceiling and their dictionary arms had fallen down pointing towards the floor (extreme).

I also asked if they "felt" a difference in the degree of tiredness between their right arm and their left. Without exception (even if there was no deflection), the subjects reported that their right arm felt more tired than their left. (I did not use this information in my study since it came from the subject's introspection and could not be overtly observed or measure.)

Test Three:

This "test suggestion" was to observe the degree of response resulting from the following suggestion:

Imagine that you cannot open your eyes. In your mind, visualize that your upper eyelids are glued to your lower eyelids and visualize that you cannot open your eyes. In a moment I will ask you to try to open your eyes, but when you try you will discover that your eyelids just stick tighter and tighter shut and all you will be able to do is raise your eyebrows. Now in your mind visualize that your eyes are stuck tight closed, but try to open your eyes now and all you can do is raise your eyebrows and your eyelids just stick tighter and tighter shut.

I recorded how well each client responded to this suggestion by assigning a number: (1) eyes opened with no difficulty, (2) the subjects struggled to open their eyes and eventually did in less than five seconds, (3) the subjects did not open their eyes although I observed that they tried.

I was also interested in finding if the subjects who responded well to my test suggestions also had a higher success ratio, over time, than those who didn't (this was not included as part of the study for credit).

To meet the requirements of this last question I needed a behavior that could be overtly observable (rather than from the subject's introspection— "I feel better than I did") to determine whether the suggestions made during the session produced the behavioral change for which the client had made the appointment. I chose smoking cessation. Smoking can be empirically observed—a client either quit smoking after a session, didn't quit, or went back to smoking after a period of time. [6]

The study showed that there was no statistical difference between the two groups in the pendulum-swinging test. Every subject caused the pendulum to swing to some degree, regardless of whether or not I used the word "sleep" during the pre-hypnotic talk.

However, there was a significant statistical difference between the "Sleep" group and the "No Sleep" group in both the dictionary-balloon test and the eye closure test; the "Sleep" group prevailed by a wide margin.

To ascertain if there was a long-term difference in the effectiveness of using "sleep now" during the induction over not using "sleep now," I contacted by telephone each of the stop smoking clients at intervals of one week, one month and six months. Of the 50 clients who were included in the study, 28 had made an appointment to stop smoking.

The bottom line was encouraging regardless of the group. 79% of the "Sleep" group and 17% of the "No Sleep" group were still not smoking after six months. Even the "No Sleep" group fared well compared to individuals undergoing nicotine substitution therapy. (In a study conducted by the Mayo Clinic Rochester, MN—reported in the November 1999 issue of the *American Journal of Public Health* in a study to determine the hazards of using the nicotine patch—subjects using a placebo patch had a success rate of 4.3%, and subjects using the actual nicotine patches had a success rate of 10.8% after 24 weeks.)

Note: We must be cognizant that the samples in my study are not representative of the general population since the samples (subjects) came from a segment of the population that considered hypnosis to be a valid method to effect a change in their behavior. If one were to randomly select fifty people off the street, the results would quite likely be different. In addition, we must take into consideration that the data obtained from the stop smoking clients may have been skewed since I, the experimenter, gathered the data and the clients may not have been willing to admit that they (or I) had failed.

---

6. The detailed data from the study can be found in Appendix V.

Considering the margin of success with the "Sleep" group, I began to emphasize "sleep" during the pre-hypnotic talk and use "sleep now" during the induction.[7]

This new approach produced better results, but I felt it still needed some refining. The biggest issue was that even with the shortened induction procedure, a session still required more than an hour and a half. So once again, I sought insight from Socrates.

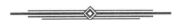

Me: I want my clients to get better results from their session while staying within the following parameters:

1. Keep a session under one hour.
2. Obtain a greater success rate with a single session if possible.
3. Discover a better way to describe the idea of visualization. The terms "visualization" and "visualize" seem a little awkward and don't quite fit the idea I want to convey.

Socrates: To achieve these objectives you will probably have to make some drastic changes in your established approach. Let's start with shortening the time for a session. Let me ask this: Which part of the session now consumes the most time?

Me: Without question, regression. Taking the client back to some past sensitizing event is the greatest time-consuming part of the session. I have cut the induction from 25 minutes to 5 minutes but each session still stretches into an hour and a half—and even more, sometimes. Not only that, but sometimes it takes several sessions before discovering *all* of the root causes of a client's unwanted behavior.

Socrates: Then it might be advisable to reconsider the value of "regressing" a client back to a sensitizing event at all.

Me: But how can I get a person to change their present behavior if I don't take them back and discover the subconscious memories that are causing them to behave now as they *don't* want to? If I am going to help people change without regressing them back to a sensitizing event, then how will they understand why they engage in self-destructive and unwanted behavior now?

---

7. At that time I conducted the dictionary-balloon test and the eye closure test to convince *me* that the client was in a state of "hypnosis." However, as my approach evolved I used these tests to convince *them* (the client) that they were hypnotized. Now I still use all three demonstrations (not tests) during my pre-hypnotic talk to validate to my client that their brain will automatically produce behavior that their mind instructs it to produce—whether they are "hypnotized" or not.

Socrates: Well, that is what I am asking you. Why *do* you have to get a client to discover an unconscious sensitizing event in order to get them to change their present behavior? Have you ever tried *not* using regression?

Me: Now that I think about it, in the past several years I have not–that is, since I met up with Eric. I will agree that if regression was not necessary it would certainly shorten the session. But if I don't use regression I am afraid that success results will significantly drop off.

Socrates: Why are you still fearful of trying something that is out of convention? We've been through this discussion before. Why do you resist trying out new ideas and schemes? You resisted the idea that it is *not* necessary to go to an imaginary scene in order to get a subject to feel peaceful. You resisted eliminating the suggestion that the subject relax every tiny muscle of their body to get their entire body relaxed and you resisted Dr. Preston's idea about there being no "altered states of consciousness." In every one of these cases, although you began with great trepidation, your effectiveness was enhanced. So why do you resist investigating an alternative approach that omits the time-consuming regression part of the session?

Me: Okay, I'll try. Maybe I can get some inspiration from my clients to figure it out.

But what can do I to achieve better results with a single session? From my study, 69% of the people who came in to stop smoking did not smoke for at least six months after a single session. I want to find a way to improve that percentage.

Socrates: Back in the 5th century B.C., *I* didn't put in writing any of my philosophies. Other people wrote down all the stuff they said I said after my death. I believed that an oral presentation was much more effective than a written one. People thought that I was a little soft in the head because I wandered around Athens babbling the same ideas repeatedly; but I also knew that for the listeners to grasp the gist of my ideas I would have to repeat the same ideas many times over. I believed that the key to getting an idea to stick was repetition. Nowadays however, with the advent of tape recorders, a person can easily record their ideas and the listener can enjoy endless repetitions until the idea is ingrained and becomes a habitual way of thinking. Isn't that what SMI was all about–spaced repetition?

Me: Yeah! I hadn't thought about applying spaced repetition to increase the effectiveness of a hypnosis session. So, what you are saying is that I should buy a tape recorder and make a recording of each session then give the tape to my client so they can listen to it, thereby reinforcing suggestions given during the session. That's a brilliant idea! I'll do it.

Now what about "visualization?" I am sure there is a better word that will convey the idea that how we "see" ourselves and "see" ourselves responding to our environment determines how we feel and act. "See" doesn't fit any better than "visualization"—both imply a visual (eye) process. I've even been using "concept" but that is just as awkward—"Create in your mind the concept that the pendulum is swinging," for example. But that is as uncomfortable as "visualize," "picture," "imagine," "think about," "create the notions," "conjure up the image," "conceive" or "believe." I've tried them all but they just don't seem to do the trick. There has to be a term that expresses the thought and conveys the same idea and has a common thread that encompasses all of those words.

Socrates: How about looking in a dictionary or thesaurus to get some fresh ideas? Or get some input from your clients?

Me: Well, Socrates, that's a good idea, too. You have presented me with some great ideas but you have also created some monumental challenges—like revamping my present approach.

So I began another adventure into unfamiliar waters in an attempt to understand and more effectively apply the hypnotic process.

CHAPTER 35

The Recording

So I went down to Radio Shack and bought a cassette tape recorder.

Let me ask *you* (the reader): What was your reaction the first time you heard a recording of your own voice? If it was like me—you were horrified!

I thought to myself, *I can't do this. I sound like my brothers, except they sound confident and self-assured when they speak. I sound tentative, insecure and my voice shakes. I may stop talking altogether if that is how I sound to other people. I don't think I can do this. I sound like I have my neck in a noose and cotton balls stuffed up my snout!*

Socrates shouted in my head, "You're dead at the bottom of a cliff so nothing can threaten you!"

Me: Yeah, that's easy for you to say. *You* never heard a recording of *your* own voice!

I took his advice and tried it again. With a few days practice I discovered that if I thought of speaking to a person rather than to a recorder, I sounded much more confident. And if I took in a deep breath before each phrase and talked from my diaphragm rather than through my nostrils, I sounded even better. It didn't take long until I began liking the sound of my recorded voice.

So I began making a recording of each session and gave it to my clients to take home and listen to so they could experience the advantage of "spaced repetition." I sent them home with a recording of the entire session from beginning to end—and that created a few problems that I hadn't anticipated.

First, the client was little inclined to spend an hour and a half listening to the entire recording—the pre-hypnotic talk, the induction, regressing back to their sensitizing events, suggestions relative to changing their behavior and waking them up.

Second, I could not find a standard blank cassette tape that could hold an hour and a half of my babbling without having to stop and turn it over. That was not only an annoyance for me while recording the session, but more so for the client who would have to open their eyes, turn the tape over and then try to get back into the mental flow of what was recorded. If self-reversing recorders had been invented at the time none of my clients had one. And some clients did not own a player and a few had never even heard of a cassette tape player, so if they were going to listen to my recording they had to go out and buy one.

Third—and probably the biggest problem—was that many of my clients had never before heard their recorded voice, either. Several clients complained that when I asked them to return back to sensitizing events and they heard their recorded voice for the first time, they immediately "woke-up," horrified!

The most logical steps for shortening the recording time and eliminating the negative response the clients experienced when they heard their own voice was to not record the pre-hypnotic talk, record only the induction, set the recorder on "Pause" during the regression, then turn the recorder back on before giving suggestions about their new behavior and the "waking up" part.

This procedure worked much better; the client was more inclined to listen to the recording because it was shorter (about 20 minutes) and they got better results with a single session. But the session still lasted an hour and a half.... *Do I dare to try leaving out the regression part of the session?* I thought to myself. *How can I do that without compromising the effectiveness of the session?*

The solution came from my clients.

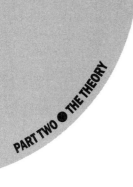

CHAPTER 36

Regression
Revisited

The idea of having to "regress" a client to some sensitizing event had become so ingrained in my approach—and because it seemed to work fairly well—I was reluctant to abandon the practice. However, I knew that if I did not have to go through the regression part of the session I could reduce the time by at least half an hour, but I just could not come up with the courage to try, nor could I think of a satisfactory way to do it. I feared that to do so would result in achieving marginal effectiveness at best. Hard as I tried to come up with a solution, my efforts were fruitless. I just could not concoct a way to negate addressing the negative influence earlier experiences had on my client's present behavior without first discovering what the experiences were. Nonetheless, as in the past, the solution came from my clients.

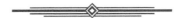

Mario wanted to stop smoking. He was a two-pack-a-day, longtime smoker; in fact, he had been smoking for 40 years and was feeling the effect it was having on his physical well-being.

"I've been smoking for most of my life and I'm fed up with it," he told me. "I've even tried some of those new nicotine patches that the doctor prescribed and they just gave me bad dreams... not only that but the patches that were supposed to keep me from smoking were four times more expensive than my smokes. It is strange that I was getting all of that nicotine in my system and still felt like I needed a cigarette. So I went back to smoking... it was cheaper."

After a little more dialog I asked Mario to sit in my recliner, and when I had finished the induction process I instructed (as was customary when working with smokers), *"Mario, return back to when you first started smoking."*

Mario came up with the "textbook" answers, "Well, back when I started smoking, it made me feel like I fit in with the less-than-academic rabble. I was a freshman in high school, the 'cool' older students smoked, and I wanted to be a part of the 'in group.' So I made off with a pack of smokes from my dad's stash and at lunch break went over to the 'smoking bridge' (just off campus) where all of the tough guys hung out, pulled out my cigs and lit up.... It only took about five minutes of puffing before I got light headed and then threw up. It turned out that chucking up was kind of an unofficial initiation ceremony into the smoking club. Everyone laughed at me but then a few admitted that they had had the same experience with their first try."

I asked, "*Mario, was fitting into the group the only reason you started smoking?*"

"Well no," he responded, "I wanted to feel older and more grown up... like my dad. I idolized my dad. He smoked like a chimney and I wanted to grow up to be just like him. Things just couldn't get any better than being out in the middle of the lake in our fishing boat on a cool summer morning and getting an occasional whiff of my dad's smoke. My dad was the best friend I had when I was growing up and I wanted to act just like him—grown up too. It is a bit ironic though; he told me that if he ever caught *me* smoking he'd beat the tar out of me."

"*Okay, so you wanted to fit into the group, wanted to be like your dad and wanted to feel older and more grown up. Is that correct?*" I asked.

"Yes, that is right," he answered.

"*Are there any other needs that smoking filled back when you first started?*"

After a few moments of reflection he said, "I had a rebellious streak in me. I loved my dad and we had a great relationship for the most part but whenever he gave me a dressing-down, by telling me what to do or what not to do, I'd rebel and do just the opposite. I think it was his telling me that he would beat me to within an inch of my life that provoked me into smoking—'He can't tell me what to do!'

"Not only that, I was a rebellious kid by nature, and smoking portrayed the image and reputation of *being* a rebel. Besides, I could get away with smoking right under my dad's nose... he couldn't tell if it was me who stank or him. It wasn't until I graduated from college that I smoked in front of him."

I could tell that Mario was reflecting back to events from his youth and after a moment he continued, "I know now that the reason Dad didn't want me to smoke was because he loved me and didn't want me to get hooked like he was—he was continually trying to break the smoking habit. I wonder how many fish expired by ingesting the tobacco from the countless packs he threw into the lake with a vow that he'd never buy another pack.

"Five years ago Dad died of lung cancer and I've been trying to break the habit of smoking ever since. I guess I *did* turn out as I wanted to—just like my dad... hooked on the habit of smoking. Just like my dad, since they were boys, I've told my sons that they would be in big trouble if I ever caught them smoking. And now they have turned out to be just like me—smokers. This cycle has got to stop some place."

With tears in his eyes he continued, "But I don't want to be like my dad any more in that respect. I want to be healthy and to be rid of this albatross. I've tried and I've tried but this habit has got hold of me and I can't break it."

As calmly as I could without reacting to his emotions I responded, *"Can you think of any other events that caused you to started smoking? Any other needs that smoking back then filled?"*

After thinking again for a minute Mario answered, "No I can't."

"Can you think of any events that have occurred since the time you started that make you feel that you need to keep on smoking?"

"Well, it gives me something to do when I'm bored. If I have to wait for someone, and I'm standing around, it just seems that I need to be doing something with my hands—you know, 'idle hands are the devil's workshop.' I can still hear my dad saying (even when I was an adult) 'Don't just stand there with your hands in your pockets, son—get busy and do something.' Smoking also seems to calm me down and relaxes me—it gives me an excuse to take a break. But I can't think of anything that it really *does* for me anymore, except make me hack my innards out in the mornings when I wake up. And something else smoking is doing for me... it's putting me in the poor house. I have even reasoned with myself: smoking makes me feel crappy, and it makes no sense to spend two bucks a day *[this was in the 80's]* to make myself feel crappy.

"And another thing: it really ticks me off when people tell me that I have got to stop smoking. It just makes me want to go smoke even more. But in spite of it all, I'd really rather be a non-smoker; it's a disgusting habit and I'm ready to stop!"

He was sobbing when he pleaded, "Can you help me? I'm desperate and I'm ready to give up these /#&^$@?> things."

I said, *"Yes, I think I can."* And to deepen the hypnotic state, and to make sure Mario was still relaxed and in a receptive state of mind, I said, *"Just take in a deep breath and hold it in while I count down..."*

After Mario had settled in again, I asked him to reason with me for a few minutes and then accept the suggestions I would be giving him—my "textbook" suggestions. *"It is understandable that back when you started smoking, it filled some genuine social and emotional needs. Smoking was cool. Smoking helped you to fit into* the "cool" group. Smoking made you feel older and more grown up like your father. Your father's smoking had been associated with enjoying his company and having fun—fishing. You were rebellious and smoking gave the appearance of being a rebel. Smoking truly filled those emotional and social needs, but somehow the rules got changed... exactly the opposite is true now. Those same needs are now filled by not smoking.

"Smoking just ain't cool no more. Nowadays, being a non-smoker you are accepted into any group—even when you are with people who still smoke there is no negative response if you choose to not smoke. In fact, they would probably envy you for having stopped.

"I don't know that you want to feel older and more grown up—you are probably through doing that by now. If you will think about it, the opposite is true. Now being a non-smoker will cause you to feel more youthful.

"Now being a non-smoker demonstrates your true independence—your rebellious nature. You are a non-smoker in spite of the fact people have been telling you that you have got to stop.

"Reason with me further: If you want to stop smoking but people telling you to stop smoking makes you smoke, then they are making you do something you don't want to do—they are making you smoke when you don't want to smoke. That's not independence or even rebellion—unless in some sinister way you are rebelling against yourself. Think of it this way, your true independence is now demonstrated by being a non-smoker in spite of the fact they want you to stop. You are a non-smoker now and it doesn't matter if they want you to stop smoking or don't want you to stop—that's independence.

"Another point: smoking never should have calmed you down or relaxed you. Nicotine is a stimulant, not a relaxant. Smoking should have keyed you up, not calmed you down. Any calming down that came from smoking did not come from the stuff in the cigarettes, it came from taking a break and the vision that smoking would calm you down. You don't need an excuse to take a break. If you feel like you need to take a break then take a break without smoking. You don't need to have a cigarette in your hand just so it appears that you are busy doing something. Busy hands—just for the sake of appearing that you are doing something, especially if what you are doing is slowly killing you—are the devil's workshop.

"Accept these suggestions: Since you now know why you started smoking and the reasons that you have more recently been smoking, there is no longer a need to smoke. Now you feel, behave and act as a non-smoker. You feel, behave and act as though you never did smoke. You behave as a peaceful non-smoker. You act like a non-smoker. You think of yourself as being a non-smoker. Smoking for you is no longer an issue. You visualize yourself as being a non-smoker. You are an independent non-smoker. It doesn't matter if people around you smoke or if they don't smoke. Other people's behavior has nothing to do with how you behave. You are free and independent and *being a non-smoker communicates your true independence. Being a non-smoker, you feel better about yourself than you ever did when you used to smoke.*

"Visualize yourself enjoying all of the benefits that just happen as the result of being a non-smoker. You wake up in the mornings with clear lungs. You have more endurance and more energy as the result of being a non-smoker. You have more money because you are a non-smoker...

"I am going to count up from one to five. When I reach the number five you open your eyes and you will feel, behave and act as though you never did smoke."

After I had counted up, Mario opened his eyes and said, "I really feel great. Right now, I feel better than I have for a long time. When I came in to your office, my muscles were all tight, I felt anxious and I felt that I really, really, needed a smoke. But now I don't. I truly feel right now as though I never did smoke.

"But all that stuff in my earlier life that we talked about I already knew and I think you knew what I was going to say before you asked—your responses seemed to have been rehearsed. It was fun to reminisce about the past and I'll have to admit that those memories were more vivid than they have been since they happened. It seemed as though I was right there in the boat getting whiffs of Dad's smoke and that I was over at the smoking bridge with the mob. That was all well and good but I already remembered all of that stuff.

"I don't know for sure what has made the difference, but right now I feel like I will never smoke again. I think it was when you told me to visualize myself as a non-smoker and to visualize all of the benefits and that it is as though I never did smoke. I think that is what did it."

After Mario left I reasoned with myself, *I think there is something in what Mario said that might hold a key to not having to regress a person back to a sensitizing event—he said that he already remembered those events. He was also insightful enough to recognize that I had heard all of those reasons for starting smoking before—he's right, maybe a few hundred times. I'm going to have to ponder this a little more and even see what Socrates thinks when I have time.*

I came up with no definitive solution or comfortable way to *not* use regression. That is, until a few weeks later.

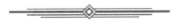

Deborah wanted to lose 85 lbs. She told me that she was desperate and would do whatever it took to shed all her excess "adipose tissue" (as she put it)—even hypnotherapy. She saw my puzzlement and explained, "I am a dietary specialist for a hospital consultant group, and 'adipose tissue'

is a 'connective tissue in which fat is stored and has distended cells through the deposition of droplets of fat' —it's kind of like 'baby fat' and the fat hibernating animals store for the winter."

She continued to explain, "I started studying nutrition initially because I have struggled with a weight problem since childhood and thought if I acquired enough knowledge about what to eat—and the bad effect that obesity has on one's health—I would be motivated to change my eating habits, but it didn't work. I've learned a lot of really neat information about nutrition, so I know exactly how I should be eating—what, how much and only three times a day—and I know that I should be exercising. I've even published a few papers on nutrition and the bad effects junk food has on good health, but I just can't stop grazing all day long. I know that I should be exercising at least three times a week but after working 9 hours a day and commuting in rush-hour traffic for another hour each way, I'm just too tired and exhausted to exercise.

"I have a little cubical in the back corner of the office where most of the time I am all by myself and no one knows that I keep a stash of junk food in the bottom drawer. I keep all of the healthy stuff sitting on my desktop."

After going through the induction I instructed, "*Deborah, return back to some event in the past that causes you to feel that you need to "graze" all day long now.*"

Deborah thought for a moment and said, "My little brother."

"*What does your little brother have to do with your munching behavior now?*"

"Mommy feeds him all the time. He is a chunky one-year-old and Mommy is saying that if he doesn't have something in his mouth all the time he is unhappy. Ever since she brought him home all she does is feed him. All she does is play with him and feed him. It makes me mad and unhappy."

Deborah was one of those subjects who returned to a past event as though she was living it, so my questions were asked as though I was there, too. I asked, "*How old are you?*"

Speaking in baby talk, and raising three fingers, she answered, "I'm three years."

I knew the answer to my next question before I asked it since there was a frown on her face and tears pouring from her eyes. "*What are you doing?*"

"I am crying."

"*Why are you crying?*"

"When Timmy cries Mommy plays with him and gives him good things to eat. If I cry maybe Mommy will play with *me* and give *me* good things to eat."

"*Is crying working? Does your mother come and play with you and give you something good to eat?*"

"No. She tells me to stop being such a crybaby. 'Can't you see I'm busy with little Timmy? You go find something to eat, that'll make you feel better.'"

"*What is happening now?*"

"I'm eating a crust of bread and Mommy is feeding Timmy some animal crackers."

"*Is eating a bread crust making you feel better?*"

"Yes it is—while I am eating. But I want Mommy to play with me. I'm not hungry but eating should help me be happy because eating makes Timmy happy and keeps him from crying."

I asked, "*What does this have to do with your grazing in the present?*"

When she answered, she switched to her grown-up voice and said, "Isn't it obvious? When I was young, I learned to eat when I was unhappy and wanted attention—eating made me happy. When I am unhappy or am not getting the recognition I think I should be getting, just like when I was three years old, I feel that I need to eat. I know I don't *need* to eat, it is just that I *feel* like I need to. If I could get rid of these feelings I think I could do loads better.

"I have always known that my eating problem was rooted in my childhood, and I remember the resentment that I felt when my mom gave Tim all of the attention. I also know that it is irrational to think I need to eat just because I am unhappy and not getting attention, but I just have this feeling—this compulsion—to eat all day long."

"*Does that mean that you are unhappy all day long or that you are not getting the attention you think you deserve all day long—or both?*"

"Don't get me wrong. I'm not an unhappy person. I have a lot of fun in my life and I have many friends. I guess it is just when I'm alone that I have the feeling that I need to eat. Now that I think of it, I suppose that I don't eat *all* day long. I don't have that feeling that I need to eat when other people are around—it's just when I am alone."

"*Tell me whatever comes into your mind when I ask you to return to the experience that causes you to feel like you need to eat when you are alone.*"

Again it took a few moments for her to come up with an answer, and then she said, "This is really crazy. It seems like I am in a lucid dream."

"*What is happening?*"

She began speaking in a very frail voice, "There are so many people and so little food."

"*What is happening? Where are you and why are there so many of you?*"

"I see myself in a prison... a concentration camp. If we could only be off by ourselves in the countryside we could find plenty to eat."

Thinking that Deborah had regressed back to a past life I asked, "*Where is the prison? What is the historical time period?*"

Tears were streaming down her cheeks and between her sobs she said,

341

"Oh, I'm in the here and now... in the present with you... I had this same kind of experience... the feeling of being some place else... when doing one of my research studies... about nutrition."

"Explain to me what this has to do with your present eating behavior."

After a few moments, her weeping stopped and she said, "I was examining what happens to people when they are deprived of proper nutrients. Part of my research involved studying the conditions in concentration camps during the Second World War. Often times when I interviewed or read the accounts of the survivors, it was as if *I* was there. I knew I wasn't there in the concentration camps, but in my imagination it was like I was there with them. It was difficult to conduct the interviews with Holocaust survivors because I was sniveling so much—it was difficult to ask rational questions at times. I could feel their hunger, their despair and their pain. At times it was as if I was there with them living their experience. I remember thinking that if we could have just been on our own out in the countryside we would be able to find *some* food... and probably, although very little, at least some of the right kinds of food. The best we got in the camps most of the time was watered down potato soup."

"What does this have to do with eating when you are alone now?"

"That is obvious. When I am alone I can eat whatever I want because I don't want to have those feelings of starving.

"Being a nutrition specialist I am self-conscious about eating unhealthy foods only when I'm with my friends and colleagues—it is kind of like being in a concentration camp—I feel like they are keeping track of every morsel I put in my mouth, so when they are around I eat very little. My coworkers are continually commenting that I should be as skinny as a rail because I eat so little. In response, I joke, 'It's because of my private research. How can a person be a real expert unless they eat a lot of all kinds of foods to determine their nutritional value—both kinds, healthy *and* junky?

"I know that what I am telling you is irrational and disjointed, but when I am alone I can eat whatever I want, but it is continuous... except when I am sleeping. I learned that when people have been starved for a long time that they need to eat small amounts—just graze! When I am alone, and awake, I have the same feelings of sorrow that I felt when reading and hearing about the plight of the concentration camp survivors so I just graze. But my problem is I don't just graze on healthy foods, it is mostly junk foods."

She stopped talking so I asked, *"Let me see if I understand this correctly. Not only do you feel like you need to eat when you are unhappy and not getting recognition, but also when you are alone? On the other hand, you don't have the feeling* that you need to eat when you are with your friends and colleagues... and the feelings have something to do with your research about concentration camps, is that right?"

"I know it sounds crazy and there seems to be no reason or logic to what I have told you. Especially when you parrot it back, it sounds even more stupid. But that is what came to my mind when you asked me to go back and to tell you whatever came into my mind. While I recalled those events, it was as if I was experiencing them and experiencing the feelings associated with those events—like I need to eat. If I could just get rid of the *feelings* I think I would be able to stop eating when I am alone or unhappy. I wish that those events would have never happened and then I wouldn't have the feeling... and then I wouldn't be so fat!"

While she was regaining control of her sobbing, I realized that what she had just said and how she had said it had triggered a flash of inspiration.

When she calmed down I asked, *"Deborah, are you telling me that all you are looking for is to get rid of the feelings that have been causing you to overeat and to feel as if those events in the past, that cause those feelings, had never happened— regardless of what the events were? And, if it was as though the events had never happened then you wouldn't have the feelings, and if you didn't have the feelings then you would not be overeating. Is that correct?"*

"I think that is what I just said."

"Then it isn't that you need to know what the events were—you just want to feel as though they had never happened. Do I have it right?"

"Yes, that is right."

"Then let me ask this. When you say that you wouldn't be overeating if you didn't have the feelings, where do you sense the feeling... the feelings that you need to eat when alone or unhappy?"

"What do you mean by 'where do I sense the feeling?'"

"You said that if you didn't have the feeling then you wouldn't feel like overeating. You must sense a different feeling when you are alone than you have when you are with your friends. What I am asking is where in your body do you feel the difference?"

"I still don't understand what you mean by where in my body do I have the feelings?"

"All of our emotions are felt physically. That's why we say I feel sad, I feel happy, I feel stressed, I feel angry. We feel our emotion somewhere in our body. A particular emotion may be felt in different places for different people, but all of our emotions are sensed somewhere in our body. Let me ask it this way, 'Right now do you feel like you need something to eat?'"

Deborah hesitated for a moment and answered, "No... because I am not alone—you are here with me."

"Where in your <u>body</u> did you 'look' to see if you had the feeling?"

"Oh, I understand now what you are asking. I looked for the feelings in my stomach, my chest and my throat... oh, and my hands."

"If those feelings were permanently removed—as if they were never there—would you feel like you need to eat just because you are unhappy or alone?"

"If I felt at all times the way I feel right now, if all of those feelings were removed whether I am alone, lonely, sad, happy, or wanting attention I think I'd have my problem licked."

"Then take in a deep breath... hold it in while I count down: 5... 4... 3... 2... 1 and exhale... And accept the suggestions that I give you now.

"The powers of your subconscious mind now and permanently remove and eliminate all of those feelings in your stomach, in your chest, in your throat and in your hands—the feelings that have been causing you to eat between times and to eat junk foods. Regardless of the events in the past—the ones that have been causing those feelings—it is now as though they never happened. Your eating behavior is now consistent with your knowledge of how you should be eating. You eat only three times a day, you choose to eat and enjoy eating healthy foods and drinks. No longer do you eat between times nor do you <u>feel</u> that you need to eat between times, even when you are alone. At each of your eating times, when you have eaten as much as you know you should eat, you feel filled and satisfied and you stop eating. Because you are eating healthy foods and drinks, you are more physically energetic so you exercise at least three times a week. Each day you use more energy than you take in by eating, so each day you lose some body fat, therefore you maintain a high level of enthusiasm about eating right and exercising.

"When I reach the number five, open your eyes and you will be wide-awake...."

Deborah opened her eyes and with a smile said, "That was a really neat experience! I feel wonderful. I didn't like all of the emotions and crying, but if I can just feel this way at all times, eating between meals would not be an issue. It's like the feelings that I needed to eat when I was alone or when I was unhappy were never there. But why did I need to go back and bring up the experience of being a three-year-old and my research studies in order to get rid of those feelings? I didn't like that part and I already knew all of those things anyway."

I responded, "Right now I'm wondering why, too."

Before Deborah left I thanked her for having been the catalyst that may be the answer to a problem I had been wrestling with for several months.

When I was alone I sat down in my recliner and headed into my inner room for a discussion with Socrates:

Me: I wonder if the answer to *not* having to regress a client back to a sensitizing event truly is that simple. Is the key to helping people change their behavior as simple as discovering where and how a client feels the emotions that have been causing an unwanted behavior and then removing the *feelings* of the emotions? Rather than the time-consuming process of taking them back to an event to discover what happened in the past that has been causing the emotion, hence producing the unwanted behavior.

I know that I am going to get a lot of flak from my colleagues when I present the idea that they don't need to regress a client to get them to change their unwanted behavior.

Socrates: You are right. It may be harder for your colleagues to let go of the old ways than it has been for you—especially when it is not their idea. Your *clients* will probably be more open to acceptance than your colleagues since most of them have not been indoctrinated as to what hypnosis is or how a session should be conducted. However, I am surprised that you didn't catch on to the idea when Mario said, "I already remembered all of that stuff (experiences related to smoking).... I think it was when you told me to visualize myself as a non-smoker and to visualize all of the benefits of being a non-smoker and that it is now as though I never did smoke. I think that is what did it." Apparently, it was the suggestions about *visualizing* himself as being a non-smoker, not the regression.

Me: I am confident that I have found the solution to my regression dilemma. I can't believe that the opinions of others have blurred my vision, and again mired me down by thinking that the "right way" is the only way. Not only do my hypnotherapist colleagues think that it is necessary to dredge up old issues in order to change behavior but the approach of traditional psychology, especially psychoanalysis, teaches that the secret to changing present behavior is to get people to divulge all of their deep, dark, hidden experiences of the past.

Socrates: It is interesting how the views of the experts cloud our creative visions. In my time (400 B.C.) and in every era before or since, the human race has accepted the suppositions of people who are in a position of authority to be true, regardless of the evidence. Remember, there is much to be gleaned from the opinions of others, but always examine their opinions and then test to see if they hold true.

Me: It just occurred to me that if I hadn't had Deborah regress back to those events I could have spared her from the anxieties and tears she experienced by recalling them—it was almost like she was reliving them.

Socrates: Take a close look at your new insight, test it and analyze the results, but just because you have come up with a possible way to reduce the time of a session does not mean that you should give up regressions altogether. Many people are curious about what happened in the past, not for therapeutic reasons but just to recall earlier experiences... even in past lives. Do not throw the baby out with the bath water just because you have finished the scrubbing. Maybe there are some cases in which regression will still hold value to the client—whether it is just curiosity or a conviction of their belief system. Regressing to events in this life or even past lives can be beneficial, interesting and entertaining for many people.

A belief in a past life or a future life for the believer gives them a sense of security, peace of mind and purpose for this life's experience. Moreover, there may be others who need to justify their present behavior by discovering what happened to them in the past. It is not up to you to decide for them what to believe or to change their convictions. If people are searching for answers, then share with them what you have learned; and if they are open to your point of view, it is sure to lead to greater refinement and clarification. On the other hand, never try to dismantle someone's belief system just to justify your own. Sure, ask questions that will cause them to examine their life and beliefs but what value is there in stripping a person of a philosophy or belief system that gives them peace and security?

Me: If it turns out that *not* having to regress a client to a past event proves to be more effective, then why shouldn't I be crying it from the rooftops?

Socrates: That is not exactly what I said. Sure, broadcast your discoveries but don't try to convince a colleague or client that their way of thinking is wrong. If your discoveries hold validity, the open-minded and the curious will embrace them, and regardless of the legitimacy and authentication of new ideas, the bigot will reject them. Only with sound logic and consistent verification will you sway the thinking of other people. So don't be too disappointed if few agree with you in the beginning. But first, you must test your newly acquired insight to find out if it turns out to be a genuine approach for getting better results with a shorter session.

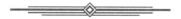

Therefore, I did. To my delight I not only saved considerable time (I could accomplish a session in an hour), but more importantly the effectiveness of a session improved! I had fewer people coming back for additional sessions and more referrals from those who had come in for a hypnotherapy session. In addition, when I stopped regressing clients I spared them from the emotional trepidation that was usually experienced when regressing them back to what was almost always a traumatic experience... not to mention the few dollars I saved on boxes of Kleenex.

As I refined my "no regression" approach, I still wrestled with a comfortable way to use the word "visualize" (or some variation of the term that would more accurately convey the concept I wanted to communicate) during my demonstrations and the session in general. Little did I know at the time that this investigation would become the core of a unique approach to hypnotherapy and possibly a new way of explaining much of human behavior in general.

CHAPTER 37

Perceptionism

It is odd how the conspicuous is perfectly apparent to everyone but the seeker. In addition, how the obvious place to find the answer sits on a bookshelf less than a few blocks away yet the searcher never takes the initiative to travel the distance. So it was in my pursuit for a better term to use, other than "visualization," when explaining how the hypnotic process works and demonstrating that it does.

Maybe it was my inadequate reading experience when I was young that limited my exposure to a variety of words and veiled the means by which to discover alternative terms, but most likely it was that I didn't know where to look that created the impasse... finding the right word to convey the idea that visualization is the key element to the hypnotic process continued to elude me.

I was forty years old before I knew there was such a thing as a thesaurus. I am reasonably sure that many readers find this absurd. I must have been absent or off on one of my daydreams on the day the teacher told the class about there being such a publication. Nonetheless, even after discovering that the lexicon existed I didn't think of using one; that is, until Socrates jogged the idea of looking in a dictionary or thesaurus to find a suitable term.

So I pulled off my shelf a copy of Webster's Dictionary and found these relevant definitions:

visualize: *transitive verb*: to make visible: as to see or form a mental image of ENVISAGE <trying to visualize a problem> *intransitive verb*: to form a mental visual image
visualization: 1. formation of mental visual images 2. the act or process of interpreting in visual terms or of putting into visible form.

Neither definition satisfied my need. So I set off to a nearby bookstore, and bought my first ever thesaurus and looked up:

visualization: [there were no synonyms]
visualize: conceive, envisage, envision, fancy, feature, imagine, realize, vision, picture, view, objectify, call up, conjure up a mental image, see in the mind's eye, see, think about, conceptualize, and concept.

So I began to try various alternative terms out on my clients. To make clear the problem, and the path that finally led to the solution of my dilemma, I'll use the pendulum demonstration to illustrate the difficulties I encountered when trying different terms. Sometimes I would use multiple terms; i.e., if one word didn't work I'd try another term. Eventually I would chance upon a word that the client could relate to and then the pendulum would start swinging in the direction they chose to visualize, see, imagine, picture, think about, conceive, see in their mind's eye, conjure up a mental image of....

When using "visualization" or "visualize" the clients would often complain, "I am not a visual person; I am more linguistic or verbal than I am visual in my thinking." Visualization also infers "seeing" with one's eyes (vision) rather than picturing in one's mind. In addition, when leading a client through the pendulum demonstration and asking them to visualize the pendulum swinging back and forth in the direction C-D, for example, I often noticed that the client was trying to make it swing by moving their eyes back and forth—trying to make it swing with their eyes. I wanted them to use their mind, not their eyes.

When I tried using "imagine," occasionally a client would exclaim that they were on the short end of the imagining scale. I remember one client telling me, "I have no imagination—at least that's what people tell me. I remember when I was a kid I had a great imagination. I even had an imaginary friend and we had all kinds of exciting adventures, but imagining got stomped out of me by my parents. 'Stop all of this pretending, it's silly to imagine things that aren't real,' I was warned time and again. I just cannot imagine the pendulum swinging because it isn't swinging. I can make it swing by intentionally moving my arm but I can't imagine that it is swinging unless it is," but when I asked him to "think about it swinging" the demonstration worked perfectly.

When I tried "picture in your mind" I often got a similar response to "visualization": "I have a hard time picturing things in my mind that I can't see with my eyes first."

"See in your mind's eye that the pendulum is swinging" often evoked the same response as "visualize" and "picture."

When I tried, "Conjure up an image of the pendulum swinging," it only conjured up the idea that some sort of voodoo is supposed to make it swing—not a mental image of it swinging.

I used "concept" for several months: "In your mind create the *concept* that the pendulum is swinging." That seemed to work more consistently than any of the other alternatives, but still didn't quite fit.

Eventually "concept" evolved into, "*Conceive* the pendulum is swinging." "Conceive" worked well for the demonstrations, but was still awkward during the pre-hypnotic talk and when giving hypnotic suggestions. For example, "*conceive* that you behave as a trim person," or "*conceive* yourself as being a non-smoker."

Out of frustration, I again consulted my thesaurus but this time looked up "concept." The synonyms were:

concept: notion, thought, impression, conception, theory, model, perception... PERCEPTION!

When perception appeared, in a flash of realization I thought, "*Perception*" *might just work. Why didn't perception long ago come to mind? Now that I think of it, perception is exactly the right term. It does not imply using one's eyes, nor does it require creating pictures in one's mind and it does not conjure up ideas of voodoo.*

I incorporated "perception" and "perceive" into the session. And the more I used them, the greater was my insight into the power the term implies; i.e., we human beings behave according to how we *perceive* ourselves and how we *perceive* ourselves responding to the things that are going on around us. In short, a person's perception *is their* reality.

To clarify my thinking and to gain a better insight into the inferences that the word "perception" can elicit, I ventured into my inner room and discussed the idea with Socrates.

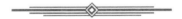

Me: Socrates, it appears that using the term "perception" or "perceive" when giving hypnotic suggestions and explaining the hypnotic process may go far beyond what is immediately apparent. Are our perceptions manifested in ways beyond those that can be overtly observed?

Socrates: In the behavioral sciences, perception encompasses a very broad range of behavioral attributes. You not only perceive with your mind (which is the type of perception associated with the hypnotic process) but you perceive with your five senses. You perceive the roughness of sandpaper with touch. You perceive music with your sense of hearing. You perceive the color red with your eyes. You perceive the tartness of a lemon with your taste buds. And you perceive the aroma of fresh rain with your sense of smell.

As you have recently observed, using the hypnotic process to bring about a change in a client's behavior requires nothing more than altering their perceptions. You change their perceptions by engaging their ability to reason, by using logic, by making demonstrations and by giving suggestions—suggestions being the process of a client perceiving with their mind that the statements you make are true.

In addition, explaining the hypnotic process merely requires demonstrating that perceptions are the key element of the process—as with your pendulum, dictionary-balloon and eye closure demonstrations. When a client perceives with their mind that the pendulum is swinging it swings in the direction they choose to perceive. When a client perceives with their mind a dictionary sitting on the back of an extended arm and balloons pulling up on the other arm, the dictionary arm sinks down and gets tired and the balloon arm floats up and feels light. After suggesting that a client perceive with their mind that their eyelids are stuck closed, when they try to open them they behave as if they are stuck.

Consider this: you rarely *falsely* perceive things with your five senses. Even then your five senses are not completely reliable, as demonstrated with your stage-show experiences—ammonia smells like perfume and lemons taste like oranges.

On the other hand, your mental perceptions are quite different. Reality is often falsely perceived and some of those false perceptions can last a lifetime—prejudices directed toward people of a different race or belief system, for example. And the improper behavior of a few can create the false perception that everyone in the group behaves improperly.

Remember always, that you can *perceive* things *with* your mind based on reality or based on false perceptions, but your brain cannot tell the difference. It, in turn, responds as if the perception is real, and consequently produces a behavior accordingly—whether the perception was founded on reality or not.

Me: That is exactly what I have concluded. In addition to that, what you just said reminds me of a subtle change that I have made in my approach that, without question, has made a significant difference in clients' receptiveness to suggestions and in their responses to my demonstrations. It's when I use "with" instead of "in."

Socrates: Please explain.

Me: I now ask a client to perceive *with* their mind rather than asking them to perceive *in* their mind. For example, "*with* your mind perceive the pendulum is swinging," instead of "*in* your mind perceive the pendulum is swinging." Rather than suggesting, "*in* your mind perceive yourself as a non-smoker," I suggest "*with* your mind perceive yourself as a non-smoker." This slight variation in wording seems to have a significant effect on a subject's aptitude for accepting suggestions. What do you think makes the difference?

Socrates: The difference is that "in" your mind is passive and is centered in one's head. Using "with" conveys the concept that they are using their mind to cause something to happen—it is more dynamic. I think that is the difference.

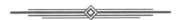

Using "perception" or "perceive" in place of "visualization" or "visualize," or any of the other alternatives, and using "with" your mind instead of "in" your mind, made a significant positive difference in both the effectiveness of a session and the ease with which I conducted the session. Seldom is it necessary to use alternative terms for a client to understand what I mean when asking them to perceive *with* their mind when conducting each of the demonstrations and in eliciting their willingness to accept my suggestions.

The more I thought about it, it became increasingly evident that a better word to describe the hypnotic process would be *perceptionism* rather than *hypnotism*. I still use the terms "hypnosis" and "hypnotism" because people would have no idea what I was talking about if I used *perceptionism* and referred to myself as being a *perceptionist*. It was in one of my inner room discussions with Socrates that the idea arose that the way to popularize *perceptionism* would be for one of us to write a book about it.

As I observed my clients' responses becoming more and more consistent with my use of "perception" and "with," I began wondering about—trying to reason out—what, in fact, is going on between the human mind and brain that causes the hypnotic process to work. How do the mind and brain communicate—what is the connection between the two? What is their language?

CHAPTER 38

The Mind–Brain Connection

The more I practiced and the greater number of clients I worked with the more conducting a session became almost automatic. Not that my focus ever strayed from each client's specific issues, but because much of the session was conducted so routinely I was afforded the benefit of being able to wonder, *What indeed is going on between the client's mind and brain and what is the connection between the two?* as I steered them through the session. I was able to converse with my client, lead them through my pre-hypnotic talk, conduct demonstrations, give suggestions and at the same time wonder what transpires between the client's mind and brain that causes the hypnotic process to work. Even so, all of my analyzing was superficial, so to understand better the deeper implications I once again consulted Socrates.

Me: Socrates, I need help examining a concept that I would like to call the *mind-brain connection*. The question I have is an extension of our last discussion. Simply put, what is the connection between the human mind and brain? What is the process by which they communicate? What is their language? I have notions about what is happening and how they mutually work and communicate, but I need to examine my ideas more closely. I want to weed out any flaws in my thinking.

Socrates: If you are going to talk about a mind-brain connection, it might be advisable to first clearly define what you mean by *mind*, *brain*, and *connection*. For simplicity, let us talk about *your* mind and *your* brain.

Me: Okay, when I think about *my* mind, I mean that part of my being that is conscious and aware—my cognition. My mind is my human ability to intentionally choose what I think about, to be aware of my environment and decide how to respond to it, to exchange ideas with other people and to analyze how the mind and the brain interact. In short, my mind is my conscious awareness.

When I talk about my *brain*, I mean the physical organ housed in my head that controls every function of my physical being. It is evident that if my brain stops working completely, all of my other body processes stop working, as well... including my consciousness.

And the connection is the process by which my mind and brain interact; how they communicate with one another—their language.

Socrates: Your thinking seems clear enough. Simply put, your *mind* is your consciousness and is at the center of your awareness, creativity, inspiration and intuition—because you are *conscious* when engaged in these activities. Your *brain* determines how you physically act and emotionally feel—your physical behavior. Is that right?

Me: That is right.

Socrates: Then it is obvious that your mind and your brain are two different things. Your brain is physical. Your mind is intangible. True?

Me: Yes, Socrates, that is correct. That is how I see it.

Socrates: Because your brain is composed of matter, your brain can be physically observed. If a surgeon opens your skull and takes a peek, in all likelihood, she will see an assemblage of the physical gray matter that is called your brain. However, no matter how hard she looks she will never observe your mind. Do you agree?

Me: Certainly, I agree.

Socrates: Then how do you "know" you have a mind if it cannot be observed?

Me: I know that I have a mind because I am aware—because I can think!

Socrates: If your knowledge of having a mind comes solely from introspection, and that knowledge is the consequence of *you* being aware, then how can you be certain that other people have a mind—if knowledge of a mind comes exclusively from introspection?

Me: That seems simple. I know that other people have a mind because we can share ideas back and forth and I can observe that they move around and accomplish things.

Socrates: I think the basis of your logic stands on shaky ground. Do you not share ideas back and forth with your computer, and does not your printer do some moving, and accomplish things? By your definition, a computer then has a mind. Is my appraisal correct?

Me: No, that is not correct at all—my computer does not "think" on its own—it is not conscious. It does not have the ability to think and, even if it could think, choose on its own what to think about. We say, "my computer is thinking" but it is not consciously thinking. It is just processing ones and zeros. I know there are numerous people who speculate about artificial intelligence, but I am completely convinced that a computer does not "think" in the same way people think. In addition, a computer doesn't accomplish anything unless human thinking is involved (the human that fashioned the computer, the person who created the programming and the human who pushed the print button). On the other hand, people, if *they* choose, can do and think things independent from what they have been "told"... often they do exactly the opposite. Not true with computers. A computer performs a pre-programmed function regardless of what a human being vocally "tells" it to do... or for that matter "tells" it where to go—something I frequently witness as I observe my secretary, Delma, talking to her computer and the printer. Delma is an excellent secretary but she is not on particularly friendly terms with her computer.

Socrates: I agree that a computer does not "think" without human participation. Nonetheless, the question is about the mind, not about thinking. By your definition, you know you have a mind because you experience being conscious. If that is the criterion for you to know there is such a thing as a mind, then how can you "know" that other people have a mind? Can you experience another person's consciousness?

Me: Well, there are a number of "mentalists" and "clairvoyants" who claim to know what other people are thinking.

Socrates: That is speculative at best. Even if there are such mystics who communicate with other minds, it is highly doubtful that they truly experience another person's consciousness. Regardless of the information they claim to convey, it is communicated by way of *their* consciousness. But that doesn't answer my question about your mind. Let me ask it differently: Have *you* ever experienced another person's mind—their consciousness?

Me: I will have to admit that I have not, Socrates. Once in a while I have a notion of what other people are thinking but I can honestly say I have never experienced another person's consciousness.

Socrates: Speculating if we can experience another person's consciousness is an interesting issue to philosophize—and is even important as a hypnotherapist; to understand that *your* mind is not *in* a client's consciousness nor does your mind directly control their mind or consciousness—but I think the question at hand is mind-brain *connection* and how the two communicate. Is that right?

Me: Right.

Socrates: Then we agree that to experience another person's mind is highly unlikely and to define another person's consciousness is tenuous at best. Therefore, you can be certain only of your own mind; you can only *assume* that other people have a mind and experience consciousness and that they are just as aware as you are.

Me: Okay, under the *assumption* that other people are as conscious and aware as I am, and they have a mind just as I do, then my question is still, what is the connection between the human mind and brain?

Socrates: For your mind-brain theory to work, two criteria must be met: First, you must be conscious. Second, your brain must be functional. Do you agree?

Me: Yes, I agree.

Socrates: Then the answer to your question is something you already know. The connection between your mind and brain, the language by which they communicate, is perception! The only way your body knows how to cause you to respond to your environment, and how to feel emotionally, is based on your perceptions. Does that seem to fit?

Me: Yes, that fits perfectly. For example, by choosing to perceive with my *mind* that the pendulum is swinging in the direction C-D, my mental perception is perceived by my physical *brain* and my brain "tells" the muscles in my arm to move, and automatically the pendulum swings in the direction C to D. Therefore, the sequence is mind-perception-brain. The connection is *perception*.

Socrates: That is correct. Your mind, by way of perception, instructs your brain and your brain produces the behavior in accordance with your perceptions. The connection is an intertwined mutual relationship between mind and brain that is geared for governing human behavior. Does that confirm your connection question?

Me: Yes, it does.

Socrates: You must also recognize that the connection works in reverse: brain-perception-mind. When you smack your finger with a hammer, your brain perceives signals from your crushed finger and your conscious awareness perceives it as pain. Do you also agree with this analogy?

Me: Yes, I do. In addition, I would like to know to what extent my perceptions control other physical processes—for example, on a cellular basis. I know that my arm moves to make the pendulum swing, but what happens at the cellular level—the cells that make up the muscles in my arm? How does my brain know which cells of my arm to collectively manipulate that in turn make my arm move in the right direction—depending on the direction I choose to perceive? Furthermore, to what extent do my perceptions interact with my neural pathways and influence my behavior biologically? To what degree do my perceptions dictate my state of physical and emotional well-being?

Socrates: Those questions are related to an entirely different discussion. But for now I think that we can agree that the connection between mind and brain is based on perceptions. For *me* to answer those other questions *you* will need to acquire additional education about the functioning of your nervous system, your brain and your mind and discover if, indeed, perceptions influence the cells that make up your biological body.

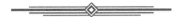

So I placed on hold my inquiry about the hypnotic process, more accurately put, I suppose, the *perception process*, and engaged my investigation in university level courses dealing with the functioning of the brain, the mind and consciousness.

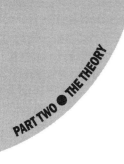

CHAPTER 39

One Mind

While delving into the influence perceptions have on our biology (cellular and neurological pathways), and how our perceptions link up with the working of our brain through scientific investigation, it became obvious that, although *consciousness* was scrutinized in each course of study, the *mind* was mentioned only in passing. However, when investigating *consciousness* philosophically the *mind* was central to the inquiry about human behavior.

In addition, many other disciplines (metaphysics, motivational speakers, success-oriented books and their practitioners) not only recognize the "powers" of the human *mind* but argue that we have a second unconscious, or subconscious, "mind" that operates, for the most part, independent of our *conscious* mind—my subconscious mind (or was it the devil) that made me do it. The more I thought about it the more I began to question the concept of a subconscious *mind*. So I engaged Socrates in a dialog concerning the issue.

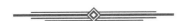

Me: Socrates, I'm struggling with an issue that clearly goes against the grain of conventional thinking of not only my colleagues; it's an idea that is also embraced by much of the general public. Nevertheless, if my thinking holds true it would certainly simplify explaining the hypnotic process and make analyzing human behavior less numinous.

Socrates: What do you mean by numinous?

Me: By numinous, I mean the mystical, supernatural and unknowable.

Socrates: Okay, go on.

Me: I'm struggling with whether there really is a subconscious or unconscious *mind*.

It is a concept that few people would ever challenge since it is so universally accepted and fundamental to the thinking of most people. In everyday conversation, people dismissively use the concept to explain their own behavior, revered motivators employ it as being the key to successful achievement, and even my hypnotherapy colleagues routinely rely on it to explain the hypnotic process. In fact, I became engaged in a spirited discussion on this very topic with my colleague and friend, Barney Howell, a highly respected hypnotherapist and director of the B. F. Howell Institute (an Arizona state-certified school for teaching hypnotherapists), and I'm quite sure he went away thinking I had lost my faculty for reasoning. In metaphysical circles the notion is fundamental to their philosophy, however, most behavioral scientists evade the idea altogether. As hard as I try to evade it, however, it will not go away. And yet, I'm finding it very hard to let go of my own preconceived notions in order to rationally consider a different way of thinking.

Socrates: So what is troubling you about the unconscious or subconscious mind?

Me: To start with, there is a minor point that I need clarified. When people make reference to a *subconscious* mind or an *unconscious* mind are they talking about the same thing? Are the terms synonymous?

Socrates: It depends on the period of history and the discipline. In the realm of experimental psychology, as you observed earlier, even the notion of a *mind*, let alone a subconscious one, is a sticky point. Nevertheless, I believe you could safely say that those who speak of an unconscious mind or a subconscious mind are referring to one and the same entity.

Me: To this point in my career, I have freely used the idea that we use our subconscious mind as a means to change behavior and to explain the hypnotic process. The problem I am having is that the concept of a subconscious *mind* implies that it is a separate entity that exists below the level of our conscious awareness—a thinking intelligence that operates on its own, and largely determines our behavior. But the more I think about it, the more it appears that we have only one mind—our conscious mind. I am thinking that there is no such thing as a subconscious "mind." How would we ever objectively confirm that we have a second mind (an un-conscious *mind*)—if it is unconscious?! It is difficult enough to get a firm handle on the quintessence of the mind, itself, let alone an unconscious one. In addition, the concept of the subconscious mind clutters up the use of, and explanation of, the hypnotic process (perceptionism).

Socrates: In order to have a discussion about whether there is or is not an unconscious or subconscious mind it may serve you to again explain what you mean by *mind*.

Me: I still define the human *mind* as being our *conscious awareness*. Our mind is a stream of consciousness that we experience as we move through time and that leaves a trail of memory that defines who we are—an autobiography of memories that are stored in our brain. Our mind is composed of our thoughts, perceptions, concepts, memories and mental images that continually flow in and out of our awareness at each moment we are conscious (remember that we are conscious while dreaming). Our mind is our aptitude to think, intentionally recall information that has been stored in our brain, imagine and choose what to think about. Simply put, our mind is our conscious awareness, and because we are conscious we humans have the unique ability to not only be aware, but to be consciously *aware* that we are *aware*... and able to analyze rationally our awareness, if we choose to. This ability sets us human beings clearly apart from the rest of the animal kingdom.[7]

Socrates: Okay, that definition gives us a foundation from which to operate, but what started you questioning whether there is or is not a subconscious or unconscious mind in the first place?

Me: It was triggered by Descartes.

Socrates: Do you mean René Descartes, who lived in the seventeenth century, who is known as being the father of modern mathematics and modern philosophy... of course you do, what other Descartes has made their mark in history! So what does Descartes have to say that causes you to question the subconscious mind?

Me: It's *dubito, ergo cogito, sum*—you know, *I doubt therefore I think therefore I am.* Quite often the "dubito" (I doubt) is left off his maxim but *I* think it is the best part—to doubt everything until all possible avenues of investigation have been exhausted and there is no possible way to *not* accept an idea, concept, theory or statement.

As you know, Descartes started out by questioning that he existed at all. He reasoned, *Maybe some "Great Deceiver" is tricking me into believing that I exist when I really do not exist.* His conclusion was, *How could I not exist since I am able to doubt (think) that I exist?* But it wasn't the doubting that triggered *my* doubting about a subconscious mind; it was the "thinking."

Socrates: Explain how *thinking* relates to there being no such thing as a subconscious mind.

---

7. All of the other members of the animal kingdom most certainly have some level of awareness, but I suspect few of them contemplate their awareness. Moreover, few instinctually recognize the concept of "self" as we humans do. There is experimental evidence that, with human involvement, some have the ability to grasp the concept of "self." An elephant looking in a mirror can use its trunk to point at a spot on its forehead, so it would seem that at some level it recognizes its forehead (self) that bears the spot, for example. However, in their natural habitat the concept probably never arises. Even if the lower animals do posses the wherewithal to grasp the concept of "self," it is highly unlikely that they spend much time pondering it. For that matter, I doubt that many human beings spend much time contemplating "self" or wondering what gives them their individual awareness.

Me: When pondering the question, *do I have a subconscious mind?* I must be thinking, and since I am thinking, *I* must exist. This leads to the supposition that my *mind* must exist, too—i.e., my conscious awareness, my ability to think. So my question is, what gives me the ability to consciously posit the questions, *do I exist? And, do I have a mind?* I must be conscious in order to ask the questions. This leads to the crux of my problem. If I am unconscious then how could I ever pose the questions? How can an unconscious *mind* ask the question and come up with the answer if it is subconscious—below the level of conscious awareness? I need to be conscious to come up with the question and I need to be conscious to comprehend the answer.

Many people contend that such questions and answers are generated by an unconscious mind, which then sends them to our consciousness in the finished form. My argument is, if I were unconscious not only would I not pose the question, but I couldn't. The point is that the only time I can ask questions and get answers is when I am conscious. So what would be the need of an unconscious *mind?*

If my mind is *not* my consciousness, then what is it? This line of reason leads to, how can I have an *unconscious consciousness*—an unconscious *mind?* My conclusion is that we don't need a subconscious mind nor do we have one.

Socrates: I know that the mystics and spiritually minded would argue that your subconscious mind is your soul or spirit. So this provokes the questions, is your soul or spirit unconscious? Or is your soul or spirit your consciousness? If it is your consciousness, then does your soul or spirit need a subconscious soul or spirit to properly function? But that is a topic for a different book.

Reason with me and answer these questions. It is apparent that you use your mind to think and that you must be conscious in order to think and to ask questions and understand answers. Do you agree?

Me: Yes, I agree. I don't remember ever asking a question or getting an answer while unconscious.

Socrates: Then why would you need an unconscious mind? Talking about an unconscious or subconscious "mind" mystifies and complicates the hypnotic process and explaining human behavior.

Me: That is exactly what I have been thinking. If we substitute the idea of a subconscious *mind* with *unconscious processes of the brain* (not a *mind*), it certainly simplifies explaining the hypnotic process and human behavior. For example, if we really want to complicate explaining human behavior then let's talk about an unconscious superego, ego and id, as in psychoanalysis; or a parent, adult, and a child, as in transactional analysis (I'm OK—You're OK). We do not need a subconscious "something" that thinks on its own. All we need is one mind (our consciousness) and one brain that responds to perceptions and that becomes conditioned to respond to a given stimulus.

Socrates: That seems simple enough.

Me: There is another issue that often comes up when I talk about there being no such thing as a subconscious mind. Can you give me an idea how to quickly refute this argument? Many people claim that they are conscious at all times since even in a deep dreamless sleep there is still brain wave activity going on, and therefore they must be conscious.

Socrates: To quickly refute that argument when it comes up again, simply ask the person what they were conscious of while they were unconscious. Just because there is brain wave activity going on why in the world would that mean that a mind is causing it?

Me: Okay, I'll do that.

Socrates: It is your consciousnesses that gives you your identity—know thy self. When you are unconscious, how would you "know" who you are? If your conscious mind gives you your identity (who you are) then when you are unconscious your self-identity does not exist. Your brain is still putting out brainwaves while it keeps everything working to sustain life, but your mind, your conscious awareness, is absent. Consciousness is everything to us humans. Unconsciousness is nothingness.

Me: Yeah, I can just hear Dr. Preston proclaiming that even when people are under general anesthesia, they still hear what the doctors are saying. "The patient is able to recall the jokes the physicians told while they were 'under' general anesthesia," he would say. The argument is that since the patient is unconscious then their unconscious mind must have heard the joke.

Socrates: Even if a patient recalls such a thing, it still does not answer the question—is there or is there not an unconscious or subconscious mind? There is scientific confirmation that while under general anesthesia there is activity going on in the auditory system as it responds to sound, but that does not mean there is an unconscious mind hearing it. The stimulus of the sound is sent to and gets stored in the cerebral cortex (not in a mind), and with the proper stimulus (the sight of the doctor or a question asked by a hypnotherapist), the patient can access that part of the brain where the memory was stored. But that happens as an every-day occurrence; i.e., someone makes a comment or you smell an aroma and it triggers memories associated with the stimulus. During brain surgery when certain areas of the cortex are stimulated with a mild electrical impulse the patient reports memories of long-past events. It is a brain that is stimulated not a subconscious mind. But it is necessary for the patient to be conscious in order to recall it.

It is like the age-old question, when a tree falls in a forest and there is no creature to hear it, does it make a sound? The answer is NO! Sure, the vibrations of air molecules still occur but "sound" is a construct of a brain's auditory system being activated by the motion of air molecules and therefore is interpreted as sound—but there must be an awareness of the stimulus for it to be comprehended as sound.

Me: That answers the question about not needing a subconscious *mind* in order to recall information from our brain, but then how do I explain to others that there is no need for a subconscious mind to power unconscious events? Many of my colleagues contend that behaviors, like keeping our heart beating, stepping on the brake pedal when the light turns red and waking up in the morning with a flash of inspiration, are a function of the subconscious mind. If there is no subconscious *mind* doing it, then what is?

Socrates: By your own definitions, *mind* requires consciousness. Why do you suppose that you need a mind to keep your heart beating, to step on the brake when the light turns red (hopefully yellow) and to wake up with a flash of inspiration? Why is it necessary to have a subconscious *mind* for those things to happen?

Me: I don't know, it is just the way people (and me, too, up until now) explain it.

Socrates: Consider this. Once your brain and nervous system become conditioned to respond to a given stimulus through repetitious exposure, the response becomes automatic, and no mind is needed—i.e., classical conditioning. In the beginning when you first learned to drive, you consciously thought about stepping on the brake pedal when the light turned yellow—you used your mind (consciousness) to understand that yellow means step on the brake pedal and you consciously took the action of doing it.

After sufficient exposures, the response became spontaneous. Once the response to the stimulus has created a neuronal pathway in your brain and your nervous system, the response is automatic—no *mind* necessary. The stimulus of the light turning yellow bypasses your conscious awareness (mind) and sends the message directly to your brain and your brain in turn automatically produces the appropriate response—you step on the brake pedal. There is no need to have a subconscious essence (a mind) to mediate the process, or to figure out what a yellow light becoming illuminated means.

Your beating heart is another function that has no need for the mind; in fact, in the short-term it does not even need your brain! For example, when a heart is removed from a transplant donor, it stops beating. When the heart is placed in the recipient, all it needs is an electrical stimulus to start it beating again. You need neither a *mind*, conscious or unconscious, nor a brain for your heart to beat. However, to *keep* it beating requires a brain (or a pacemaker)—but still not a mind.

In the case of the flash of inspiration, whether upon waking up or while engaged in a routine task, the creation of a new idea is generated by unrelated unconscious memories getting "mixed up" with each other and a new idea flashes into your conscious awareness. (Remember that memory is *stored* in the brain, not in a mind.) And it is necessary to be conscious in order to conceptualize the new idea. There is no need for third party involvement (a subconscious mind).

Does any of this make sense?

Me: Yes, I understand and agree with your arguments.

Socrates: I want you to understand clearly that I am not suggesting that there are *no* processes going on in your brain below the level of your conscious awareness. What I am saying is that those processes are *not* happening because of a second "subconscious" *mind*. They happen as the result of brain functions, and the hypnotic process provides a way to use a client's *conscious awareness* to interact with their *brain*. When working with a client you are *not* communicating with a subconscious mind, you are communicating with their conscious awareness, which in turn interacts with their brain. When giving suggestions you use words to create in the client's conscious awareness perceptions that are sent to their brain and their brain responds to the perception—no need for an intermediary mind.

So instead of talking about a *subconscious mind* being involved, talk about the communication that goes on between your client's conscious awareness and their brain. By doing so, it clearly simplifies explaining the hypnotic process and human behavior in general.

During your pre-hypnotic talk, you demonstrate how perceptions drive the hypnotic process. That is to say, the communication between mind and brain are the perceptions that are sent back and forth between the two entities. Perceptions that are received by your brain automatically trigger a response, depending on the nature of the perception.

Is my understanding of what you have been thinking correct?

Me: That is correct. That is how I see it.

Socrates: In addition, your brain sends to your conscious awareness information that has been stored in it in the form of past perceptions. Memory is a process of retrieving perceptions that have been stored in your brain and, at times, sending a flash of inspiration to your conscious awareness as normally unrelated perceptions get intertwined with each other. It would appear that those flashes of inspiration are the consequence of those stored memories interrelating with one another as the brain goes through its normal processing function. It is not an unconscious *mind* that is doing the processing; it is a process of the brain.

Once again, think of it this way. By divorcing from the equation the idea that human behavior is powered by a subconscious mind, and replacing it with the idea that behavior is a function of the *brain* that responds to perceptions, you simplify the explanation of the hypnotic process. Simply put—one mind and one brain that interact and communicate by means of perceptions.

Me: I agree. From my studies on the brain and consciousness, two things are evident. First, behavior is the product of the interaction of billions of neurons and trillions of synapses in our brain and this interaction constitutes the root of every aspect of our behavior; and second, perceptions are the means of communicating. In addition, I learned that the term *perception* not only refers to mental perceptions but also is a term by which neurologists describe the process that individual living cells use to "know" how to behave.

As I consider the process that goes on between our mind and brain it is evident that the communication happens only in the present—in this instant of NOW.

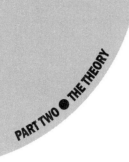

PART TWO ● THE THEORY

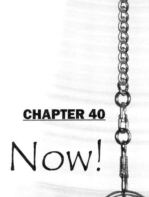

CHAPTER 40

Now!

Over the past few decades, the concept of "NOW" has become an essential part of my approach in helping people attain the behavior or state of being for which they made an appointment. It all started in the late 80s with Mark.

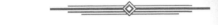

"Mark," I asked, "why do you want to stop drinking?"

"It's messing up my life, probably shortening it and holds the likelihood of my landing up in jail," he replied.

Mark was a highly successful public personality whose name would be recognized by many.

I asked, "How often do you drink, and what do you drink when you drink?"

He responded, "I started drinking back when I was 16 years old."

I interrupted him, "I didn't ask why or when you *started* drinking, I asked how often you drink and what you drink when you drink... if you want to expand on why you want to *stop* drinking it would be helpful, but why you started drinking is unimportant."

Taken a little aback he answered, "Until I was divorced six years ago, I drank only occasionally when I was out with my college drinking buddies, but now, since she left me, I go through more than a six-pack of beer every evening. I don't drink during the day and I never drink when I am around my family—parents, ex-wife, siblings or children. I can go on a two-week vacation with my family and not drink at all... I don't even think about having a beer. I live alone now and I doubt my family even knows I drink—even when I was married I covered it up pretty well... I thought."

I queried further, "What motivated you to give up drinking now? And why did you think of 'hypnosis' as a way to accomplish it?"

He answered, "Well, there are several reasons that I want to stop drinking but only one that made me think of hypnosis as a way of doing it.

"Using hypnosis as a way to stop drinking never entered my mind until I happened upon one of my old drinking pals that I hadn't seen for several years. I suggested that we swing by the pub and have a cold one or two, and he refused. 'I am a non-drinker now,' he told me. 'You've got to be kidding,' I responded. 'You were probably the best drinker in the crowd! How did you do it and what made you stop?'

"My friend went on to tell me that after he got a couple of DUI's, spent some time in jail, and his wife told him that she didn't want any of their kids to become a drunk like their dad, he thought he'd better stop. He said that he joined AA but didn't have much success, but then he went to this crazy hypnotist guy in Tempe, Arizona and hadn't had a drink since.

"He gave me your calling card and I've been packing it around in my wallet for the past nine months, but yesterday I got a real shocker: Johnny, another one of my old drinking buddies, died of liver disease. He was my age, only 46 years old. I visited him at the hospital the day before yesterday and he said the doctors told him it was his drinking that did it. And the next day (yesterday), he was dead. I called you right after I heard.

"Another biggie for wanting to stop drinking is that occasionally I'm out on the road after having several drinks. I've never had a DUI but it scares me to death to think of the consequences if I were to run a red light or miss a stop sign and kill or maim someone... or myself. In addition, if I were to get a DUI it would destroy my life. My credibility would be compromised, my standing with my associates would be shattered and my relationship with my family would be ruined. I've done a good job of covering it up with my family, but I don't want my boys to think that it's okay to drink... oh yeah, and I don't want to die young like Johnny did."

I responded, "I am sorry for the loss of your friend. It is understandable that something like that would shake someone out of their apathy and prompt them to take action."

He said, "You're right. Not only that, when I've had a few beers I lose my motivation to get things done. When I drink, or even think about drinking, I feel guilt, self-condemnation and I'm ticked-off at myself because something (beer) is controlling my behavior.... I *know* that my life would be so much simpler and more rewarding and meaningful if I didn't drink, but knowing this doesn't seem to make it any easier."

I said, "Let me ask you this. Except when vacationing with your family, how long have you gone without drinking?"

Mark said, "Oh, in the past several years I've made it for a month a couple of times but I fall off the wagon and I feel even worse about myself. Over the years, from time to time, I've gone to AA meetings and I have their twelve-step program down pat, but living up to my commitments is something else.

Besides that, to stand up before a group of people and tell them that I *am* an alcoholic doesn't make sense. Being an alcoholic is what I *don't* want to be. They also preach that all I need to do is to just take it one day at a time, but sometimes that "one day" seems like a very, very long day. That's my problem. At the end of the day is when I usually cave in—one full day seems so long.

"When I visited with Johnny in the hospital he asked me what *I* would do if I knew I had only one day left to live. He might have had a premonition it was *his* last one. At that moment, I was so insensitive and out of tune with what he must have been experiencing that I just blew it off by telling him that he was still a young man and would probably outlive me.

"However, since he passed away, it seems that's all I can think about. I have been thinking... *If I had only one day left on this earth, how much of it would I want to spend being drunk?* My predicament is that thinking about dying just makes me feel depressed and makes me want to drink even more, especially when I think that I have to go for a whole day without a drink.

"Last night it was as though I needed to celebrate since apparently this wasn't my last day. Maybe tomorrow will be my last one but today isn't. I'm not supposed to think about tomorrow, according to AA philosophy... besides, I thought, *I'm going to the hypnotist tomorrow and I'll stop drinking then.* So I jumped in my car, drove down to the convenience store and picked up *one* 6-pack. I usually buy two 6-packs—never a 12-pack—because I rationalize that this way, I'll drink just one pack tonight and have nice cold one in the fridge when I get home tomorrow night. But it seldom works out that way. Most of the time the next morning all twelve are empty."

Something that Mark said earlier created an incisive spark of enlightenment, so I said, "Give me some feedback about one day being too long. How about if you took not drinking a 'half-a-day at a time'—would it seem easier?"

"I haven't thought of it in those terms," he said, "but maybe it *would* be easier if I thought of not drinking a half-a-day at a time."

"Then would taking it an 'hour at a time' make it seem even easier?"

After thinking about it for a moment Mark said, "I think you are playing with my mind, but if I thought that I only had to go for one hour without drinking, not drinking would seem even easier—I don't *know* for sure that it would be, but right now I think it would *seem* easier."

I said, "Well, you are right. I *am* playing with your mind. I think that is the reason you made an appointment to see me—to juggle things around in your mind so it seems easier to *not drink* than it is to drink... and as a result, feel good and good about yourself for having stopped drinking for good. Is that right?"

Mark said with a hint of reservation, "That is right but I thought I'd need to be hypnotized before you started fiddling around with my mind."

I chuckled and said, "Then let's talk about this process that is *called* hypnosis...."

After going through my pre-hypnotic talk and conducting my three demonstrations (pendulum, dictionary-balloon and eye closure), I returned to the topic of reducing "being a non-drinker" to an even shorter period of time.

I said, "Earlier you agreed that being a non-drinker would be easier if you took it an hour at a time rather than a day at a time. Do you still agree with that idea?"

"Based on what you have demonstrate about my brain responding to what I perceive, yes, I really believe that thinking all I need to do is be a non-drinker for an hour at a time would make it much easier."

I asked, "How about five minutes at a time? Would that be even easier?"

He agreed, "Yes."

"How about a minute at a time? If you thought about being a non-drinker for only this minute—taking it only a minute at a time—would it seem even easier?"

He again considered my logic and said, "If I thought all I needed to do was to not drink during this minute, it would be even easier," he agreed. "But then what happens when this minute is over... doesn't a different minute start?"

"You are right, it does, however I thought you were going to take it *this* minute at a time—not a sequence of minutes. When this minute is past, then the next minute becomes *this* minute. Does that make sense?"

"I guess it does. So what you are saying is that when I am on my way back to my apartment from work, and I drive by the convenience store and I keep in mind the idea that at this minute I don't drink and this minute I behave as one who doesn't, I'll drive right by and *not* pull in and pick up a couple of six-packs? Or if I am sitting around on Sunday afternoon watching the Arizona Cardinals lose again, and the Budweiser commercial comes on, I won't run over at half-time and pick up some beer to help me deal with my frustrations?"

I said, "Yes, as you put it, if you for this minute *behave* as one who doesn't drink, which includes not buying beer, then obviously you are a non-drinker. What do *you* think? If you take it a minute at a time, regardless of what is going on, who you are with, what you are doing, or what the score is, wouldn't it be much easer to not drink?"

"I think you might be right—if I take it a minute at a time."

So during the session I gave suggestions to Mark that centered on being a non-drinker "a minute at a time," and that in *each* minute he would be aware of enjoying the end-result benefits of being a non-drinker. *"You perceive yourself in this "minute" as experiencing and enjoying high self-esteem, having and maintaining good health, driving safely and possessing peace of mind when out on the road (no longer concerned if a police officer is tailing you). In this minute you are grateful that you are serving as a role model for your boys. You enjoy the experience of being healthy and engaged in a lifestyle that leads to living a long, peaceful and healthy life... all as the result of being a non-drinker in this minute!"*

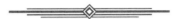

A year later (on the anniversary of his being a non-drinker), Mark called to tell me that he hadn't had a drink since he left my office. However he confessed, "There were a few times that I almost caved in, but when I remembered that all I needed to do was just take it "this minute at a time," all of the feelings and thoughts about drinking evaporated."

I remembered Mark immediately, not only because of his public name recognition but because in almost every session since he was in my office the year before, I had used the concept that he inspired. And I've continued to use it in almost every session since.

I congratulated Mark for his achievement but went on to explain, "You were the catalyst that triggered the development of a powerful concept that has made a considerable difference in helping my clients to achieve the behavioral change for which they came to see me. By incorporating into each session the idea that you inspired, not only has the change been easier, but it has significantly enhanced the likelihood of their desired change being permanent." I added, "Maybe one minute at a time is still too long. Why not take it a single 'now' at a time!"

After Mark had left my office a year earlier, I ventured into my inner room for a discussion with Socrates to think through the idea that popped into my mind during the discussion about Mark being a non-drinker a minute at a time.

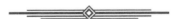

Me: Socrates, when working with Mark, why did I stop at "a minute at a time?" Why not take it "a second at a time" or a "half a second at a time?" How short a time could I have reduced the interval to and still had it make sense? Or is it like the principle that if you move half of the distance to the wall, and then once again move halfway to the wall and keep on moving halfway to the wall you will never reach the wall; if you just keep on moving only half the distance with each move, you will get very close but never actually get there?

Socrates: Not at all! At least if you consider it from a physics and quantum mechanics point of view. The *quantum* part of quantum mechanics means that matter, space and energy exist in discrete tiny *quantities*. A quantum leap, for example, means that the energy state of an atom does not "slide" up and down the energy scale but rather "leaps" from one state of energy to another state. This leads to the fact that there is no energy state between each leap.

Length also comes in a discrete distance. In physics, the shortest measurable distance in space is called Planck length (10^{-33} centimeters). Between each distance, there is no space. Therefore, when you move one-half of the way to the wall on the last leap you *reach* the wall. At 10^{-33} centimeters you have arrived, since there is no distance beyond.

There is also Planck *time*, which measures each tick of time at 10^{-43} seconds. Between each tick of time there is no time! So "now" happens with each tick. To put "now" into perspective, there are more ticks of "now" in one second than there have been seconds since the formation of the solar system—4.5 million years.

Me: That is an extremely short period... so short, in fact, that this "now" is gone.

Socrates: So why not have your clients take it a "quantum tick" or each "now" at a time?

Me: That is a great idea. I could have suggested to Mark that he need be a non-drinker only "a now" at a time, and being a non-drinker would be been even easier.

Socrates: If you will closely think about it, behavior, thoughts, events, and actions exist only in this instant of now. It is only with your mind that you perceive of things existing outside of now—memory and speculation of future events. The events that led to writing this book do not exist in this instant of now. The writing of this book exists only in the now that it takes to think of what to say and the instant that it takes to push a computer key—the now in which you typed each previous letter of each word does not exist, the letters exist but the act of typing it doesn't. In addition, tasks that you *will* accomplish in the future do not exist in this tick of time—they exist only in your imagination. You are stuck in the instant of each now!

I know that there is endless speculation about time *being* or *not being* linear. On the other hand, it has been confirmed that the passage of time varies with respect to high speed and the intensity of gravity. It's fun to debate and to contemplate these issues but in your everyday life (which is the modality you deal with in your profession) things do not happen in the future nor do they happen in the past. And time, with respect to the velocity and the gravity of the earth's pull, ticks on—one tick after another—at a predictable constant rate! At this moment in history, there has been no concrete physical demonstration that time is *not* linear—only mathematical functions that support other notions and are of no practical use in your day-to-day life. Even if time is something other than linear, we have not learned how to change past or future events in the present—in this now.

The bottom line is, if we take care of this instant of now (for example, not drinking in this tick of now), somehow "now" turns out to be forever! But your clients don't have to be concerned about forever, because they can't get out of *now*, and from now on just happens!

Me: It appears to be paradoxical. This tick of now is very, very short, but it seems that it is always now, yet it turns out to be forever....

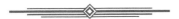

I have found that by incorporating the concept of "now" into my pre-hypnotic talk and suggestion part of a session, it has had a profound positive effect on the psyche of my clients. I ask, "In which 'now' had you planned to be a non-drinker? If you are going to be a non-drinker, you must do it in *this* now."

Or asking a person who has a fear of flying, "In which 'now' had you planned to be at ease about flying? In this 'now' as we sit here in my office, you are perfectly safe. In each 'now' when you are on the way to the airport, you are safe (as safe as you can be when out on the roads). In each 'now' as you board the airplane, you are safe. In each tick of 'now,' as you are quickly traveling to your destination, you are safe. The time to experience fear and anxieties about being killed in a plane crash is when the captain's voice comes over the intercom and says, 'We've lost all of our engines and we are going down'—that is the 'now' to feel panic and fear! But don't mess up a gazillion other 'nows' by worrying about an event that isn't happening and is less likely to happen than being in a car crash on your way to and from the airport."

It appears to me that one of the biggest problems many people have relative to being peaceful and having peace of mind is that they are "living" outside of "now" with their mind. Since our brain and nervous system cannot distinguish the difference between what is real and what is *perceived* to be real, when we are re-living tragic past events or imagining tragic future events, our brain causes us to feel emotionally as though the perception *is* reality—in the present.

The key word is "perception." This leads us to the final chapter of my book. There are a few appendices that follow if the reader is interested, but the story ends with chapter 41.

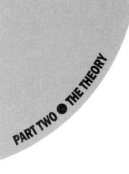

CHAPTER 41

Perception
Revisited

Why do many people harbor prejudices and hatred towards other people, yet others show friendship and acceptance of people who are physically and culturally different and hold dissimilar beliefs from their own?

Why do some people have peace of mind while others, aware that peace of mind is more favorable, seldom experience it?

Why are there so many different forms of government and political persuasions, yet most people are convinced theirs is the best?

Why do we applaud the new guy on the home team, when last season he was on an opposing team and we jeered him? Why do some people hate Chevrolets and love Fords, and vice versa, knowing that either satisfactorily fills their intended function—transporting people and goods?

Why do some people have a fear of bugs, mice, crickets or nonpoisonous snakes, even though they know they are not harmful, while others play with them, have them for pets and enjoy examining their behavior?

Why are there gangs that treat members of rival gangs brutally, knowing that it will only return retaliation and harm, while other people are willing to put their lives on the line to interact with both sides in an attempt to reduce violence?

Why are there so many religions and belief systems, and so many factions within each, although each was founded for the same reason—to bring to its believers purpose for this life and hope for a favorable requital when they move on—yet each one subscribes to different sets of theological philosophies, rituals, ordinances, ceremonies, rules, standards and principles?

Why are there people willing to follow unethical leaders even in the face of dire consequences, and others willing to follow leadership that engages them in noble causes that may result in even more dire *personal* consequences?

Why do we tend to believe in, cling to and enjoy traditions, rituals, ceremonies and customs (the tooth fairy, the Easter bunny, Santa Claus and Groundhog Day) knowing all the while that that is all they are—traditions, rituals, ceremonies and customs?

Why are some people successful and others not, yet each possesses the same opportunities and level of education?

Why do some of us, knowing that a behavior is self-destructive, continue to engage in it while others seemingly with no effort, engage in healthy and uplifting behavior?

The answer to these questions, and a never-ending array of others, boils down to one fundamental principle— what we believe to be good, bad, right, wrong, true, false, valid or real is determined by how it is perceived!

As I trekked along my adventure of using hypnotherapy to help people change how they act and feel, it became increasingly evident that our behavior is largely dependent on our perceptions—how we perceive ourselves and how we perceive the world around us. Our self-perceptions (how we perceive ourselves engaging other people and events that take place from moment to moment in our daily life) determine who we are, how we behave and what we believe.

I am convinced that regardless of the approach (hypnotherapy, psychotherapy, counseling, messages preached from the pulpit, coaching or friends talking to friends), the way to effect a change in a client's, parishioner's or friend's behavior is to simply instigate a change in their perceptions. And this is why I no longer think of the hypnotic process as being hypnotism but rather "perceptionism!"

I define *therapeutic perceptionism* as being *any* approach that successfully facilitates a change in a client's perceptions that leads to the behavioral change the client is seeking. There is also entertainment perceptionism—an approach that causes a stage-show volunteer to perceive himself or herself behaving in a way the stage-show hypnotist chooses for them. The *process* is the same. In one case (therapeutic), the client chooses the behavior, while in the other case, someone else (the hypnotist—or perceptionist, if that ever becomes an everyday term) chooses the behavior.

It is relatively easy to measure the overt behavior and emotional results of perceptionism by observation and introspective feedback from clients (smoking cessation, weight loss, freedom from stress, removal of phobias and inhibitions, etc.). The hard part is grasping the neurological process that causes a perception to be converted to physical and emotional behavior and to determine the extent our perceptions play in our biology. For years I wondered, *Could our perceptions interact with our neurological network and accomplish things like maintaining good health, accelerating healing, slowing down the aging processes, maintaining clarity of mind into old age and hastening postoperative recovery, as well as changing counterproductive attitudes and intolerance?*

My suspicion was yes. But I had neither the means nor the inclination to launch a full-scale investigation on my own. So at Socrates' advice, I immersed myself in numerous university level courses and programs of study relating to neurology, genetics, human anatomy, functions of the brain, theories of consciousness and human behavior. It turns out that the term "perception" is fundamental to understanding and explaining the underlying principles of these disciplines and that, indeed, our mental perceptions do impact not only our day-to-day actions and emotions but our biology as well.

It had been over thirty years since I was engaged in structured courses of study, so some of what I previously learned had become obsolete, especially in the area of brain functions, neural science and genetics. With the advent of brain imaging equipment (fMRI [f = functional] and CAT scan) and countless well-controlled studies, brain researchers and neuroscientists have a reasonably clear understanding of which areas of the brain are primarily used when a person is engaged in a given physical or mental activity. In addition, in the past few decades, the electrical and chemical processes by which neurons interact have been refined and, of course, understanding the workings of genetics has expanded exponentially.

Of the copious points of view presented by various researchers and professors, I have selected a few that lend credence to my theory of "perceptionism." In a very broad use of the term, perception is central to explaining human behavior, the driving mechanism behind the hypnotic process (perceptionism) and the key to helping people live healthier, peaceful, prosperous, happy, fulfilling and purposeful long lives.

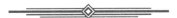

I learned that the term "perception" not only applies to visual and mental perceptions (the mental processes that interface the mind and the brain) but is an idiom used to explain how living cells communicate with other cells and how an individual cell "knows" how to react to its environment. Human brain cells kept alive in a lab Petri dish can *perceive* the difference between a nutrient and toxins, for example—they move towards nutrients and away from toxins.

I learned that "areas" of the human brain, although each has its own primary function, interact with each other (left and right brain interaction, for example) as we engage in a given mental or physical activity. We have up to 100 billion neurons (brain cells) and 100 trillion synapses (brain cell connections) in our head that are waiting to act when they *perceive* they are needed. I also learned that throughout our life we *do not* grow new neurons in our cerebral cortex when we learn, as was once thought.

I learned that learning and memory occur at the synapse. We do continue to create new synapses and neurological pathways for cognitive learning and acquiring new physical skills, but most often we use existing neurons and create new pathways when we learn a new behavior or comprehend a new concept.

I learned that behavior is caused by the communication that goes on between, and within, each cell of our body via a vast network of neurons, synapses, their various sensory capabilities and a combination of a variety of chemicals that are in and around them.

I learned that the composition of body chemistry plays an essential role in maintaining good health, in how we feel emotionally and perform physically. Our body chemistry significantly influences how well we learn, recall and deal with our physical world.

I learned that physical addictions (the result of ingesting chemicals) and psychological addictions (the result of engaging in respective physical and mental activities) involve the same brain mechanisms—endogenous reward system. fMRI's show that the same areas of the brain "light up" in both types of "addictions."

I learned that a sequence of neuronal events occurs when our brain *perceives* stimuli from various organs throughout our body, our five senses and our mental perceptions. Once our brain perceives a given stimulus it triggers a sequence of neuronal events that result in a physical, mental or emotional experience.

Neurons communicate with each other by *perceiving* information received from their up-line connected neighbors that triggers an electrical current within the neuron, which then sends the same information to their down-line connected neighbors. Neurons are not actually connected with each other (they do not touch), but rather information is conveyed from one neuron to the next by sending or receiving different chemicals over a synaptic gap (a very tiny space between each neural connection). The nature of the message is dependent on the composition of the chemicals that leap across the synaptic gap. When the next neuron perceives a chemical that exactly fits one of its receptors, it sends the same message to the next neuron. This information follows neuronal pathways that eventually (almost instantly) end up causing us to feel and behave according to the original perception that triggered the sequence.

Mood altering drugs, whether legal or illegal, either replicate natural chemicals (neural transmitters) or block them from reaching a neighboring neuron's receptors. In either case, an artificially-induced action (or inaction), cognition, sensation or emotion is experienced.

I learned that when various organs in our body *perceive* a need for the chemicals for which they are designed, they manufacture and release them into the biochemical mix to sustain a natural, normal balance of body chemistry, thus maintaining a healthy physical, cognitive and emotional state of being.

I learned that the single component that upsets our normal chemical equilibrium more than any other factor (outside of artificially-induced chemicals—i.e., drugs) is stress! When the normal balance of our body chemistry gets upset, it alters the flow of information between neurons and consequently, our mental, emotional and physical well-being gets upset. In addition, if the normal equilibrium of our body chemistry is out of kilter, healing slows down; our immune system is impaired and our cognitive processes are altered.

I learned that living cells and neural pathways are dormant until they *perceive* a stimulus from an outside source. For example--using my pendulum demonstration to illustrate--the cells that compose the muscles in your arm are inactive (dormant) until you mentally perceive the pendulum swinging. Your mental perception is a stimulus to which the cells (neurons) in your brain respond by sending messages to the muscle cells in your arm. When the cells of your arm that are involved in swinging a pendulum collectively *perceive* the message they expand or contract in exactly the right way to result in the behavior (your arm moves) that causes the pendulum to swing in the perceived direction.

It is theorized that cancer cells in our body remain dormant until they are stimulated by an outside source—chemicals that are ingested, injected, produced by or from adjacent active cancer cells or that are created by stress and anxiety.

I learned that our brain is very plastic (resilient, workable, flexible) and if one area is not used for its intended purpose, it can be used for some other function. For example, a blind person uses area 17, the area of the brain primarily used for vision, to enhance the acumen of their auditory system.

I learned that the process of *human* conditioning is most often different from that of animals. Experimental animals start with a natural instinctual behavior (Pavlov's dogs' instinctual reaction to the aroma of food was to salivate), and then a stimulus (the sound of the bell), with repetition, becomes paired or associated with the instinctual behavior that was already in place.

Other animal conditioning occurs just by hit or miss—a rat running around in a Skinner box by chance hits a lever that provides a reward—and eventually with accidental repetition an association is established between hitting the lever and being rewarded.

Although we human beings sometimes become conditioned in those same ways, most often our conditioned behavior requires cogitation, not instinct or chance. As mentioned in an earlier chapter, we do not come into this life's experience with the instinctual behavior of stepping on the brake pedal when a light turns yellow, nor do we just by chance hit the brake pedal when the light changes. We had to use our cerebral cortex's cognitive ability to figure out that the illumination of a yellow light means step on the brake pedal. With repetitious exposure, the action becomes automatic—a habit.

I learned that many lower forms of animal life (those who have no cerebral cortex) rely solely on their instinct to enhance the likelihood of survival. They do not think, plan or remember; they simply respond to a given stimulus.

On the other hand, *our* large cerebral cortex gives us the ability to think out a plan of action beforehand and then *choose* to act (or not act) accordingly. Planning is a process of *perceiving* a situation or need and then *perceiving* the action that is necessary to successfully deal with the situation or fulfill the need, and at times, come up with a never-before-thought-of way to accomplish it—creative thinking.

True, some creatures have the ability to figure things out. Gorillas stack boxes to reach bananas attached to the ceiling of their cage, a cat or dog can figure out how to work around obstacles to find hidden a toy, however this ability is in direct proportion to the size of their cerebral cortex and their body mass. For us humans that ratio is comparatively huge. So for all practical purposes, planning and following through with our plan, is a unique human quality—obviously, we sit on the very top of the cognitive totem pole.

Another unique quality that we humans have is to *intentionally* go against instinctual, conditioned or learned behavior. We are the only creatures that can *intentionally choose* what to think about.

Only we humans can *intentionally* choose our perceptions, and as a result, enjoy or suffer the consequences of our perceptions. This, then, may explain why there are so many different cultures, lifestyles, political parties and religions among humans and so few variations in behavior within the population of other species. We have the ability to choose our perceptions and they don't.

This brings us back to the question of why then, despite so many diverse cultures among humans, is there so much consistency of behavior and beliefs within each given culture? Why do most people cling to *their* religious, political and social convictions, and disparage other people's convictions... and do so without considering the possibility that another person's lifestyle and beliefs may be valid, too?

It all boils down to their perceptions.

I believe it is a relativistic problem. A verifiable truth from the orientation and perception of one person can be verified to be false from a second or third person's orientation and perception, yet all three are simultaneously true. It is like the pitch of a train whistle that is moving toward one person is perceived as being higher than the pitch of the same whistle moving away from another person, while the conductor of the train hears yet another pitch—the Doppler effect. Which pitch is the true tone? All three are the true tone relative to the position and perception of the "hearer" and motion of the whistle, but each observer can verify that his is the true pitch, and therefore conclude that any different pitch from the same whistle must be false. A person living in a given culture tends to believe that his or her cultural view and belief orientation is appropriate and the true one, and in so doing, is led to conclude that someone else's is false–but both (or all three) can be true depending on the perception of each.

This leads to the most important lesson I learned, and the answer to the set of questions (and thousands more) posed early in this book and at the beginning of this chapter. Whenever we perceive a new concept, engage in a new physical task or accept a new philosophical or religious belief, the perceptions of the concept, task or belief create neural pathways in our brain, and the more a neural pathway is used the more it is strengthened and, consequently, the more a behavior, opinion or belief becomes ingrained. Another person's belief system and way of behaving, although contrary to our own, may be just as valid as ours; it is just that our perceptions are different. Of course, the ideal scenario would be that *everyone's* behavior, opinions and beliefs were identical, but that is not human nature and would only stymie creativity and progress, and make this life a very boring proposition.

I learned that some of our behaviors have little to do with rational thinking, logic, knowledge, or wanting or trying to behave in a given way. True, probably 95% of our perceptions are consistent with rational thinking, logic, knowledge, physical reality and what we are trying accomplish, but it is that remaining 5% against which we struggle–false perceptions.

I learned that our brain does not care about the behavior it produces–our brain is completely impersonal. Our brain doesn't care if the behavior it produces is constructive, rewarding, healthy, peaceful and insures freedom, or if it produces behaviors that lead to misery, degradation, poor health or imprisonment. Our brain uses the neural pathways that have been created, and strengthened over time, and causes us to feel, act and believe accordingly.

Once the pathway has been established, each subsequent time the same mental or physical task is engaged the pathway is strengthened. Eventually, that behavior or way of thinking or believing becomes so strong that it is difficult to get out of the "rut" that was created by continual use and can restrain us from even considering that some other way of behaving, thinking or believing may hold credence.

If neural pathways ("ruts") produce a behavior that leads to good health, peace of mind, a sense of well-being and positive results, then there is no need to change them—they are good. On the other hand, if ingrained pathways produce behavior that leads to poor health, self-destructive behavior, fear, anger and negative results then it might be well to work on establishing new pathways. The problem is that when we try to break out of a negative rut it *seems* so hard, and the perception that it has to be hard reinforces the neural pathways so it seems all the harder to change our behavior, so we give up and continue to use the same old pathways. Ironically, calling up memories of the perceptions that created an unwanted way of thinking or behaving only strengthens the neural pathways.

I struggled to find a way to 1) clearly present the implications of creating and strengthening new neural pathways, 2) describe how those well-traveled pathways lock us into a behavior or belief system (whether rational or irrational, rewarding or self-destructive) and 3) explain how to disentangle ourselves from the unwanted ones. So I engaged Socrates, who came up with the allegory of the ruts.

Socrates' Allegory

THE RUT

Socrates: In a distant land, where rain prevails and the ground is most often waterlogged, there is a network of unpaved roads. At the end of some of those roads lie stores of riches.

A lone traveler, after many attempts, has found a pathway that leads to a stash that meets his needs.

When he arrives at his destination, he loads a measure of riches and returns to his home. When his recently acquired stock has diminished, he repeats the trek and acquires an additional supply.

The first time the traveler's conveyance moves over the trail, its wheels leave an imprint in the soft ground. The next time the imprints become grooves. With repetition, the grooves become furrows and finally, the furrows become ruts that reach nigh to each wheel's hub.

In due course, the goods at the end of his route dwindle. However, rumor has it that there are treasures elsewhere in the land to be garnered and all one need do is choose a likely trail, proceed to its end, and discover if at its terminus riches reside. But to venture off into the unknown, with scant certainty of what lies at the end, is a frightening consideration, so the traveler persists with his familiar comfortable but rutted path.

Eventually the traveler realizes that his reserves have dropped off and scarcely meet his needs, and with great longing he attempts to change his course. He has often noticed un-rutted trails that cross his well-traveled route and conjectures that, surely, at the end of at least one must lie new riches. But his attempts to embark upon a new course are foiled because of the depth of the ruts that his travels have excavated from continuous use and the difficulty of getting out of them.

Out of desperation, desiring to explore a new route, the traveler seeks the advice and assistance of a well-schooled expert who has learned various theories for extracting travelers from their rutted trails and is schooled in advising them how to find and embark on alternate paths. The standard approach for helping others find a new direction is to accompany the seeker of a new route over the rutted trail and point out the branches that may lead to new riches—but the seeker already knows of these paths, he has seen them many times. Because the learned one has only theoretical knowledge and no personal experience of extracting one out of a rut, the best he can do is point out the branches and speculate how to accomplish the task of getting unstuck. Ironically, the more the seeker and the learned one visit the route, the deeper the ruts become and the chance of launching a new direction only becomes more remote.

Then one day while covering the distance alone, having given up on the advice of the well-schooled expert, the traveler happens upon a second traveler whose course is perpendicular to his own and whose wheels easily span and cross over the ruts in which he is trapped. After hailing the stranger, he explains his dilemma of being stuck in his self-made ruts and the difficulty of finding a way to get out of them.

The second traveler explains: "Early in my experience of traversing the territory, from time to time I found myself in your same predicament. I soon learned that trying to extricate myself out of the old established grooves in an endeavor to change my course proved useless so long as I wallowed in the same old ruts. However, after several unsuccessful attempts, my familiarity with the terrain grew, and by combining my own reasoning with the sound advice from experienced travelers, I learned to abandon the old trail at its onset, to start afresh from whatever point I happen to find myself and establish a new un-rutted route. Once I blaze a new pathway, it is *as though* the old deep, rutted, unwanted passage was never there. It isn't that the old trail no longer exists, but with the passage of time it erodes and is less obvious. Nevertheless, I know if I were to choose to set upon an old course again, in short time I would find myself stuck in the same old worthless ruts. Now I choose to set my course in some different direction that circumvents the old depression, which keeps me from falling back into the old ruts that lead to exhausted riches. And for that matter, I keep a sharp eye out so I don't find myself stuck in someone else's ruts."

So the traveler took the advice of the experienced traveler, returned home and set out in an entirely different direction, and with time discovered riches at the end of several trails which led to living an abundant rounded life by drawing on a variety of riches, rather than relying on the goods of a single trail.

Me: That is a great metaphor and I think that I understand its implications, but go on to explain how it is analogous to human behavior, prejudices, irrational activities, political and religious biases and conditioned behavior. I know that at times I get stuck in a rut of unwanted behavior or thoughts, and that only by engaging in some other task or thinking about something positive have I been able to extract myself. Nevertheless, go on to explain the implications of your allegory.

Socrates: The analogy is based on perceptionism and how our perceptions create neural pathways in our brain that, in turn, determine how we act, feel and believe. After all, isn't that what this book is about—perceptionism?

The riches at the trail's end are the hopes, desires and longings we have for financial security, good physical health, comfort, recognition, the respect of others, self-fulfillment, happiness, self-esteem and peace of mind—our riches.

The unpaved roads are the undeveloped neural pathways in our brain that are primed for establishing the behaviors, knowledge and attitudes that are necessary in order to attain our riches. Neural pathways are initiated by the perceptions that are created as we learn new tasks, concepts or beliefs.

Arriving at the destination represents neural pathways that are established by having discovered the behaviors, concepts and beliefs that lead to attaining our riches. The diminishing of the newly retrieved riches after arriving back home is the atrophy that occurs in neural pathways if they are not used by practicing a physical task or revisiting newly discovered concepts.

The imprints, grooves, furrows and eventually ruts are neural pathways that are strengthened with each use of that pathway and that, with repetition, become so strong they become a habitual (rutted) way of behaving, thinking or believing.

For instance, each time a smoker goes through the ritual of lighting up, the neural pathways associated with the behavior are strengthened and over time become so strong that it seems hard to break the habit. Each time a person perceives himself or herself as being worthless the neural pathways associated with feeling worthless are strengthened and it seems difficult to shun the feeling.

Me: These examples of neural pathways are associated with negative behaviors and emotions. Doesn't it hold just as true for positive actions, feelings and beliefs, as well?

Socrates: Of course it does, but I believe in your profession you seldom encounter a client who wants to get out of ruts that produce positive, up-lifting results.

Me: That is true. Go on explaining your allegory.

Socrates: The dwindling of goods at the trail's end is analogous to discovering that an established habit or way of thinking or believing no longer fills our needs or we come to the realization that our behavior, thoughts and beliefs are unproductive, limiting or self-destructive.

The rumors of other riches represent the neural pathways that have arisen from realizing that we possess the ability, qualities and attributes to advance new and better ways of acting and thinking, but have not yet learned how to use them.

The un-rutted trails that traverse the rutted one are the ideas that have surfaced from learning new concepts, gleaning ideas from others, observing the means that have led others to achieving their riches (material substance and self-enrichment) and imagining the possibilities of achieving the same.

The fear of venturing off into the unknown trails represents precisely that. These are the neural pathways that have been formed by being told (or that have been created by our own perceptions) that we can't or shouldn't take chances or venture off into uncharted waters. The neural pathways that are created by hearing: Be careful, don't do anything rash, what will people think of you if you mess-up, don't say or do something that will upset people, you will end up in hell if you don't believe as I do, you will never amount to anything worthwhile, don't stick your neck out.... If these neural pathways are deeply rutted, when accessed they create fears, anxieties, self-doubt and feelings of worthlessness that are paralyzing and keep us from taking action, so we just revert back to our comfort zone and familiar way of acting, thinking, believing and feeling.

The well-schooled expert represents a person who is stuck in his or her own ruts and gives only advice that is based on what others think, but presents no definitive plan of action or acceptable means for a person to change their behavior.

The knowledge that the first traveler already possesses (i.e., the knowledge that there are other pathways) corresponds to the concept that most people already "know" what they should be doing (or shouldn't be doing) and have a suspicion that their thoughts are responsible for their unwanted behavior, limitations and emotions, but have not discovered the means by which to change them.

Well-schooled advice givers are also those who do not apply their advice to themselves but continue to advise others based on only learning or hearsay. Well-schooled teachers and preachers are the bigots whose own neural pathways are so deeply ingrained in a given approach, philosophy or belief system that they are imprisoned, limited and constrained to a very narrow view of life and held back from experiencing or discovering a vast array of possibilities.

The real irony is in the regressive approach to therapy. Each time a thought, behavior or perception is revisited, the neural pathways with which they are associated become all the more strengthened and the behavior or way of thinking is even more indelibly worked into the neural pathways and fabric of their worldview. Since our brain and nervous system cannot distinguish the difference between a real experience and one that is perceived to be real, rerunning past events only reinforces existing pathways.

The second traveler whose wheels span and easily cross over the first traveler's ruts is a person (well-schooled or not) who has, through personal experience and experimenting with new ideas, created neural pathways that produce confidence in the plasticity of the brain-led creativity. He or she has not only learned ways to help people change their unwanted behavior but can *show* them how to do it. He or she is a person who understands that neural pathways are never completely eradicated (except in the case of stroke, surgery, brain injury, disease and death) and knows that if once again they engage in an old behavior or way of thinking they will find themselves stuck in an old unwanted behavior—stuck in the clutches of the old neural pathway.

It is like the recovering alcoholic who knows if he or she takes *one* drink, they fall back into the habit of drinking. Or the reformed smoker or drug user who thinks… just *one* smoke or *one* hit won't hurt. Well, it does! Engaging in such an act revisits the neural pathways that had been established by their old habit and they are suckered back into their old rutted habitual activities.

The wise traveler also represents a person who is willing to consider the thoughts, advice, and actions of other people, but exercises a healthy skepticism to ensure that he doesn't become stuck in someone else's rut. The wise traveler is one who freely examines the thoughts, actions, beliefs and ways of life that are based on hearsay, mysticism, unverifiable evidence and inconsistent philosophies. I emphasize that he is still free to investigate such things but exercises caution so he doesn't get stuck in a behavior or belief system that would restrict him from exploring other possibilities.

Me: And is choosing to set a new course at the onset similar to my approach of *not* digging up old issues or wallowing around in past experiences? Is it a process of discovering how clients desire to act and feel and showing them how to take it from where they are at the present time and then, by giving positive suggestions, painting in their mind the perception that they *are* as they choose to be?

Socrates: Yes it is. There is no need to go back over old neural pathways in order to establish new ones. Regressing a client back to past events only strengthens those neural pathways and makes it even more difficult (and may take several sessions) to ignore the old neural pathways and create new ones.

The process of establishing a new neural pathway is a procedure of ignoring the old ones and establishing new ones. New neural pathways are easily established by using sound logic, demonstrations and positive suggestions to paint in the mind of your client perceptions that their chosen behavior is how they behave *now* and the perception that they *are* now enjoying the end result benefits of the new behavior. Once again, since our brain and nervous system cannot distinguish the difference between an actual experience and one that is perceived to be real, the more the new pathway is visited by actual experience, or is perceived with the client's mind, the stronger the new favorable pathway becomes. The more the favorable way of behaving and thinking is engaged, the sooner the behavior or way of thinking becomes habitual.

Nevertheless, always keep in mind that much of a person's behavior is the result of being stuck in *good* ruts.

Ruts of healthy eating, being physically and mentally active, or having a philosophy that engenders peace of mind and benefits oneself and others are good ruts. Stuck in a rut of doing good deeds, serving others, maintaining a positive attitude, reading good books, seeking new knowledge, and engaging in healthy debates or worthwhile activities are other good ruts in which to be stuck.

When rutted neural pathways lead to happiness, good health and the well-being of self and others, then travel them often. On the other hand, if ruts lead to misery, unhappiness, low self-esteem, fear and the degradation of others then it may be time to set out on a new pathway.

Nonetheless, even a good rut can have grievous consequences if a person becomes obsessed with that rut only and ignores the possibility that other pathways may lead to meaningful rewards. This is the downfall of closed and narrow-minded people, for example; i.e., bigots.

On the other hand, when a traveler sets out on a diversity of trails, his life is filled with a variety of riches. So it is with a person who explores a variety of concepts, philosophies, disciplines and possibilities... they discover riches they would not have otherwise experienced or known.

Me: It appears that by creating a clear perception in the mind of my client, thus creating a new neural pathway, the resulting behavior can be immediate. And that it is not necessarily the perception of the *behavior* that causes the change but rather a perception of the end result. It is apparent that our brain has the capability to figure out the behavior that causes an end result benefit to occur, once it receives the perception of the end result.

Just to illustrate, most of the time when a smoker walks out of my office they feel and act as though they never smoked. So apparently, a new neural pathway was established during the session that produced the *behavior* that led to end result *benefits* of being a non-smoker. But the curious part is that by suggesting the end result benefit of being a non-smoker (not the behavior of being a non-smoker) *"Your lungs are fresh, clean, strong and healthy"* their brain function invokes the neural processes that lead to the *behavior* that causes the end result perception to become actuality—having fresh, clean, healthy lungs.

Socrates: It would seem that that is true. Your client does not need to be concerned at all with how their brain "knows" how to create the neural pathways that produce the behavior of being a non-smoker any more than they needed to be concerned with how their brain "knew" how to manipulate the muscles in their arm to make a pendulum swing. In both cases, it is the perception of the *end result* that caused the behavior that, in turn, produced the end result.

Me: So it all boils down to this: Our brain holds the potential for creating a truly *limitless* number of neural pathways—you can always create a new one, the same as there is no number so great that you can't add one more. New pathways are created each time we engage in learning a new physical task or we mentally perceive a new concept. Each time a physical task or perception is engaged, the neural pathway associated with that task or perception is strengthened and over time *becomes* a physical habit or a habitual way of perceiving things. Established neural pathways determine our physical action, our emotional state, how we respond to different stimuli, our opinions and our belief system—basically, who we are. Is that correct?

Socrates: That is correct.

Me: Furthermore, if we are dissatisfied with our present state of being—our behavior, our emotions, our way of thinking or who we are—then the process to change any unwanted condition is to establish new neural pathways that are associated with a favorable state of being. In addition, we do not have to ferret out old pathways before we can establish new ones. True?

Socrates: True.

Me: And finally, (relative to helping my clients make a change in their state of being) since their brain cannot distinguish the difference between a real experience and one that is perceived to be real then the process of establishing new neural pathways (hence a new behavior) is to simply create new perceptions. Furthermore, this is accomplished by using logic, sound reasoning, demonstrations and suggestions.

Socrates: Yes, that is correct.

Remember, your conscious experiences leave a trail of memory that defines who you are—your autobiography. It may not necessarily be accurate because we sometimes falsely perceive things; nonetheless, *who* you are, *how* you act, *how* you emotionally feel and *what* you believe is the sum total of your perceptions to this point of your life's experience. How could it be otherwise? If you are dissatisfied with your present state of being, all that is needed is to establish and reinforce new neural pathways by creating new perceptions and revisiting the desired ones often—perceiving with your mind the desired behavior is how you behave now.

Moreover, when helping other people change their behavior, the process works at its optimum level when your client's body is relaxed and in a conscious sleep state, where their mind is focused *only* on the suggestions that are given and that are perceived as being true "NOW." This *is* the "hypnotic process"—the process of perceptionism.

The End

"Tell me one last thing," said Harry. "Is this real? Or has this been happening inside my head?"

"Of course it has been happening inside your head, Harry, but why on earth should that mean it is not real?"

J. K. Rowling, *Harry Potter and the Deathly Hallows*

APPENDIX I

STRUCTURE OF A TYPICAL PERCEPTIONISM SESSION

This appendix is a narrative of my *present* approach of conducting a "perceptionism" (hypnotism) session from start to finish. I say *present* approach because how I now conduct a session will (with more experience and experimenting) undoubtedly be "tweaked" from time to time, and who knows, maybe radically transformed if a more effective approach becomes apparent.

This example session is an actual session with a real client, whom I will call "Judy." Judy made the appointment to overcome her fear of leaving her home by herself or even going out to the end of her driveway to collect letters from her mailbox (agoraphobia).

Although the organization of all my sessions is essentially the same as the one presented here, every session is tailored to meet the needs of each client and the issue for which the client made the appointment.

The dialog in the **left column** below is a re-creation of Judy's session just as it happened as I communicated my thoughts, perspectives and suggestions and as *she* commented and responded.

In the **right column** are explanations, experiences, thoughts, feedback from clients and my own introspections that are intended to explain, clarify and defend the dialog on the left.

The session actually begins the moment a client calls to make an appointment. Everything I say (or Delma my secretary says) to a perspective client paints in their mind a perception of what to expect as the result of the session. For example, if I tell a client that their issue can probably be resolved in a single session, the likelihood of it taking a single session is significantly enhanced. On the other hand, if I tell a client it is going to take a half dozen sessions to resolve their issue, then it probably will.

The session is divided into four segments:

- The Pre-Hypnotic Talk
- The Induction
- The Suggestions
- The Awakening

In addition, each segment is broken down into several sub-divisions that deal with the specific concepts I want the subject to grasp as they relate to using *their* mind and brain to achieve the behavioral change they are seeking.

After Judy arrived at my office and the preliminaries were taken care of (introductions and filling out the confidential information intake form), I asked her to sit on the other side of a small desk that facilitated looking directly into each other's eyes, and we began:

The Pre-Hypnotic Talk

Clarifying the <u>Client's</u> Reason for Making the Appointment

Session Transcript	Annotation
Me: Judy, why do you want to get over your fear of leaving your home? It would appear that you *do* have the ability to leave your home because you are sitting here in my office. I can understand that it may have been no easy task, but you made it. What is the real reason you want to resolve this problem?	*The reasons a person would want to resolve their agoraphobic behavior are obvious, but I wanted to hear her unique issues. I used the phrase, "get over your fear of leaving home," because that is how she described her condition when she filled out her information input form.*
Judy: I just want to live a normal life. I want to be out and about, and to go and visit my family and friends without being whacked-out from the trauma of just getting there. I want to be able to go shopping, to the movies or to the doctor without having to medicate myself silly just to get out the door.	*As a client expresses their reasons for having made the appointment, I make a mental note of what they say and how they say it, so I can use <u>their</u> terminology during the pre-hypnotic talk and when I give suggestions relative to changing their behavior.*
It took everything I had to get here today—especially without taking any medication, as you asked me to do. On the way here, I tried to persuade my husband to turn around and take me home where I would feel safe—he refused. Even right now I feel like I want to get out of here and go home... can you help me?	*If a person is taking medication for anxiety-related problems, I ask if they think they could make it to my office without using their medication. I do this for two reasons. First, I have found that if a person is "doped-up" they make a very poor subject. Second, I want to demonstrate to them that they have the power to feel good without using medication.*

Me: Yes, I am sure I can. And by the way, those were all the right answers you gave. I was looking for the wrong answer.

Had I not been completely confident in the perceptionism process and that I could show Judy how to use her mind-brain powers to change her behavior, I would not have said "yes."

Judy: What would have been the wrong answer?

Me: The *wrong* answer would have been, "Someone else is telling me that I have to get over it and they *sent* me here!" If you had said that, I would have sent you back out the door and asked you to send *them* in and I would "hypnotize" them so how you are doesn't trouble *them*.

*If I have any suspicion that a client has been "sent" in, and that that is the sole reason for them being in my office, I terminate the session and then ask them to call back when **they** are ready to change their behavior independent from what other people think.*

The only reason that I can think of that you should get over your fear of leaving your house is that *you* think you should, and have decided that it is time... and *you* have chosen hypnotherapy as a way to do it.

If someone calls and wants to make an appointment for someone else, with few exceptions, I ask them to have the other person call and make the appointment. I have no intention or desire to help a person change just because someone else wants them to change.

Judy: I know that it would please my family and that they would be happy for me if I didn't have this problem, but I'm not doing it because of them; I'm doing it because of me. I really want to *not* have these anxieties. I want to be over it.

Pleasing other people may be a motivating factor for change, but I have found (much to my disappointment) if that is the sole reason, the session is most likely destined for failure.

Discovering the <u>Feelings</u> Associated with the Behavior

Session Transcript	Annotation
Me: When you think of the feelings associated with your fear of leaving the house, where in your body do you sense the feeling?	*When dealing with emotional issues, I ask the client questions about where they "feel" their unwanted emotion early on in the session so later on I can refer to those body "places" as I demonstrate to the client how their brain knows how to eliminate or create physical and emotional "feelings."*
You see, all of our emotions are felt physically, we "feel" them somewhere in our body. Where do you *feel* your fear—your anxiety?	
Judy: I feel it in my stomach, my chest, my shoulders tighten up and my hands get sweaty—like they are right now. Oh yes, and I clench my teeth.	*People experience their emotions differently. Judy's response is typical for anxiety issues, but sometimes the feelings are unique to a client—my toes curl up, for example.*
Me: If you didn't have those *feelings*, if those feelings were removed, do you think you would be able to leave your home and enjoy being out and about?	*I am interested in removing the emotional "feelings" associated with the condition, not finding the "core events" that precipitated the condition.*
Judy: I haven't thought of my emotions as being felt in my body but now I realize I do feel my anxieties physically. Obviously, if I didn't have the feelings, I wouldn't have the anxiety or fear.	*Most people have never thought to examine where they feel their emotions (good or bad). Take a moment and examine where in your body you "feel" your happiness or anger.*

Why "Hypnosis?"

Session Transcript	Annotation
Me: Why did you think of "hypnosis" as a way to get over your fear of leaving your home?	

Judy: Well I've tried everything else. I tried counseling, psychotherapy, I talked to my minister, I've prayed, I even tried acupuncture and nothing seems to help.... And all the doctors and psychiatrists want to do is feed me more pills.

Then last week a new hairdresser came in to do my hair. He said that he came to you several years ago to get over his fear of heights. He told me that he can now drive up and down steep windy canyon roads with hundred foot drop-offs and even look over the edge of the Grand Canyon without feeling sick to his stomach if he wants to. He said it was easy, but I don't think getting over my problem is going to be easy. I've really tried hard to keep calm when leaving the house. Besides, right now, I'm really apprehensive about being hypnotized.

Me: Well then, for the next few minutes I want to talk to you about the process that is *called* hypnosis and get rid of any false perception you might have about it.

I still use the term hypnotherapy or "hypnosis" rather than perceptionism because a person would have no idea what perceptionism is and what a perceptionist does—until they have been through one of my sessions.

Most clients have apprehensions about being "hypnotized" if they have not previously had the experience. It is interesting how many clients say, "I thought of hypnosis as a last resort."

Having been in practice for almost four decades, a substantial part of my business comes by way of first, second, or third hand referrals—"my brother told me his friend's mother came in to see you." Quite often a client from twenty or thirty years ago will refer a person. There is something to be said in favor of practice longevity.

There are textbook definitions of hypnotism: a trancelike state that resembles sleep but is induced by a person whose suggestions are readily accepted by the subject. Even so, every hypnotist that I know or read has his or her own definition.... So why should I be any different?

The reason that I say "*called* hypnosis" is because I really don't "know" what "hypnosis" is. However, I know that there is a process that is always going on up in our head that is *called* hypnosis and that we can use that process to change how we feel and how we act. I also know that *you* possess the ability to use the powers of your mind and brain to remove and eliminate your fears and anxieties about leaving your home. However, exactly what "hypnosis" *is* has not been precisely defined or universally accepted.

I define the phenomenon that is call hypnotism as being perceptionism—a natural process by which the human brain produces a behavior when a suggestion is perceived as being factual, while the subject is in a conscious state of sleep.

Behavior produced by our perceptions is our natural mind-brain mode of operation while we are conscious; it is just that the process is compelling when the subject is in a sleep state and, necessarily, conscious of the suggestions.

I do not perceive "hypnotism" as being a static state of mind but rather a dynamic interaction between the human mind and brain.

A Different Approach to Hypnotherapy

Session Transcript

Me: My approach to "hypnosis" is different from other hypnotherapists out there. One difference is that I don't think we need to spend any time whatsoever rummaging around in the past in order to change our present behavior.

Annotation

As I discussed in Chapter 41, we do not have to discover the neural pathways associated with a given behavior in order to establish new ones. New neural pathways are created by creating new perceptions. By establishing new self-perceptions, and revisiting them, the new neural pathways associated with a desired behavior are strengthened and the old ones atrophy.

Judy: That makes me feel better already. That's all the psychologists wanted to do. Most of the time I left feeling worse than I did before I went in because all we did was talk about miserable past stuff.

It is surprising how telling a client that we don't need to visit past issues immediately puts them at ease, thus opening their mind to what is being said.

Me: I think that is why most hypnotherapists want to see a client several times and why traditional psychology takes forever—going back and dredging up old issues and sometimes dredging up issues that were not even an issue before they got dredged up. Then they have to deal with those issues as well.

We can't change anything that has happened in the past... darn it! It is over. It is done. It is completed.

Have you seen the movie *The Lion King?*

Most clients consciously know the events that are associated with their unwanted behavior. I am convinced that those events do not have to be revisited nor do we need to uncover new ones. Having a client regress back to a "sensitizing event" can be interesting and even entertaining, but it has been my experience that doing so only gets in the way of quickly changing present behavior. Also, revisiting past issues only strengthens the neural pathways associated with the issue and makes it all the harder to ignore.

Judy: Yes I have, but it's been a long time.

Me: Do you remember the part when the monkey whacked the lion on the head with a stick? The lion said, "Jeez, what did you do that for?" and the monkey answered, "It doesn't matter, it is in the past."

*Using this "Lion King" story effectively makes the point that past events really don't matter as far as our present emotional state is concerned. Certainly we should learn from past experiences, but **reliving** the negative ones only conjures up the emotions associated with them.*

Judy: Yes, I remember that now. That's really quite funny.

Me: My approach is kind of like that. The closest I'll come to dealing with past issues is to suggest that, *Regardless of what the events were in the past that created the perception that there is something threatening about leaving your home, it is now as though the events that created those perceptions never happened as far as your emotions are concerned now.*

Using this approach (no regression) has most certainly increased the effectiveness of a session as well as simplified it–to say nothing about significantly shortening it.

Judy: I like that idea. I haven't thought about it that way, but if all of those things that were dug up during my counseling and psychotherapy sessions would have never happened, how could they affect me now?

This was one of those occasions that a client came up with a better way of expressing a concept than I had been using. It is so simple. If an event had never happened, or if it is as though it had never happened, how could it affect our present behavior?

Me: That is an excellent way of putting it. You did a better job of expressing it than I did!

Conscious State of Sleep

Session Transcript

Me: My view of the hypnotic process is different from that of other hypnotists and probably most people who have ever experienced the process.

Probably the greatest false perception people have about hypnosis is that they think while hypnotized they are supposed to be unconscious and not know what is going on. That is not true at all. If a person while hypnotized was unconscious, how

Annotation

The only exposure most clients have had to hypnosis is from what they've observed at stage-shows, or have seen on TV shows and in movies. Most people, because of appearances, think the hypnotized person is unconscious.

*In addition, many think that while hypnotized they lose control, and that the hypnotist holds power over them and can **make** anyone do anything that the hypnotist chooses.*

would they know what the hypnotist was saying? And that's the reason a hypnotist cannot *make* someone do something that would violate their basic moral or ethical standards—because they are always conscious and aware and would reject any suggestions that would go against their standards.

But the hypnotist *can* get people to do things that they *normally* wouldn't do, as long as it doesn't violate their standards. Like in those stage-show comedy acts with hypnosis. People *normally* don't go around barking like dogs and clucking like chickens just because someone suggested they would.

And people don't *normally* get rid of their anxieties about going out of the house just because someone (me, the hypnotherapist) suggested that they would. Everyone who comes into my office is looking for help to do something that they *normally* don't do or *haven't* been doing—like enjoying being out and about doing things... True?

Judy: That is true. I *normally* don't do that!

*It has been my experience that for a session to be effective it is essential that these issues be addressed early in the pre-hypnotic talk before they are brought up by the client. Once the false perceptions about the process have been settled, the client is free to focus their attention on what is being said rather than **wondering** about such issues.*

*I have heard my colleagues say, in an attempt to assure their client that they will not violate their standards, "A hypnotist cannot make you do something that you **normally** wouldn't do."*

*It seems to me that that is the very purpose of the session—to help the client behave in ways that they **normally** have not been behaving. In Judy's case, although she said she wanted to be normal (like other people), **her** normal behavior for years was feeling anxious about leaving home.*

Me: Another difference in my approach from other hypnotherapists is that I don't think a person goes "*into* hypnosis" or "*under* hypnosis!" But rather, hypnosis is a natural process that is *always* going on in a person's head... it is just that the process works best, for making a change in their behavior, when they are in a *sleep* state.

You can be asleep but still aware and conscious—as in dreaming. While you are dreaming a dream you are *not* unconscious... are you?

Judy: I don't know. But when I am dreaming I'm asleep, aren't I?

Me: That's right. You *are* asleep, but you are also conscious of what is going on in your dream *while* you are dreaming it... and even remember it sometimes when you wake up. So that must mean that you can be both at the same time— asleep and conscious. True?

Judy: True.

Me: If a person was unconscious, how would they know what the hypnotist was saying?

Judy: They wouldn't.

My colleagues and I have wonderful debates about this issue. I understand what they mean when they say "under" or "into" hypnosis but it looks to me like the subject is in a sleep state. They argue that the subject cannot be asleep because they are sufficiently conscious to understand and carry out suggestions and even engage in conversations. My rebuttal is, what's wrong with being asleep and conscious at the same time? Sleep is not necessarily a state of unconsciousness... as in dreaming.

Mind-Brain Connection (Perceptionism)

Session Transcript	Annotation

Me: I am convinced that our *brain* will automatically produce any behavior our *mind* instructs it to produce.

Well if that is true, then I am sure the next question is, *how do you get your mind to tell your brain to produce the behavior you want?* I mean, how do you say to yourself, *I'm going to get over being anxious and fearful about leaving the house for good*...and then automatically be rid of your anxieties about leaving your home for good?

Judy: I don't know. How do I do that?

Me: If what I am saying is true, I am sure the next question is, what are the instructions your mind sends to your brain and how do you get them in there?

Well, the messages your mind sends to your brain are *not* the things you say to yourself. If what you *said* to yourself were the instructions to your brain, you wouldn't be sitting here in my office—you would already be over your anxieties... true?

Judy: That is true. I've told myself a thousand times that I'm going to stop being anxious and get on with my life. That didn't seem to work very well.

*For the sake of brevity, I use the statement, "our brain will produce **any** behavior our mind instructs it to produce," however it is not completely accurate and needs some clarification.*

*We do have physical and mental limitations, so we can't experience **any** behavior. I toyed with, "within the bounds of our physical and mental limitations our brain will produce any behavior..." (which would be more accurate), but it very often led to a lengthy discussion and distracted from the flow of the session.*

Self-talk doesn't work... unless our words create a perception that what we are saying is true in the present. Our brain does not understand words; it only understands the perceptions that words create. Unfortunately, often times what is said does not produce the perception that the words were intended to create. Words do not determine behavior, only the perceptions that words create affect our behavior.

Me: The instructions your mind sends to your brain are not the things that other people say to you. If they were, *for sure* you wouldn't be sitting here. And the messages are not even what you are thinking. The messages, the instructions, your mind sends to your brain are the *perceptions* that are created by what you say to yourself, what other people say to you and what you think.

The problem is this: in an attempt and desire to change our behavior, the things that are being said can produce exactly the opposite perception!

For example, what *really* comes into your mind when you say something like, "*I'm going to get over my anxieties for good?*"

Judy: What comes to my mind is, *Who am I kidding? I've said I'm going to get over this a thousand times and not much happens. Even if I do get over it, it will only be temporary. But maybe I will be over it when all the kids are gone from the house and I don't have to be here to keep them safe... maybe. Besides that, I've had this problem for years so it will probably take years to resolve it.*

After many years of observation, experimenting, research, scrutinizing the opinions of others and studying the workings of the human brain, I am convinced that our brain does not understand words; our brain understands and responds to our perceptions.

Me: *Those perceptions* are the messages to your brain, not what you said.

By the way, how old are your children?

Judy: My daughter is 20 and the boys are 22 and 24. They are all off to school and doing very well.

It is not necessary to discover how she acquired the perception that being home keeps her children safe in order to change her behavior now.

Me: If your children are all away to school, why do you feel that you need to be home to keep them safe?

During the suggestion segment of the session, I will suggest, "Since your children are grown up and away, you no longer feel that you need to be at home to keep them safe."

Judy: I know it sounds silly, but that is one of the things that comes to my mind when I think about leaving the house.... What if my children need me? I know that they can call me on my cell phone if they need help but it doesn't get rid of the feeling that I need to be home to keep them safe.

Irrational behavior has nothing to do with logic or reasonability. Judy's knowing that her perception was silly did not get rid of her irrational anxiety, nor did the knowledge that they could reach her by cell phone if they needed her change her anxieties about leaving home.

Me: What comes to your mind when someone else says to you something like, "Come on Judy, just calm down and relax, there's nothing to be fearful of so just get over it?"

Judy: What comes to my mind when people say that is, *Don't you think that that is how I want to be? When you tell me to just get over it, it just makes me angry. I don't have any control over it, I feel that you are criticizing me so it just makes it worse. Why can't you be a little more understanding and supportive? I feel bad enough already so why don't you just shut up and leave me alone?* That's what comes to my mind when other people tell me to just get over it and get on with my life.

Me: Again, your *perceptions* are the messages to your brain, not what was said.

What I am saying is this—and see if I have this right. In your attempt and desire to be and feel secure, peaceful, comfortable and confident when being away from your home, the things *you* have been saying and the things *they* have been saying *did not* produce the self-perception that *now* you are secure, peaceful, comfortable and enjoy being out and about on your own. Because if you had been perceiving yourself that way *now* you would have automatically been behaving and feeling that way, without having to put forth any effort at all, other than perceiving that that is how you are *now*.

Judy: Yes, that is exactly right. I have not been perceiving myself that way. That is exactly what I am looking for.

*I believe that we **all** have a negative reaction when people "tell" us what to do, especially when we already know we should be doing it.*

Pendulum Demonstration

Session Transcript

Annotation

Me: I want to demonstrate to you that what I just said *is* true.

I want to demonstrate that *your* perceptions are literally instructions to your brain and that your brain in turn will *automatically* produce the *behavior* that causes the perception to become physical reality, without you having to put forth any effort whatsoever, except perceive it.

To make this demonstration, just slide up closer, brace your elbow on the desk, and take this pendulum and hold it right over the middle of the crosshairss.

Now with your mind perceive that the pendulum *is* swinging in the direction C to D and it will automatically swing C to D (giving Judy time to create the perception and observe the results).

Now with your mind perceive that the pendulum *is* swinging in a circle. You decide which way you want the pendulum to swing and perceive that it *is* swinging in the direction that you choose (again giving Judy time to perceive and observe).

After placing a sheet of paper (on which is drawn a crosshairss) on the table in front of the client I <u>show</u> them exactly how I want them to hold the pendulum—elbow on the desk, hold the pendulum ¼" above the center of the crosshairss so it can swing freely (Chapter 32 page 313).

Now perceive that the pendulum *is* hanging perfectly still right over the center of the cross.

I want to demonstrate to you that your perceptions are instructions to your brain only when conceived of as being true *now* and in the present.

*I emphasize, "Your brain produces the **behavior** that causes the perception to **become** reality." It isn't perception itself that causes anything to occur, it is the **behavior** (the movement of their arm) that causes it to swing. The perception is just a message to their brain that in turn brings about the behavior.*

Without exception, once the client creates a perception of the pendulum swinging, it automatically begins swinging in the direction they perceive.

Judy: What is making this happen?

Me: We'll talk about that in just a moment.

I want to demonstrate that your perception instructs your brain to act only when thought of as true *now* and in the present.

Instead of perceiving that the pendulum *is* swinging C to D, perceive that sometime off in the future, it is *going* to swing in the direction C to D... and you will see that nothing happens at all.

If you are perceiving it is going to swing sometime off in the future, to your brain, that means that now it isn't swinging. That's like thinking, "I am <u>going</u> to get over my phobia of going away from the house." If you are *going to get over it,* that means that *now* you haven't.

*I cannot emphasize strongly enough the importance of perceptions being conceived of as being in the present (in this instant of **now**) for perceptionism to express its full power.*

*We exist in this millisecond of **now**. Our brain cannot cause any behavior or emotion to occur outside of **this** instant. Events that happened in the past or that will happen in the future do not exist! In our memory past events exist, and in our imagination we can conceive that they are going to exist, but in physical reality they are non-existent except in this moment of now.*

Now change your perception from it is *going* to swing, to it *is* swinging in the direction C to D, and it will automatically swing in the direction C to D.

Judy: There it goes. Now it is swinging!

Me: Continue to perceive that the pendulum *is* swinging C to D. I want to demonstrate that your words are meaningless to your brain. Your brain only responds to your perceptions.

While perceiving that the pendulum *is* swinging C to D, say to yourself over and over, "A to B, A to B," but still perceive C to D... and you see that what you are saying has nothing to do with your behavior. Your brain does not understand words. Your brain only understands and responds to your perceptions... true?

Judy: That is true, but how does that work?

Me: I'll answer that question in just a moment, but first I want to demonstrate that it is *you* that is making it swing, not *me*.

Now without me saying anything, you decide some direction for it to swing and perceive that it is swinging in the direction that you choose (giving Judy time to choose, perceive and observe the results of her perception).

Judy: I didn't believe that I could make it swing on my own, I thought it was *you* that was doing it. That is really, really strange—incredible. What makes it work?

*I remember the moment it dawned on me that words all by themselves are meaningless to our brain. As with many other flashes of understanding, this concept was triggered by one of my clients who said, "I was trying to make the pendulum swing by **saying** the letters and nothing happened, but the instant I "saw" it swinging it began swinging in the direction that I imagined it swinging.*

Words have meaning only when they create the perception that the words represent.

I ask the client to choose a direction on their own so they know that it is not me who is making it swing. It is interesting how many people think I have a magnet hidden under my desk that I use to manipulate the swinging or that it is my mental powers doing it.

Me: Now pay attention and reason with me for a moment so you clearly understand the implications of what just happened... it was the movement of your arm that made it swing.

Judy: No it wasn't! I was trying to hold my arm still.

Me: I know you were, but that is the very point of the demonstration: consciously you were trying to hold your arm still and trying to keep the pendulum *from* swinging. You were not even aware that it was your arm that was making it happen.

Well apparently, your brain didn't care what you were trying to do on a conscious level; your brain only understood and responded to your perceptions.

Your brain doesn't care that you have been trying to get over your fear of leaving your home. Your brain doesn't care if you *never* leave your home. Your brain doesn't care if you are out there confidently and comfortably doing things and going places.

Your brain only understands and responds to your perceptions.

If a client does not grasp the concept that their perceptions are instructions to their brain and that their brain sent messages to the muscles in their arm and that it is their arm movement that made the pendulum swing, then the remainder of the session will be meaningless.

Arm movement can be very apparent or barely noticeable, but either way the client is seldom aware of the movement.

For over three decades and over 27,000 clients, every time the pendulum begins to swing I still wonder what is truly going on. What is the interaction between our mind (our consciously chosen mental perceptions) and our brain that makes the muscles in our arm extend and contract in precisely the right way so our perceived end-result (the swinging of a pendulum) becomes observable actuality?

No matter how much I search and delve into the insights gleaned from countless studies and ideas conceived by brilliant minds, the underlying process (the actual energy forces–the mechanics) of how it works still eludes me.

Up until now, your brain has been producing behavior that you *didn't* want because you have been perceiving that there is something fearful about being away from your home.

The perceptions that you have this phobia you can't get over and that it has got to be hard to get rid of your anxious feelings have been the messages to your brain. Your brain doesn't care what you are trying to do or wanting to do, it only responds to your perceptions.

How much effort did it take to make the pendulum swing?

Judy: Well, it didn't take any effort—none!

Me: None Judy, is how much effort it takes to be peaceful, confident, comfortable, and even enthusiastic about being out and about—none, once your brain gets the instruction—and the perception is established in your brain that that is how your are now.

Judy: It can't be that easy, can it?

Me: Yes, I believe it can be that easy.

Reason with me further. You did not perceive your arm moving (the behavior that made the pendulum swing), you chose to perceive the end-result—the *pendulum* swinging, right?

It is easy to demonstrate that our perceptions are transformed into physical behavior, but why they are remains hidden. However, the fact that we don't fully understand why the process works doesn't keep us from using it... any more than not knowing why gravity works keeps us from using it.

Many hypnotherapists (and psychologists) argue that it has to be hard to affect behavioral changes in their clients—and even project that perception. I will admit that some cases are more difficult than others, but I know that by communicating the perception that it is easy to change our behavior, it tends to make it easy.

411

Judy: That is true. I was not even aware that my arm was moving.

Me: My question is this: How does your brain know how to take a perception of a pendulum swinging up there (pointing to Judy's head), do some kind of processing and know exactly which muscle in your arm to manipulate to make it swing in the right direction—the direction you perceived?

What a curious occurrence. How many times have you practiced making a pendulum swing by perceiving it swinging?

Judy: I can't remember ever even thinking about it, let alone trying it.

Me: Now this is the idea I want you to grasp. You perceived the pendulum swinging (the end-result) not the behavior that made it swing (your arm moving); all your brain needed was a perception of the end-result. Nevertheless, your brain needed the end-result perception *first* and that it is true *now*, and you didn't need to be concerned about how your brain knew the *behavior* to produce that caused the perceived end-result to become reality... the behavior (the movement of your arm) just happened!

Our brain is completely impersonal. Our brain does not care about the behavior it produces. Our brain only responds to the perceptions it receives, be it perceiving the need for more oxygen in our blood stream (causing us to breathe more deeply), perceiving the need for antibodies to combat an illness or perceiving a pendulum swinging. It is only our consciousness that gives us human beings the capacity of caring or knowing that we care... but our **brain** *doesn't care.*

Before I developed confidence in "perceptionism," I made "test" suggestions after the induction part of the session to convince **me** *that the client was "hypnotized."*

Later on I gave the same "test" suggestions to convince the **client** *that* **they** *were "hypnotized."*

Now I use demonstrations (the same instructions I used as tests) during the pre-hypnotic talk to demonstrate to the client that their perceptions determine how **they** *act and feel.*

So later on in the session I will give you suggestions relative to your being and feeling secure, confident, peaceful and enjoying being out and about. By perceiving that that is how you are *now*, you don't have to be concerned at all about how your brain knows how to cause it to happen, any more than you needed to be concerned about how your brain knew it was supposed to move your arm to make a pendulum swing.

Does that make sense?

Judy: Yes, it does, but it seems so simple.

"Perceptionism" Process

Session Transcript	Annotation
Me: In a minute I will have you sit in my recliner and I will lead you through a mental process to get your body into the conscious state of sleep (in which you are still aware) where this process works for changing your behavior.	By explaining to the client what to do later on in the session, I am literally giving them **Suggestions** on what to do later on in the session. When the time comes to do what was suggested they automatically do it. Instructions (which are really suggestions) that are given to a client early in a session (relative to what to do later on) are as valid as any suggestion given after the induction. Actually, the pre-hypnotic talk is part of the induction process. And for that matter, it appears to me that most of the perceptionism ("hypnosis") happens during the pre-hypnotic talk.
But to get into the conscious state of sleep in which your brain is open to receiving suggestions, all you need do is to perceive that what I am saying is true *now*.	
So when I suggest to you, *Now your legs, your arms and your entire body is relaxed*, with your mind perceive that it is true—every muscle *is* relaxed and every nerve of your body is relaxed.	

413

When I ask you to *Relax your mind now*, perceive that your mind is open and receptive to the suggestions that I give. Having a receptive mind is as simple as letting go of your analyzing, by choosing to perceive that what I am saying is true *now*.

And when I say to you, *Relax and sleep now*, perceive yourself as *being* in a deep peaceful sleep. That is, your body as being in a deep peaceful relaxed sleep, although at every moment you are aware of my voice and what I am saying.

Then when I give you suggestions relative to you *being secure, peaceful, confident, comfortable, at ease and feeling good* when away from your home, perceive that that is how you are *now!*

By painting in the mind of the client, as I go through the pre-hypnotic talk, the perception that the behavior they are seeking is easy to achieve and that they are now in possession of the behavior they are seeking, their brain causes it to happen.

Near the end of the pre-hypnotic talk, I ask the client how they are feeling compared to how they felt before they came into my office. Usually they report that they feel relaxed and have none of the negative emotions, physical feelings or urges they had **before** *coming in.*

The Importance of NOW

Session Transcript

Annotation

Me: Judy, have you ever wondered how long NOW is?

Judy: No, I have never before wondered how long *now* is, but it can't be very long.

Me: Well you are right... *now* is not very long. It is so short that this one is gone. However, somehow you can't get out of now.

But what I am wondering is, in which *now* had you planned to be peaceful about being away from your home?

Refer to Chapter 40 for insight into how I arrived at the importance of **NOW.**

Judy: Well it would appear to me that if I am going to do it at all I am going to have to do it in this *now!*

Me: You are right. To enjoy being peaceful and secure about being away from your home and out there doing things without feeling anxious, you must do it in this *now*. By having the self-perception that right now you are secure; that right now you enjoy being out and about, regardless of what you are doing, whether you are with someone or alone; that right now you are peaceful ... somehow right now turns out to be forever. From now on just happens. But you don't have to be concerned about forever, because you can't get out of *now!*

Does that make sense?

Judy: It does make sense. But until now I haven't thought about *now* that way. If I can keep in my mind the idea that all I need to do is just take it *one* now at a time it ought to be easy. I guess that the only time I should feel anxious is when there is truly something to be anxious about right now, instead of worrying about what might happen in some future now or what happened in some past now.

Dictionary and Balloon Demonstration

| **Session Transcript** | **Annotation** |

Me: Judy, let me make another demonstration.

I want to demonstrate to you that your behavior (how you feel and how you act) is not determined by what you know, or what you want, or what you are trying to do, but rather, how you feel and how you act is determined by your perceptions.

To make this demonstration, just put your arms out in front of you like this (showing her to put her arms straight out at shoulder level with palms down) and close your eyes.

With your mind, perceive that on the back of your right hand and wrist is balanced a big dictionary—you know how heavy a dictionary would be sitting out on your extended arm like that. Now, with your mind, perceive that that dictionary is pushing your right arm down now, lower and lower. The muscles in your right arm and shoulder are getting heavier and heavier, more tired and fatigued, the weight is pushing your right arm down now lower and lower.

Now with your mind, perceive that your left arm is floating up in the air. With your mind perceive that there has been tied around your left wrist a giant bunch of helium-filled balloons like you would see at a carnival—a giant bunch of balloons pulling your left arm up higher and higher. All of the muscles in your

Early on I had the client perceive trying to hold up a "bucket full of water," rather than a dictionary balanced on their hand and wrist—thinking that a clenched hand would make their arm more tired by itself. I also put the bucket in the hand of their weak arm, reasoning that it would tire more quickly, but in a discussion with Socrates, it became apparent that if the process works, I don't need to resort to any kind of trickery. So now I have the client place both arms out straight with both hands open and put the dictionary on the back of their dominate arm. I determine whether they are right-handed or left-handed by observing which hand they use to fill out their information sheet and use for the pendulum demonstration.

*The dictionary-balloon demonstration is, for me, the most compelling of the three. The other two demonstrations (pendulum and eye closure) could be accomplished by a client **intentionally** moving their arm to make a pendulum swing or **intentionally** keeping their eyes closed. We "know" how to do those things intentionally—we know how to do them as often as we like. But how often do we **intentionally** cause one arm to "feel" tired and the other one not tired?*

left arm and shoulder are relaxed now, but those balloons are pulling your left arm up higher and higher.

Now open your eyes and look where your arms are. (And when she did, she saw that her right arm was lowered, and her left arm was raised.)

Put your arms down now, reason with me again for a moment, and answer a few questions.

Did your right arm feel more tired than your left arm?

Judy: Yes it did.

Me: And you were probably trying to hold your arms level...true?

Judy: Yes, that is true.

Me: Well the point of that demonstration is that *just now* you were feeling, behaving and acting as though something was real that wasn't real. Both arms were out there the same period of time, they should have been the same degree of tired. You are even right-handed, aren't you?

Once we understand that our brain "knows" how to cause an arm to feel tired and the other one not tired (by perceiving a circumstance that in **physical** reality would bring it about), then we can create other perceptions that in physical reality would produce other behaviors and feelings that we choose to experience.

Our brain cannot distinguish the difference between a real event and one that is perceived to be real. Our brain "knows" how to cause us to feel fearful and anxious or how to cause us to feel secure and peaceful, depending on our choice of perceptions. The same as it knows which arm to make feel tired and which one to make feel not tired... depending on which arm gets a dictionary and which one gets balloons.

The amount of deflection from level in the client's arms is immaterial (sometime it is large and other times barely discernable). The point is that their brain produced the "feelings" of tired and not tired.

How we feel and act is determined by our perceptions and not necessarily physical reality. Most of our day-to-day perceptions are based on what is actually real, so most of our feelings, actions and emotions are rational and appropriate. The problem arises when we are falsely perceiving circumstances, hence our actions and emotions are irrational and inappropriate.

Judy: Yes I am.

Me: That is the reason I put the dictionary on your right arm... so you wouldn't have an excuse.

Judy chuckled.

Me: Now listen to me closely. Your brain not only knows how to make one arm feel tired and the other one not tired, your brain knows how to remove and eliminate all of the feelings of stress, anxiety and panic attacks that you used to experience. When I say used to experience ... Do you have any of those panicky feelings right now?

Judy: No, right now I really do feel relaxed and feel no anxiousness at all.

Me: As I remember, at the beginning of this discussion, you said that you felt anxious about coming to see me, anxious about being here, anxious about being "hypnotized" and anxious about being away from your home. What seems to have made the difference? Why is it that you were anxious then and now you are not?

This is the very crux of perceptionism. Our brain truly knows how to create sensations or eliminate them, depending on our perceptions. Our behavior is largely determined by how we feel—physically and emotionally. By causing a change in a client's self-perceptions, their brain creates or removes how they feel and consequently how they behave.

Asking Judy how she feels right now confirms some important aspects of the session:

- *It confirms to her that she has the ability to be away from home and peaceful at the same time*

- *It confirms to me that she has been paying attention and has comprehended what I have been saying*

- *It signifies that she is an excellent subject*

Judy: Well, I'm not sure. It is just that when you talked about being peaceful and secure *now*, my muscles began to relax and my anxieties left. That's really strange! Right now I feel peaceful and relaxed and I didn't take any of my pills earlier so I could get here—curious! Even my hands are relaxed and dry.

Me: It wasn't the talking that caused you to be relaxed, it was that the talking has changed your perceptions.

And Judy, it is no more difficult for your brain to permanently eliminate the feelings of anxiety than it is for it to do it *right now*, regardless of what you are doing or where you are.... It is always now!

Eye Closure Demonstration

Session Transcript	Annotation
Me: Let me make one last demonstration.	*This demonstration is very powerful and sets the stage for the induction and suggestion segments of the session.*
I want to demonstrate to you that the thing that makes things seem to be difficult and hard to do is perceiving that we can't do it.	
What I am saying is that it could have always been as easy for you to be as comfortable and peaceful when away from your home as you are right now. It is just that up until now you have been perceiving that you *couldn't* be peaceful and comfortable when away from your	*At the end of the demonstration, when I ask the client to perceive their eyes are open **now**, many say, "I really thought I was going to be able to open my eyes **while** you were telling me that I **wouldn't** be able to, but when I tried, and I couldn't open them, I was truly astounded."* *Every time this demonstration is successful, I, too, am astounded.*

419

home, so you haven't been. It isn't that you couldn't have been peaceful, it is just that you have been behaving *as though* you couldn't be.

To make this demonstration, just close your eyes again. *With your mind perceive that now your upper eyelids are stuck to your lower eyelids and the perception that now you can't open your eyes. In a moment I am going to ask you to try to open your eyes and when I do, try, but all you will be able to do is raise your eyebrows. The harder you try to open your eyes the more they will just stick tighter and tighter shut.*

With your mind, perceive that now your eyes are sealed, they are stuck tightly closed, but try to open your eyes now and they will just stick tighter and tighter shut.

(Judy's eyebrows raised with all of the appearance of trying to open her eyes.)

Me: Now, not trying to open your eyes any more, leave them closed, reason with me again and answer a few questions. Did you try to open your eyes?

Judy: Yes, I really did try.

Me: Why didn't they open?

Judy: I don't know why. They just wouldn't open.

*Occasionally when a client opens their eyes, I know that either they did not create the perception of them **being** sealed or that being unable to open them constituted a threat.*

*So I say to them, "Some people feel threatened if they can't open their eyes. I'm not trying to show you that **I** can stick your eyes shut, all I want to do is demonstrate that as long as you are perceiving that you can't open your eyes, you don't open them and **you** make something that should be easy, difficult."*

Then I lead them through the instructions again but add, "Give yourself a reason for your eyes to be stuck. Perceive that your eyes are taped closed, or super glued, or zipped closed."

Usually the second time works.

*Occasionally the client says, "No I **didn't** try."*

*When I ask **why**, their answer is generally, "Because I thought they would open and I didn't want to be disappointed or disappoint you."*

So I go through it again and emphasize "try" but still perceive them stuck. This usually works, too.

Me: I don't know *why*, either. All I know is that my words created in *your* mind a perception that you couldn't open your eyes, and your brain produced the behavior so you *didn't* open your eyes and that right now you are making something that should be easy, difficult, true?

(Judy once again tried to open her eyes.)

Judy: Yes, that is true.

Me: Now to make something that should be easy, easy, Just change your perceptions from "your eyes are sealed" to "they are open," and they will open easily *now*.

(Judy's eyes popped open.)

Me: Now *really* reason with me. Once you established in your brain the perception that you *couldn't* open your eyes, you *didn't* open your eyes. It isn't that you couldn't have opened them, it is just that you didn't open them.

I mean, all of the muscles were still there to open your eyes. You still knew how to open your eyes and you still had the ability to open your eyes. You had no limitations whatsoever to have just opened your eyes. It is just that as long as you had in your mind the perception that you *couldn't*, you *didn't*, and you made something that should have been easy, difficult. But the instant you changed your perceptions and perceived them as open, you got out of your own way and then what should have been easy became easy...True?

I truly do not know why perceiving one's eyes are stuck keeps a person from opening them.

*I do know, however, that it is the perception of them being stuck that somehow instructs their brain and causes them to not open, but it is beyond my comprehension to understand **why**!*

It is interesting to observe the various expressions clients display when their eyes pop open. It is also curious that their eyes do not open until I say now.

No doubt the reader has noticed that I constantly ask the client to "reason with me," and that it is most often followed by "true?" or "does that make sense?" This practice has several benefits:

- *It captures their attention*

- *If what I am saying is reasonable to the client they are very likely to accept suggestions related to other concepts.*

- *If they acknowledge in the affirmative I know that they grasp the concept and if they respond in the negative, I can restate it differently*

- *I want them to understand that they are involved in the process and that I'm not "telling" them what to do or think*

421

Judy: That is true.

Me: Reason with me further: It isn't that you couldn't have been peaceful and comfortable when away from your home, it is just that, up until now, you haven't been, because you have been perceiving that you couldn't, so you weren't, and you have been making something that should be easy, difficult.

So that is all we will be doing during the remainder of the session: changing your perceptions from, "it is frightening to be away from your home," to "being out of the house is not only easy but enjoyable."

My demonstrations (not tests) are conducted to reveal to my clients that they have the power to change their behavior simply by changing their self-perceptions.

Only if I am convinced that the client has grasped and understood the concepts related to "perceptionism," and has successfully accomplished the three demonstrations, do I proceed to the suggestion segment of the session.

If a client is unable (or unwilling) to accept, comprehend and carry out the instructions of the pre-hypnotic talk, it is highly unlikely that they will accept, comprehend and carry out suggestions relative to the behavioral change for which they made the appointment.

Judy: That sounds great!

Me: Then sit over in my recliner and we will proceed.

The Induction

After a client is seated in my recliner, I explain to them that I will be making a recording of this part of the session that they will take home to listen to for reinforcing the suggestions (strengthening neural pathways). And that during this part of the session all they need to do is perceive that what I am saying is true now. Then I ask them to close their eyes and make themselves comfortable. (Note: Words that are italicized and in bold are words that I emphasized.)

Session Transcript

Annotation

Me: Judy, just make yourself comfortable, and with your eyes closed, take in a deep breath now....

Hold it in, and to yourself count down from five to one and then exhale... (Giving the client time to take in a deep breath and time to count down and to exhale.)

Now take in another deep breath, hold it in, count down and then exhale....

And now just one more time....

And now breathing normally, just relax **now**... and **sleep now!** Drifting down into a deep peaceful sleep now.... aware of my voice at every moment, but continuing to drift into a deeper and deeper **sleep.**

And with your mind, perceive that what I am saying is true **now.**

Every muscle and nerve of your entire body **is** relaxed. Search around throughout your entire body for any physical tension or tightness, any nervous tension or stress. If you can find any remaining place in your body, let it all go **now.** You *are* drifting down now into a deeper and deeper **sleep.**

I have the client take in breaths of air because that is what most of us do, anyway, when we want to relax–it is a behavior that is associated with relaxing (a conditioned behavior).

By having the client do the "counting down," it forces them to get involved in the process–it turns their attention inward.

Also, I can tell how well the client is paying attention by observing if they follow the instructions. If a client does not hold their breath in while they count, I know that they are not listening or following my suggestions, so I will ask them if they are listening. Then I lead them through the instructions again until they get it right.

If a client is unable to follow these simple instructions, it is unlikely that they will grasp or carry out suggestions that are given later on.

As I explained in Chapter 31, the purpose of the "induction" is to get the client relaxed and peaceful– every nerve relaxed and every muscle relaxed. Taking a person off into an imaginary setting only lengthens the session and does not directly cause a client to relax and be peaceful.

Perfectly free and able to adjust your body in any way at any moment, if you feel a need to, so you remain relaxed and comfortable and secure. You are perfectly aware of my voice at every moment, but continuing to drift into a deeper and deeper **sleep**.

And, if you feel any stress, tension, or nervous or physical tightness remaining in your hands....

With your mind, search and see if you can find any stress, nervousness or physical tightness in your hands....

Or in your arms....
Or in your shoulders....
Or your neck....
Or in your head...
Or jaw....
Or your throat....

If you can find any stress, nervousness or physical tightness remaining in any of those places, let it all go **now**, by perceiving that

I have found that if a client adjusts their body, loosens their clothes or removes their shoes when I give this suggestion, it is an indication that they are paying attention, accepting my suggestion, and consequently, an excellent subject.

*If at any time I suspect that a client has fallen into an **unconscious** sleep and is not comprehending what I am saying, I will give my recliner a little nudge and ask them to pay attention.*

I am convinced that for a session to have successful results it is imperative for the client to be conscious at every moment and willing to perceive that each suggestion is true. If the client is not conscious of a suggestion, the suggestion is meaningless and has no affect, whatsoever, on changing their behavior.

After I ask a client to search in each body part to "see" if they have any stress in that area, I give them a few seconds to examine that part in order to "see" if there is any physical tightness or any nervous tension or stress.

*The first time through, I am **not** asking the client to let go of the stress or tightness, I am just asking them to "see" if they can find any.*

*The second time through is intended to cause it to happen by perceiving that every muscle, nerve and cell **is** relaxed.*

every muscle, every nerve and every cell is relaxed **now**, in your hands....

your arms....
your shoulders....
And your neck....
And in your head....
And jaw....
And throat....

Drifting into a deeper and deeper *sleep now...* aware of my voice at every moment but continuing to sink into a deeper and deeper *sleep... **now***!

Or, if you feel any stress, nervousness or physical tightness remaining in your chest, with your mind examine your chest and see if you can find any stress, nervousness or physical tightness remaining in your chest....

Or your upper back....
Or your stomach....
Or in your lower back....
Or in your hips...
Or legs....
Or feet....

If you can find any stress, nervousness or physical tightness remaining in any of those places, rather than trying to make it leave, perceive with your mind that every muscle, every nerve, every cell *is* relaxed **now**, in your chest....

*By perceiving it as true **now**, (muscles and nerves relaxed) the client's brain takes over and, with the same ease that it took to make the pendulum swing, causes every muscle to relax and every nerve to relax.*

*Also, the more often I can systematically work into the session the suggestions, "**sleep**" "**sleep now**!" and "**now**," the deeper their conscious state of sleep becomes.*

After experimenting with a few hundred clients, I concluded that by breaking the "examining" and "relaxing" suggestions into two segments, the client was able to grasp, understand, and carry out the suggestions more readily—reaching a deeper relaxation and conscious sleep.

I also experimented with starting at the client's feet and then working up to their head and then down to their fingers. I don't think it makes any difference, it is just that starting with the client's hand is the sequence that I initially learned, so I continue using that method.

Your upper back....
Or in your stomach....
Or in your lower back....
Or in your hips....
Or legs....
Or feet....

Drifting down now into an even deeper, peaceful, comfortable, calm, quiet, secure, relaxed *sleep... now.*

And your mind is relaxed **now.** The only thing mattering now is my voice, what I am saying, and perceiving that what I am saying is true **now.** My voice is continuing to relax you deeper and deeper.

And accepting the suggestions that I give **now.** For what I say, Judy, is true.

I believe that most of the "induction" takes place during the pre-hypnotic talk. I go through this "formal induction," first, because the client is expecting a formal induction, and second, so the induction will be on the client's recording for when they listen to it for reinforcing the suggestions—to strengthen the neural pathways in their brain.

The "induction" takes about five minutes.

The Suggestions

Although it rarely happens, if a client does not appear to be relaxed and show signs of being in a peaceful state of conscious sleep after going through the "induction," I do not proceed with the suggestion segment of the session. If I suspect that they are not completely relaxed, I pick up their arm at the wrist and let it fall to the arm of the recliner. If their arm feels heavy and when I let it go, "plops" down to the chair arm, I know that they have accepted my suggestions. If they "help" me pick up their arm, I know that they have not accepted my instructions. In this case I will go back over the induction suggestions again and this time through, ask if they are perceiving (or if they can imagine) that what I am suggesting is true. If they say no, I terminate the session. Seldom does that happen.

When I am convinced that the client is accepting my suggestions, I say:

Session Transcript

Me: Judy, there are powers and there are processes at work in you—the same ones that made your arm make a pendulum swing just by perceiving it swinging. The same powers that caused one arm to feel tired and the other one not tired, just by perceiving a dictionary and balloons. The same powers that kept your eyes from opening as long as you perceived them sealed. And also the powers that allowed your eyes to easily open the instant you perceived them as open... and then what should have been easy, became easy.

Those same powers and processes now produce the behavior, and consequently the end-result benefit, of being peaceful, confident, comfortable and secure while at home, when leaving your home, when being away from your home, or when thinking about leaving your home.

It is as if that is how you have always been... **now**. That is, peaceful, confident, comfortable and secure before leaving your home, when you leave your home and after leaving your home.

And regardless of what the events were in the past that created the false perception that there is something to fear about being away from your home, it is **now** as though the events that created those false perceptions never happened.

Annotation

When developing the suggestion segment of the session, I frequently asked clients, after the session was over, if referring back to the demonstrations conducted during the pre-hypnotic talk helped strengthen their willingness to accept suggestions, or distracted them from accepting suggestions. Without exception, clients said that it increased accepting suggestions and gave them confidence that the session would be successful. Therefore, I continue to include it as a part of the suggestion segment of the session.

I learned to include **before, during** and **after** from a client who came in for painless childbirth to whom I had suggested that she would feel no pain during delivery. Two years later, she returned because she was pregnant again. She told me that after her session, the remainder of her pregnancy and delivery was "a piece of cake," but the moment the delivery was over, she felt pain. "If you would only have suggested that I would be comfortable after the delivery, as well, I don't think that would have happened," she said.

If the "core events" that created an unwanted behavior would never have occurred, obviously they would have no effect on our present behavior. And since our brain has the ability to cause us to behave, feel and act

427

as though something is real that isn't real (dictionary and balloon demonstration), then suggesting that it is as though past events never happened, the client behaves as though they never did.

Regardless of what the events were that created the perception that staying at home would keep your children safe, it is now as though those events never occurred.

Early in the session, Judy mentioned that staying at home seemed to keep her children safe. When I asked her **why**, she said, "It is irrational to think that way but that is what came to my mind." I didn't need any more information about the issue, but I did make a mental note of her answer.

It is very understandable that when your children were young, being at home gave both you and them a sense of safety. Now that they are grown-up, capable adults, they are safe whether you are at home or away from home.

No longer do you feel a need to stay at home to keep them safe.

Whether this was a "core issue" or not doesn't matter; it only mattered that she mentioned it. So I included suggestions about it no longer being an issue—"it is as though the events that created the perception never occurred."

The powers that are in your mind and brain now, and permanently, remove and eliminate all of the feelings—the negative emotions—that used to keep you from comfortably and confidently leaving your home. You are confident and comfortable whether you are away from your home with other people or by yourself.

The powers that are in you now and permanently, eliminate the feelings in your stomach and your chest, the tightness in your shoulders and hands and cause the muscles in your jaw to remain relaxed, regardless of what you are doing.

I emphasized **negative** emotions since it seems to me that we ought to keep and enjoy the positive ones.

When I say "emotions that used to keep you from leaving your home," it implies that now they no longer do.

You now enjoy going places and doing things away from home.

Now you visit your family and friends as often as you choose with peace of mind and confidence. You love going shopping and to the movies now. Your self-esteem, and the esteem others have for you, continue to increase for having overcome an issue that at times seemed impossible to overcome.

You are confident, secure and peaceful regardless of whether you are at home, leaving home, thinking about leaving home or out and about. It is now as though that is how you have always been... **now**.

And at any time, in any place and for any reason, should you sense any of those old feelings starting to creep back in, you are able to, and do, remove and eliminate them easily and immediately just by taking in a deep breath and while exhaling saying to yourself, Judy, relax **now** and be at peace.

That short exercise and phrase are instructions to your brain to remove and eliminate all of the stress and anxiety and produce a sense of well-being and peace–the same sense of peace that you are feeling right now. You will still have plenty of physical energy, motivation and enthusiasm. But by taking in a deep breath and while exhaling saying to yourself, Judy, relax **now** and be at peace, those powers in your mind and brain produce a self-

Here my suggestions refer back to the behavior and emotions that Judy, at the beginning of the session, said that she wanted to experience. The suggestions are stated in the present tense (in the now) as if they are true and she is experiencing them at every moment of her day-to-day life.

Suggesting to a client, "You are **going** to be peaceful," is really a suggestion that now they are not peaceful.

But it is fine to suggest that something is **going** to happen sometime off in the future if a specific time or event is attached to the suggestion–when I snap my fingers, you will bark like a dog, for example.

I insert this suggestion at the end of the suggestion segment of the session so a client can recreate, at any time, the same peace and sense of well-being that they experience right after the session is over. Without exception when I ask, "How do you feel?" (at the end of the session) the client reports that they feel relaxed and peaceful–wonderful!

This exercise (taking in a deep breath) and reciting the incantation while exhaling (relax now and be at peace) is the culmination of many attempts to create for my clients a mantra to remove stress, anxieties or unwanted behavior, should they arise.

I have had many clients tell me that by doing the exercise and speaking

confident peacefulness that allows you to behave at your optimum level–a state of peacefulness in which you just keep getting better and better and better in every way.

the mantra, they were able to make it through situations that would have otherwise created anxiousness or would have caused them to "cave in" and revert to their unwanted behavior or attitude.

The Awakening

Session Transcript

Annotation

Me: I am going to count up from the number one to the number five. When I reach the number five, open your eyes and you will be wide awake feeling refreshed and wonderfully well.

It has been my experience that a client will more readily accept a suggestion if I tell them what I am going to suggest before giving the suggestion. "I am going to count up from one to five. When I reach five..." Then I count up.

You now follow and carry out the suggestions that I have given.

One.... You are beginning to come up now, the strength and energy is returning to your body, not nervous energy at all, just physical energy, for every nerve and muscle of your entire body remains relaxed, peaceful, calm and comfortable.

*Many of my colleagues count **up** whether "hypnotizing" a client or waking them up. I like to count **down** (actually have my client count down) when leading a client into a conscious state of sleep and count up when waking a client up.*

Two.... You are coming up now. Your mind is clear and your body is refreshed, following and carrying out the suggestions I have given.

The suggestions are simply.... You are confident, secure and peaceful when leaving your home, when away from your home and when in your home and thinking about leaving your home. You are free now to go and come as

By recapping the suggestions, it not only reinforces the suggestions (thereby strengthening the neural pathways) but I can reduce the suggestions to very concise statements. I try to make these suggestions as close as I can to the benefits the client expressed they were wanting at the beginning of the session when I asked why they made the appointment.

you please. You enjoy being confident and peaceful while shopping, going to movies and visiting family and friends. It is as though that is how you have always been... **now.**

Three.... You are beginning to wake up now. And within you there is a sense of peace, a sense of well-being, even a feeling of joy and happiness, feeling wonderfully well, a great burden has been lifted from you **now** and you enjoy all of the benefits that just happen as a result of being peaceful, secure and confident when leaving and away from home... **now.**

Four.... You are waking up **now.**

Five.... And, WIDE-AWAKE!

How do you feel?

Judy: I feel great. I really do feel peaceful and relaxed.

Me: If you felt this relaxed and peaceful at all times, would you have any difficulty leaving your home?

Judy: I am sure I wouldn't. It has been a long time since I have felt this good

Me: How you feel right now is the *real* you. This is your base, natural, normal state of being. Feeling anything different from how you feel right now was the result of *false* perceptions.

*In addition, I emphasize **now.** As mentioned earlier, it appears to me that our brain responds only to perceptions that are conceived of in this instant of **now.***

These suggestions are given to specifically instruct the client how they "feel" when they open their eyes, as well as once again reinforcing the benefits that occur when the suggestions are carried out.

This answer is typical after a client wakes up.

I engage in a short, relevant conversation after the session while the CD recording goes through its "finalizing." Getting into a discussion about some topic not related to the session seems to distract from the effectiveness of the session.

431

But should you start having any of those old feelings, you can eliminate them just by taking in a deep breath and while exhaling saying to yourself, *Judy, relax and be at peace.* That exercise and mantra are instructions to your brain to produce the same peacefulness that you feel right now. Or you can listen to this recording I made of your session at any time you want... except when you are driving!

Judy gave a smile and a chuckle.

Me: How long did that seem?

Judy: I don't know... maybe five minutes.

Me: When you listen to this recording you had better plan about 20 minutes. However, don't you feel like you have just had a good sleep?

Judy: Yes I do. I have been having trouble sleeping, too. I guess I didn't mention that.

Me: Well you can get a lot of sleep if you get your body relaxed. So something you might do is to re-record this CD and on the copy leave out the part when I count up and say *Wide awake,* and then listen to it when you go to sleep at night. You will get a whole night's worth of this same quality of sleep and wake up in the morning refreshed when your alarm (or your mental alarm) goes off.

I often think of Richard's advice about what to do after the sale is closed: "Shut up and leave." So as quickly as I can, I shut up and send my client out the door... of course, only after collecting my fee.

It is interesting that few clients get the time for the suggestion segment right. It is either "just a few minutes" or "it seemed like hours." Either way they always report "feeling" as if they just had a nice long nap.

The reason for making a recording of the session is to reinforce the perceptions that each suggestion was intended to create. Some clients never listen to their recording. On the other hand, some listen to their recording every day for months, not necessarily because they need the reinforcing, but because they like the relaxation and peaceful state of mind they experience when they do. Of course, each time the client listens, and perceives that the suggestions are true **now***, the neural pathways associated with the suggestions are strengthened.*

Judy: That's a great idea. When you said you were going to count up and I'd be wide awake, I remember thinking, *I'd rather just stay here for a while longer.*

Me: Well, you can stay there for the whole night by leaving out the "wake up" part. Besides that, all of the suggestions will be reinforced by doing so.

Note: A week later, I received a call from Judy and she reported that although she thought about being anxious when leaving home, she didn't *feel* the anxiety. And when she used her mantra and deep breath exercise, the thoughts of anxiousness "just evaporated and I walked out of the house with no difficulty." She also reported that by listening to her re-recorded CD (without the wake-up suggestions) she was now sleeping the whole night through.

APPENDIX II

PERCEPTIONS INFLUENCE AND INTERACT WITH NERVOUS SYSTEM AND MUSCULAR BEHAVIOR

I am in awe of the influence our perceptions have on our nervous system and our muscular behavior. It appears that our perceptions strongly influence, and even control, nearly all aspects of our physical being.

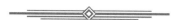

Shirley made an appointment to stop "shaking." She was 78 years old and avoided going out in public because she was so self-conscious about her condition.

Her husband brought her to my office and filled out my information intake form. Shirley was unable to because of her shaking. As I looked at the information sheet, it was evident that John's hand wasn't all that steady, either. I think he was in his 80s.

Shirley explained that she had no control over the condition except when her hands were sitting in her lap and when she was resting. She demonstrated her problem by attempting to raise her hand up to her head as if combing her hair. As soon as her hand left her lap not only did it begin to shake, but her arm made large gyrations and I feared that she might slap herself in the face or poke out an eye.

"I went to my family doctor, she sent me to a neurologist, who sent me to a brain specialist for evaluation—CAT scan, x-rays and an MRI. He sent me to a psychiatrist who gave me a prescription that made me sick to my stomach. The specialists' final conclusion was that I start shaking when attempting to make fine muscle movements with my hands and arms. They could find nothing wrong with me except that I start shaking when I try to make fine muscle movements with my hands and arms—now isn't *that* brilliant?" Shirley was very sharp for a 78-year-old and had a wonderful sense of humor

When I asked her how long she had had the condition she told me it started about two years earlier and that she could not identify anything in her life at that time that could be attributed to the onset of the malady. "One day I just woke up and went in to fix my hair and I noticed that my hand was shaking a little bit. Nothing like it shakes now, but enough to make me anxious, so I went to my doctor," Shirley told me.

She went on to say, "It seemed that after visiting each of the specialists it just got worse. Especially when they would tell me that they could find nothing wrong that could cause the disorder and that there was nothing they could do about it so just go home and deal with it... So I pretty much stopped going to specialists. I know it gets worse when I'm stressed out, anxious and self-conscious about people noticing my shakiness... Sometimes just thinking about it starts the shaking—look at them." She held her hands out and sure enough, they were trembling.

When I asked her why she thought hypnotherapy would help her when all of the other approaches hadn't worked, she answered, "Doctor Jacobson, one of the few doctors that seemed to really care and whom I have confidence in, suggested that I call you. I think she has a few other patients who came to you to stop smoking."

As I began going through the first part of my pre-hypnotic talk, (the process works when in a conscious state of sleep and that our mind controls our brain by way of perceptions) I noticed that not only did Shirley's hands stop shaking, but also her arms seemed to relax and her shoulders drooped a little. When I got to the pendulum demonstration, I was a little reluctant to ask her to hold the pendulum, thinking that she may not be able to hold her arm still enough for it to be successful. I remember debating with myself; *Shirley looks a lot more relaxed than she was when she came into my office. If she is able to hold the pendulum still long enough for the pendulum to swing at least a little, it may give her confidence that I might be able to help her. On the other hand, if she can't hold it still at all, it may blow all possibilities of proceeding with the session. I'll take my chances and do the demonstration,* I decided.

So I said, "Shirley, I want to make a demonstration that will involve letting your arm relax. I am confident that you will be able to participate in this little demonstration because you look much more relaxed now than when you first came in. Just slide your chair a little closer to my table and take this pendulum like this." I showed her how to brace her elbow on the table and hold the pendulum over the center of the crosshairss.

Without any hesitation Shirley slid up to the table, took hold of the pendulum and held it over the center of the crosshairss. She didn't seem to notice that she was not shaking at all. It turned out that Shirley was successful in every aspect of the demonstration!

I said (as I always do after the demonstration but giving no hint that I noticed that her arm and hand didn't shake), "Shirley, that was your arm moving that made the pendulum swing."

With a typical response Shirley said, "No it wasn't, I was holding my arm still." And a shock of realization dawned on her and she cried, "I *was* holding my arm still! I didn't shake at all!"

I replied, "That is right, but still, it was your arm moving that made the pendulum swing... and you were not even aware that it was moving, true?"

"Okay, but why didn't I shake? Let me try that again."

She took the pendulum and held it over the center of the crosshairss and exclaimed, "How am I doing this? I haven't been able to hold my arm this still in years. I don't believe it."

I continued with the pre-hypnotic talk and when I came to the dictionary-balloon demonstration, once again I had reservations about having her hold her arms out in front of her, since earlier it seemed that she had no control at all when showing me her condition.

So again, I took my chances and said, "I want to make another demonstration that will require you to be relaxed, but it will also involve holding your arms out in front of you like this." I showed her what I wanted her to do, with *my* arms. "Do you think that you might be able to do that for just a few minutes?"

She thought for a moment and said, "Well, the other demonstration worked, so sure, I'll try it."

After Shirley stretched her arms out in front at about shoulder height (without shaking) I suggested, "*Close your eyes and with your mind perceive that sitting on the back of your right hand and wrist is balanced a big dictionary....*"

Shirley responded perfectly to the suggestions—her right arm went down and her left arm floated up with no evidence of shaking. And when I said, "Now open your eyes and look where your arms are" she did, and said, "How did *that* happen?"

I said, "I don't know. I only know that by perceiving a dictionary balanced on your right hand and wrist and perceiving a bunch of balloons pulling up on your left arm, your brain caused you to behave and act as though there was a dictionary and balloons there. Not only that, but didn't your right arm feel more tired than your left arm?"

Shirley answered, "Well, yes, it did... and I don't think I did any shaking, either."

"I didn't see any shake while you had your eyes closed," I said.

Shirley asked, "Do you think that maybe I will be able to comb my own hair now?"

"I think so. Why don't you try mimicking combing your hair."

Shirley did so without shaking at all and seemed to have complete control of her movements.

I continued with my pre-hypnotic talk and when I came to the eye closure demonstration I said, "Maybe, Shirley, the only reason that up until now you have not been able to take control of not shaking is that you have been perceiving that you couldn't control it.

"Let me lead you through one last demonstration. I want to demonstrate to you that if you perceive you can't do something that you really can that should be really easy, your brain causes you to behave so you don't and you make something that should be easy, difficult."

"Just close your eyes and with your mind perceive that now your upper eyelids are stuck to your lower eyelids...."

When I asked Shirley to try to open her eyes, it appeared that she was really trying. When I asked her to perceive them open, they popped open.

Shirley said, "What made that work? I really tried hard to open my eyes but they just wouldn't open."

I replied, "That's right, but it isn't that you couldn't have opened your eyes, it is just that as long as you perceived you couldn't, you didn't, and you made something that should have been easy, difficult.

It isn't that you couldn't have been rid of your shakiness; it is just that up until now you haven't because you have been perceiving that you couldn't be rid of your shakiness. And just like with your eyes, the instant you change your perceptions you get out of your own way and then what should have been easy *becomes* easy.... It really is easier to not shake."

During the suggestions segment of the session I suggested to Shirley, *"Regardless of the events that created in your mind the false perception that you couldn't or shouldn't be relaxed and have control of the smooth movement of your arms and hands, it is now as though those events never occurred. Now you easily and comfortably comb your hair, brush your teeth, write checks and feel comfortable when around people. It is now as though you never did shake."*

After the session when John pulled out their checkbook to pay for the session Shirley said, "Here, let me do that!" She did, and her husband was astounded... as was I.

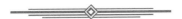

How Shirley went from having no control over the shakiness and movement of her arms, to write a check with no difficulty in less than hour, I cannot explain. Nevertheless, it is evident that somehow her perceptions interacted with her brain, and that, in turn, interacted with her nervous system and muscles and removed the malady.

A couple of months later, Shirley's hairdresser made an appointment to stop smoking and told me that until recently, she had not seen Shirley in several years. "Shirley had stopped coming because she was so self-conscious when out in public because of her shakiness; but when she showed up for her appointment last week she was confident and calm without a sign of a shake."

APPENDIX III

AN UNCHANGEABLE PERCEPTION

As described in Chapter 41, strong neural pathways that reside in our brain are the result of years and years of repetitive exposure to a perception; consequently it is understandable that those pathways would become deep-seated, thus forming staunch convictions and beliefs. So staunch, in fact, that even in light of reason, logic and positive proof that the person's convictions are bogus, their irrational perceptions and behavior persists.

Nevertheless, neural pathways are initiated by a *single* experience and can influence a person's behavior over a lifetime. Witnessing or being involved in a serious accident or the unexpected death of a loved one can change a person's perception of the world in which they live, for example.

Neural pathways can also be initiated by perceptions created by a statement, command or rebuke from another person. For instance, being ruthlessly scolded in front of his or her peers can severely alter a child's self-perception and that perception can be strengthened over a lifetime if the child mentally relives the event repeatedly.

On the other hand, suggestions that are perceived by a client or a stage-show volunteer create neural pathways that can be strengthened with time and can produce a healthy, rational way of life. However, occasionally a neural pathway initiated by a suggestion can produce irrational conduct, convictions and beliefs that are difficult to change so long as the person clings to the perception... Such was the case with Tara.

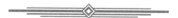

A friend, Michael, hired me to do a stage-show presentation at his wife's birthday party to which about 20 guests were invited. To discover which of the guests would make good stage-show subjects, I led the entire group through a very short pre-hypnotic talk that included the dictionary-balloon demonstration and the eye closure demonstration. I observed which of the guests responded best to the "test" suggestions and selected three "volunteers." I call them volunteers, although it was *me* who chose them.

One of the three volunteers was a woman, Tara, whose age was hard to gauge—somewhere between 25 and 50—because of her unusual dress style and large, round glasses that magnified her eyes to twice their size. Her attire seemed bizarre because it was in such stark contrast to the other guests, whose dress was stylish and sleek. I remember thinking, *Tara's garb would not be at all unusual if I were performing for a group of fortunetellers and séance mediums.*

Tara turned out to be a very good subject and because of her uniqueness proved to be the star of the show. However, one routine I suggested created a perception that she was unwilling to relinquish.

"Tara," I suggested, "when I snap my fingers you will open your eyes and feel an urge to visit the restroom. You will stand up and take a step in the direction of the restroom, but your left foot will be stuck to the floor due to the fact that there is an elephant standing on your shoe. You will see the elephant and attempt to move it off your left foot by heaving your weight against its leg. You will feel the roughness and hairiness of its leg and comment on it. On your third attempt to extricate your foot, you will be successful and head off to the restroom. However, just before you reach the hallway the elephant will grab you around the waist with its trunk and hold you back from reaching the hall. You will use your creativity to discover a way to disengage yourself from the elephant's clutches. After you free yourself, you will proceed to the restroom. Upon returning, the elephant will be gone and everything will be back to normal."

My mistake, as it turned out, was that I didn't know what Tara's "normal" was.

[Snap!]

Tara opened her eyes and gasped, "Where the heck (she didn't say heck) did this elephant come from? Michael, which way is the restroom?"

Michael pointed toward the hallway.

Tara stood up, took a step in the direction Michael had indicated, stopped dead in her tracks and said, "This blooming (she didn't say blooming) elephant is standing on my shoe and I've got to go to the bathroom." She hauled back and with all of her weight, but to no avail, heaved against the un-seeable obstacle. Obviously flustered, she stood back, looked again and exclaimed, "Get off my shoe you darn (she didn't say darn) rough-skinned, bristle-haired, stinking pachyderm."

With that, Tara pulled back again, made another heave against the imaginary object, bounced off once more and shouted, "I don't know how you got in here or why you are standing on my shoe, but you had better lift up your foot or I'll jab you in the rump (she didn't say rump) with my wand." Her foot stayed fastened to the floor as if an elephant *was* standing on it.

"Well then, if that's how you are going to be..." Tara squatted down, flung her arms around a make-believe elephant leg, hefted it up like an Olympic weightlifter, and slid her foot from under a pretend elephant foot.

All of the other guests were guffawing at the sight as Tara stood up, dusted off her hands and headed toward the restroom.

It was as if a giant hook caught her around her middle just before reaching the hall. Tara jerked back and cried out, "What the heck (she didn't say heck)!

Get your slimy, snaky nose off me. I warned you earlier.... I can't reach your rump but I can reach your nose!" With that, Tara extracted a wand from a fold in her dress and jammed it into the nostril of an imaginary trunk. It seemed to have done the trick since, without a whimper, Tara disappeared down the hallway.

I later learned that Tara was a self-proclaimed witch/magician, and was there to perform a few tricks of her own.

And a very curious thing happened after Tara returned from the restroom—which is the point of this story. When Tara reappeared she said, "Where *is* the beast? I've never been that close to an elephant before. What an unusual experience! Did you get a whiff of him, he really stunk... and the hair on his leg felt like wire brush bristles bristles. How did you get him in here? There's no door large enough to fit him through. Sure, *I* can conjure rabbits or chickens out of a hat... but an elephant!" Tara turned to me and said, "I thought you were a hypnotist, not a wizard!"

The guests seemed as interested in Tara's response as entertained by the routine. I tried to explain to her that it was all imagined, "There was no elephant, he didn't stand on your shoe and you didn't jam a wand up his trunk. It was an illusion, not reality. Ask the guests if they saw an elephant if you don't believe me."

She did, and of course, the guests confirmed there had never been an elephant in Michael's front room.

She was unconvinced, "Well, what kind of a joke are you guys playing on me? It's a conspiracy! Why would you want to play a trick on me? I know that I saw, felt and smelled an elephant and nothing you can say will change my mind. I don't know how you got him in here. I know that he could not have fit through the door, so he must have been conjured. I don't know which one of you did the conjuring but you possess some very convincing 'magical' powers."

Tara refused when I asked her if I could give her suggestions that would undo her false perceptions. "Why would I want to *not* have this experience be real and remember it? How many times does a person have an elephant grab them around their waist and get it to let go by sticking their wand up its nostril? I will never have another opportunity do that for as long as I live...."

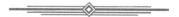

After this occasion, the few times Michael and I crossed paths, invariably the topic of Tara would come up and our conclusion was always the same— Tara is a single-minded mystic who, for reasons of her own as it relates to conjured elephants, is living in a mythical, delusional world. In fact, Michael confessed that with time, her conviction continued to become all the more intense and her tales about the event more bizarre. "That hypnotist guy was *really* a great wizard in disguise who shrunk the elephant by using a powerful reductive charm so he could get it through the door—only a really powerful wizard could have pulled that off."

Michael said, "Tara is truly convinced there was an elephant in my front room and actually believes in all of this magic stuff." If the event had been more recent, I would have thought she'd been strengthening her neural pathways by reading too much Harry Potter.

Regardless of the event that initiates a new neural pathway, whether it be from our culture, a tragic event, what other people say to us, or in Tara's case a single suggestion, every time the event is revisited (relived in our mind, be it continual study of a topic or relived in our imagination) the neural pathway is strengthened. Moreover, over time, it is locked into our lifestyle, our conviction and our worldview. Regardless of how hard one person tries to change another's convictions (perceptions) they have little chance; that is, until the other person discovers a need for change and is open-minded enough to consider other possibilities.

APPENDIX IV

ELIMINATING THE ADVERSITIES OF STRESS AND ANXIETIES

Innumerable studies have shown that chronic stress and anxieties:

- Kill brain cells
- Damage the cardiovascular system
- Reduce the immune system's ability to fight disease
- Decrease DNA repair mechanisms thus increasing the likelihood of cancer
- Are linked to Alzheimer's disease
- Disrupt body chemistry
- Reduce learning and recall
- Inhibit rational thinking that leads to making poor decisions

Without question, the most compelling characteristic of perceptionism (the hypnotic process) is its power to remove stress. Physical relaxation and a mental state of well-being keep body chemistry in balance and are the foundation upon which perceptionism is based. In my opinion, whether we call it psychotherapy, counseling, talking through problems with friends, prayer, hypnotism or perceptionism, if at the end a person's stress and anxieties have been removed the process that brought it about is the same—the person's self-perception has been changed.

However, it can work the other way. If a session, visit or prayer creates perceptions of hopelessness, misery, injustice, despair or helplessness, then the stress and anxieties are intensified, not removed. I believe this is the problem with a regressive approach to therapy.

It is interesting how often clients who made an appointment for stress-related issues (agoraphobia, panic attacks, anxieties, chronic worrying etc.), and who have been through traditional counseling and therapy, say that when leaving their counselor or therapist's office they feel worse than they did before they went in for the session. I think that the reason this happens is that the session was spent rehashing events of the past, finding fault with someone else's behavior or talking about issues that the client has no control over.

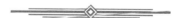

My secretary was off for the day so I was sitting in the receptionist area when T.J. stepped in. After introducing himself he said, "I've been walking past your office door for several months on my way to visit my psychiatrist. Every time I see your sign I wonder if hypnotherapy could help with my condition.

My wife dropped me off early on her way to a job interview so I have an hour to kill before my appointment with the doctor. Do you have a few minutes to tell me a little bit about hypnosis and if it could help with my anxieties?"

I did have a few minutes so I said, "Yes."

When I asked him why he was seeing the psychiatrist he said, "I have lupus. I am a type "A" personality—I've been going full-bore for my whole life and my M.O. is to stress out. Now that I have lupus I'm in pain most of the time, I have high blood pressure and they tell me that if I don't get a handle on my stress I have six months or maybe a year to live. I'm so stressed out and anxious about my condition I can't do my job right, and I'm on medical leave and am about to lose the job for good if I don't get this stress and anxiety under control. The psychiatrist is giving me antidepressants and the doctors are giving me blood pressure and pain pills, but I am still anxious and I still hurt."

Lupus is an autoimmune disease that can be fatal. It attacks the body's cells and tissue, resulting in inflammation and damage to tissue. It can affect any part of the body but most often the joints, skin, internal organs and nervous system. The sequence of the disease is unpredictable with periods of flare-ups alternating with remissions. After questioning T.J. for a few minutes, he admitted that there was a direct correlation between his flare-ups and his level of stress and anxieties.

T.J. was an exceptionally good subject. Over the next six years I saw him professionally four times, each for a different issue (T.J. was one of a very few clients that I occasionally interacted with outside my office).

During the first session we dealt with getting rid of his stress and anxieties and removing much of his pain. As he left my office he said, "So this is what it feels like to be relaxed and peaceful... and right now my joints don't hurt at all." T.J. religiously listened to the recording I made of his session, and over the next few weeks stopped using his antidepressant medication and his pain pills, and went back to work.

The second time I worked with T.J. (about six months later) he reported that since our first session he had greater mobility and his lupus seemed to have halted its progression and may have even reversed. He left my office a non-smoker.

The third session was at the hospital four years later. The lupus had affected his joints (kind of like arthritis does) and it became necessary for knee replacement surgery. T.J. called me from his hospital room and said, "Can you come over to the hospital and hypnotize me to get rid of the pain from the surgery? The pain drugs don't seem to be working and I'm afraid to have them increase the dosage."

So I posed as his minister, pulled the curtains around his bed and gave him a "blessing." T.J. had asked about using hypnosis to help his condition and was told by the staff, "Here at Desert Samaritan Hospital we don't let in 'charlatans or quacks.'" Immediately after going through the induction, T.J. relaxed and his pain vanished. I also gave him suggestions that since he was comfortable and relaxed that healing would occur more quickly—which happened.

The fourth session was two years later. T.J. was scheduled to have his other knee replaced so he called me beforehand. When he came in for the session he reported the "blessing" session had helped significantly, and that he left the hospital that afternoon and completed his physical therapy in half the expected time. So for this session I gave similar suggestions to those I had given him during the "blessing" session but also suggested that during the surgery there would be less bleeding. A month later T.J. called (the only time he had called to report on his success) and said, "The surgery was a success. I'm through with my physical therapy and after the surgery the doctor told me that it was really strange how there was almost no bleeding during the procedure. My blood pressure is good, and for the most part over the past six years (since we had our first session) I've been a type 'B' personality—peaceful, calm and purposeful in taking care of things rather than reacting. The early effects of my lupus are still there (swollen joints) but I have relatively good movement in my joints and there is seldom any pain. But best of all... I am still alive!"

I have lost track of T.J. over the past 15 years so I don't know his present state of being, but I think of him often.

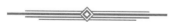

I am still amazed at T.J.'s recovery and improved state of health. I believe that a great deal of his enhanced state of physical and psychological well-being was the result of removing his stress and anxieties. I am convinced that when we are in a peaceful state of mind and our body is relaxed, body chemistry is balanced so all of our natural healing processes can work at their optimum strength and our immune system performs at its most advantageous level.

APPENDIX STUDY DATA

TESTS DATA

Pendulum Demonstration (during pre-hypnotic talk) Data:

	GROUP	
Amount of swing	Sleep	No Sleep
No swing	0	0
Slight swing (less than 1")	6	7
Large swing (more than 1")	19	18

Dictionary-Balloon "Test" (after the "induction" procedure) Data:

	GROUP	
Deflection from original position	Sleep	No Sleep
No deflection from original position	0	8
Slight deflection (less than 3")	13	9
Large deflection (more than 3")	12	8

Eye Closure "Test" (after the "induction" procedure) Data:

	GROUP	
Degree of ability to open eyes	Sleep	No Sleep
Eyes opened with no difficulty	2	10
Struggled to open	11	11
Could not open their eyes	12	4

✳ ✳ ✳ ✳ ✳

The categories for which to determine the effectiveness between the "sleep now" and the "no sleep now" are as follows. Note: If a subject had gone back to smoking they were not included in the next survey call. All of the participants who had gone back to smoking I invited back for a no-charge session to see if I could discern why most of the clients had stopped and they hadn't.

Survey results one week after the session:	GROUP	
	Sleep	No Sleep
Lit up a cigarette right after leaving my office	0	2
Had gone for three days but started again	1	3
Had not smoked since their session (one week)	13	9

Survey results one month after the session:

	GROUP	
	Sleep	No Sleep
Had started smoking again after the first week	1	1
Were still not smoking	12	8

Survey results six months after the session:

	GROUP	
	Sleep	No Sleep
Had started smoking again	1	3
For six months had not smoked	11	5

BIBLIOGRAPHY

Books

John D. Barns, *Secrets of Sympathetic or Animal Magnetism* (Published in 1773, Webster Brothers)

Claude M. Bristol, *The Magic of Believing*

Jill Bolte Taylor, *My Stroke of Insight*

Steve Chandler, *Shift Your Mind*

Dale Carnegie, *How to Win Friends and Influence People*

George Estabrook, *HYPNOSIS: Current Problems*

Arnold Furst, *Post-Hypnotic Instructions*

Napoleon Hill, *Think and Grow Rich*

Maxwell Maltz, *Psycho-Cybernetic*

Earl Nightingale, *The Strangest Secret*

Michael D. Preston, *Hypnosis: Medicine of the Mind*

Norman Vincent Peale, *The Power of Positive Thinking*

Richard M. Pico, *Consciousness in Four Dimensions*

Plato, *Euthyphro, Apology, Crito* (Translated by F.J. Church)

Plato, *The Republic of Plato* (Translated by Francis MacDonald Cornford)

Melvin Powers, *A Practical Guide to Self-Hypnosis*

University Level Courses from *The Teaching Company*

Biological Anthropology: An Evolutionary Perspective: Course No. 1573 (24 lectures, 30 minutes/lecture). Taught by **Barbara J. King**, The College of William and Mary, Ph.D., University of Oklahoma

Biology and Human Behavior: The Neurological Origins of Individuality, 2nd Edition: Course No. 1597 (24 lectures, 30 minutes/lecture). Taught by **Robert Sapolsky**, Stanford University, Ph.D., Rockefeller University

Biology: The Science of Life: Course No. 1500 (72 lectures, 30 minutes/lecture). Taught by **Stephen Nowicki**, Duke University, Ph.D., Cornell University

Birth of the Modern Mind: The Intellectual History of the 17th and 18th Centuries: Course No. 447 (24 lectures, 30 minutes/lecture). Taught by **Alan Charles Kors**, University of Pennsylvania, Ph.D., Harvard University

Consciousness and Its Implications: Course No. 4168 (12 lectures, 30 minutes/lecture). Taught by **Daniel N. Robinson**, Philosophy Faculty, Oxford University; Distinguished Professor, Emeritus, Georgetown University, Ph.D., City University of New York

Great Ideas of Philosophy, 2nd Edition: Course No. 4200 (60 lectures, 30 minutes/lecture). Taught by **Daniel N. Robinson**, Philosophy Faculty, Oxford University; Distinguished Professor, Emeritus, Georgetown University, Ph.D., City University of New York

Great Ideas of Psychology: Course No. 660 (48 lectures, 30 minutes/lecture). Taught by **Daniel N. Robinson**, Philosophy Faculty, Oxford University; Distinguished Professor, Emeritus, Georgetown University, Ph.D., City University of New York

Great Minds of the Western Intellectual Tradition, 3rd Edition: Course No. 470 (84 lectures, 30 minutes/lecture). Taught by **Dennis Dalton, Alan Charles Kors, Robert H. Kane, Phillip Cary, Louis Markos, Darren Staloff, Robert C. Solomon, Jeremy Adams, Jeremy Shearmur, Kathleen M. Higgins, Mark Risjord, Douglas Kellner**

Philosophy of Mind: Brains, Consciousness, and Thinking Machines: Course No. 4278 (24 lectures, 30 minutes/lecture). Taught by **Patrick Grim**, State University of New York at Stony Brook

Theory of Evolution: A History of Controversy: Course No. 174 (12 lectures, 30 minutes/lecture). Taught by **Edward J. Larson**, University of Georgia, J.D., Harvard University; Ph.D., University of Wisconsin at Madison

Understanding the Brain: Course No. 1580 (36 lectures, 30 minutes/lecture). Taught by **Jeanette Norden**, Vanderbilt University, Ph.D., Vanderbilt University School of Medicine

* *The Teaching Company* is a Chantilly, Virginia company that produces recordings of lectures by nationally top-ranked university professors and high-school teachers. These courses are sold on DVD, audio CD, Audio Download, etc. *The Teaching Company*, 4840 Westfields Blvd., Suite 500, Chantilly, VA 20151   Phone: 1-800-TEACH-12 (1-800-832-2412); Website: http://www.teach12.com